Hormones, gender
and the aging brain

The significance of hormone action in psychiatry has long been studied, but only very recently has this study included the psychiatric effects of hormones on the aging process. This is the first clinical reference to address the hormonal basis of mental disorders in older people. Hormones influence a wide range of states and conditions, from pain tolerance and anorexia to attention, mood, immunity, cardiovascular and cognitive function, schizophrenia and Alzheimer's disease.

Written by an eminent team of psychiatrists, psychologists, geriatricians and neuropharmacologists, this book brings together established information and recent findings in four sections:

- an overview of the basic science of neurosteroids
- sex difference and the roles that cortisol, thyroid hormone, and the sex steroids estrogen, progesterone, dehydroepiandrosterone and testosterone play in common mental disorders and pain sensitivity
- psychoneuroimmunology in relation to age
- sex differences and hormones in psychotropic drug metabolism in the elderly.

Clinicians and researchers alike will value this comprehensive review of a complex and sometimes controversial area of psychiatry.

Mary F. Morrison is Assistant Professor of Psychiatry and Internal Medicine at the University of Pennsylvania School of Medicine and is the recipient of a career development award to study the role of estradiol in mild to moderate depressive disorders in aging women.

Hormones, gender
and the aging brain

The endocrine basis of geriatric psychiatry

Edited by

Mary F. Morrison

Departments of Psychiatry and Internal Medicine,
University of Pennsylvania, Philadelphia, USA

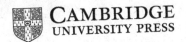

CAMBRIDGE
UNIVERSITY PRESS

CAMBRIDGE UNIVERSITY PRESS
Cambridge, New York, Melbourne, Madrid, Cape Town, Singapore, São Paulo

Cambridge University Press
The Edinburgh Building, Cambridge CB2 8RU, UK

Published in the United States of America by Cambridge University Press, New York

www.cambridge.org
Information on this title: www.cambridge.org/9780521653046

First published 2000
This digitally printed version 2007

A catalogue record for this publication is available from the British Library

Library of Congress Cataloguing in Publication data

Hormones, gender, and the aging brain : the endocrine basis of geriatric psychiatry /
[written by Mary F. Morrison . . . et al.].
    p.   cm.
Includes index.
ISBN 0 521 65304 5
1. Geriatric psychiatry.   2. Aged–Diseases–Endocrine aspects.   3. Aging–Endocrine
aspects.   4. Aged–Mental Health.   I. Morrison, Mary F. (Mary Frances), 1958–
RC451.4.A5   H67   2000
618.97′689–dc21   99–045853

ISBN 978-0-521-65304-6 hardback
ISBN 978-0-521-04173-7 paperback

Every effort has been made in preparing this book to provide accurate and up-to-date information
which is in accord with accepted standards and practice at the time of publication. Although case
histories are drawn from actual cases, every effort has been made to disguise the identities of the
individuals involved. Nevertheless, the authors, editors and publishers can make no warranties that
the information contained herein is totally free from error, not least because clinical standards are
constantly changing through research and regulation. The authors, editors and publishers therefore
disclaim all liability for direct or consequential damages resulting from the use of material contained
in this book. Readers are strongly advised to pay careful attention to information provided by the
manufacturer of any drugs or equipment that they plan to use.

To my husband, Mickey, and my son, Nathaniel

Contents

Part III   **Effects of hormones and behavior on immune function**

Part IV   **Hormones and gender differences in psychotropic drug metabolism**

Contributors

Dr Dewleen G. Baker, Psychiatry Service, University of Cincinnati, USA

Dr Mary H. Burleson, Department of Social and Behavioral Sciences, Arizona State University West, USA

Tanya J. Fabian, Department of Pharmaceutical Sciences, University of Pittsburgh, USA

Dr Loretta M. Flanagan-Cato, Department of Psychology, University of Pennsylvania, USA

Dr Thomas D. Geracioti Jr, Psychiatry Service, University of Cincinnati, USA

Dr Robert B. Gibbs, Department of Pharmaceutical Sciences, University of Pittsburgh School of Pharmacy, USA

Dr Julie Akiko Gladsjo, Department of Psychiatry, University of California, San Diego, USA

Dr Ronald Glaser, Institute for Behavioral Medicine Research, Comprehensive Cancer Center and Department of Medical Microbiology and Immunology, Ohio State University, USA

Dr M. Jackuelyn Harris, Department of Psychiatry, University of California, San Diego and Psychiatry and Psychology Services, San Diego V.A. Medical Center, USA

Dr Robert Heaton, Department of Psychiatry, University of California, San Diego, USA

Shelley C. Heaton, Department of Psychiatry, University of California, San Diego, USA

Dr Dilip V. Jeste, Department of Psychiatry, University of California, San Diego and Psychiatry and Psychology Services, San Diego V.A. Medical Center, USA

Dr John W. Kasckow, Psychiatry Service, University of Cincinnati, USA

Dr Janice K. Kiecolt-Glaser, Institute for Behavioral Medicine Research and Department of Psychiatry, Ohio State University, USA

Dr Patricia D. Kroboth, Department of Pharmaceutical Sciences, University of Pittsburgh School of Pharmacy, USA

Dr Laurie A. Lindamer, Department of Psychiatry, University of California, San Diego, USA

Dr James W. McAuley, Departments of Pharmacy Practice and Neurology, Ohio State University, USA

Dr John E. Morley, Geriatric Research, Education and Clinical Center, St Louis Veterans' Administrative Medical Center and Division of Geriatric Medicine, Saint Louis University Health Sciences Center, USA

Dr Mary F. Morrison, Departments of Psychiatry and Internal Medicine, University of Pennsylvania School of Medicine, USA

Dr James J. Mulchahey, Psychiatry Service, University of Cincinnati, USA

Dr Jane S. Paulsen, Department of Psychiatry, University of Iowa, USA

Dr Teresa A. Pigott, Department of Psychiatry and Behavioral Sciences, University of Texas Medical Branch at Galveston, USA

Dr Marta Pisarska, Department of Psychiatry, University of Cincinnati, USA

Dr Bruce G. Pollock, Geriatric Psychopharmacology Program, University of Pittsburgh Medical Center and Department of Psychiatry and Pharmacology, University of Pittsburgh School of Medicine, USA

Dr Eva Redei, Department of Psychiatry and Behavioral Sciences, Northwestern University Medical School, Chicago, USA

Ajit Regmi, Department of Psychiatry, University of Cincinnati, USA

Dr Victor I. Reus, Department of Psychiatry and Center for Neurobiology and Psychiatry, University of California, San Francisco, USA

Dr Susan Robinson-Whelen, Veterans' Administration Center of Excellence on Healthy Aging with Disabilities, Houston, Texas, USA

Dr Steven P. Roose, Department of Psychiatry, College of Physicians and Surgeons of Columbia University and the New York State Psychiatric Institute, USA

Dr Stuart N. Seidman, Department of Psychiatry, College of Physicians and Surgeons of Columbia University and the New York State Psychiatric Institute, USA

Suresh G. Shelat, Institute of Neurological Sciences, University of Pennsylvania School of Medicine, Philadelphia, USA

Dr Wendy F. Sternberg, Department of Psychology, Haverford College, Haverford, Pennsylvania, USA

Dr Gabriel K. Tsuboyama, Department of Psychiatry, Cornell Medical Center, New York Hospital, USA

Kathryn Tweedy, Department of Psychiatry, University of Pennsylvania School of Medicine, USA

Dr Owen M. Wolkowitz, Department of Psychiatry and Center for Neurobiology and Psychiatry, University of California, San Francisco, USA

Dr Kristine Yaffe, Departments of Psychiatry and Neurology, University of California, San Francisco and the San Francisco Veterans' Administration Medical Center, USA

Preface

Two of the great mysteries of life for those beyond the age of 30 are: Why do we age? What can we do about it? The idea of 'successful aging' has captured the interest of researchers in the biological and social sciences as well as the interest of the public. While our hopes for our retirement years focus on unencumbered time pursuing interests and adventures with leisure, we fear that changes in our physical and emotional/cognitive integrity, brought on by the aging process, may get in the way of realizing those hopes. The process of aging holds many risks, including medical illness, pain, and living with disability. Our fears may focus on the loss of self and others to new onset psychiatric conditions such as depression, anxiety, psychosis, and cognitive disorders. The high prevalence of medical comorbidity in the aged and the biology of aging create especially challenging issues in geriatric mental health.

This book begins to clarify the growing body of knowledge on the hormonal causes and treatment of mental disorders among the elderly. The interplay between endocrinology and psychiatry has a long and fascinating history, but only recently has research into this area included the elderly.

Here, perspectives on the role of hormones in mental function in aging are presented in four sections: basic science overview; endocrine aspects of mental disorders in aging; psychoneuroimmunology; and pharmacology. A first chapter by John Morley comprehensively integrates the endocrine changes in aging with the behavioral effects of hormones that have received less attention. An overview of the anorexia of aging and the involvement of hormones and nitric oxide is presented.

The book's first part also reviews the basic biosynthesis and pharmacological interactions of neurosteroids. Loretta Flanagan-Cato reviews the basic mechanisms of hormone effects in the brain, with an emphasis on the biosynthesis, the site of action, and the diverse cellular mechanisms employed by hormones that affect neuronal function.

Part II, Chapters 3 through 12, integrates basic sciences research with clinical data in reviewing the common mental disorders in aging populations and their relationship to hormonal changes. Mood disorders, changes in cognitive function including Alzheimer's disease, anxiety disorders, schizophrenia, and chronic pain, are influenced by hormonal changes.

In Chapter 3, John Kasckow provides a synopsis of recent research into the role of the hypothalamic–pituitary–adrenal (HPA) axis in geriatric populations, reviewing both basic and clinical research. The chapter discusses alterations in the HPA axis that occur with normal aging and relates these to alterations in cognition and mood in the elderly. Chapter 4, by Gabriel Tsuboyama, summarizes the characteristics of the aging thyroid axis and the role of the thyroid axis in geriatric major depression.

Chapters 5 and 6 are devoted to the role of estrogen in depression in aging women and the role of testosterone in depression in aging men. A growing body of evidence implicates the reduction in circulating estrogen in the pathophysiology of mood disorders, Alzheimer's disease, osteoporosis, and heart disease in aging women, and estrogen replacement has led to therapeutics research with important public health implications. But the effects of declining testosterone levels in aging men are less understood. Stuart Seidman provides an overview of research into the link between testosterone levels and depression in men, as well as an overview of research into the neurovegetative, cognitive, affective, and sexual effects of exogenous testosterone administration.

In Chapter 7, Owen Wolkowitz examines current data regarding the effects of dehydroepiandrosterone on mood and cognition in the elderly, particularly its possible efficacy in treating neuropsychiatric illness in the middle-aged and elderly.

Chapters 8 and 9 focus on the role of sex steroids in cognition in aging populations. In Chapter 8, Kristine Yaffe reviews the differences in cognitive functioning between aging men and women and the role of estrogen and testosterone. Estrogen replacement has been linked to a decreased risk of Alzheimer's disease. Robert Gibbs summarizes the recent animal research pertaining to potential mechanisms by which estrogen may help to reduce the risk and severity of Alzheimer's related dementia in women. In particular, estrogen has beneficial effects on the cholinergic neurons which project to the hippocampus and cortex and are involved in memory.

Gender differences exist in the clinical course of schizophrenia and anxiety. Even in the elderly, these gender differences are thought to be at least partly mediated by gonadal hormones. In Chapter 10, Laurie Lindamer analyzes ongoing research into the role of gender on specific aspects of schizophrenia, including the interaction of dopamine and estrogen. Difference in time of onset of illness and clinical course in schizophrenia may be related to the presence of estrogen in women. In Chapter 11, Teresa Pigott reviews anxiety disorders in aging population and data suggesting that sex steroids may play a role in the increased prevalence of anxiety disorders in women throughout the lifespan.

Chronic pain is a significant problem in aging populations and in many people pain both causes and is exacerbated by depression. Less commonly appreciated is the fact that men and women experience pain differently. In Chapter 12, Wendy Sternberg examines the role of hormonal mechanisms in acute and chronic pain in the elderly, including how sex steroids may explain some of the sex differences in endogenous pain inhibition. The clinical implications of a novel pain mechanism in female rodents is discussed.

Part III provides an understanding of the field of psychoneuroimmunology in relation to aging. In Chapter 13, Mary Burleson summarizes estrogen's immunomodulatory effects and estrogen-related differences in cardiovascular and neuroendocrine reactivity to brief stressors in women. She includes research on estrogen's effects on immune reactivity to stress, and speculates on the possibility that estrogen may moderate hormonal and immunological responses to stress through alterations in sympathetic nervous system reactivity and through regulation of corticotropin-releasing hormone. In Chapter 14, Eva Redei investigates sex differences in regulation of immune function at the cellular level. She explores the hypothesis that common genes are involved in certain autoimmune diseases and mood disorders. Aging and hormone replacement therapy may affect the expression of these genes since many of them are known to be regulated by estrogen.

In Part IV, Chapters 15 and 16 review the influences of gender, hormones, and aging on the metabolism of drugs. Older women are the greatest consumers of all classes of psychotropics, with evidence indicating that the elderly in general, and women in particular, experience a higher frequency of adverse drug reactions. Information on gender differences in pharmocokinetics is minimal, however, and rarely being used in clinical practice, according to Bruce Pollack. In Chapter 15, he reviews the research on the effects of endogenous and exogenous estrogens on the metabolism of psychotropics and gender and on gender-related differences in the half-lives of psychotropics. Finally, in Chapter 16, Patricia Kroboth reviews data that demonstrate that aging and ovarian hormones, specifically progesterone metabolites, affect benzodiazepines levels either by altering drug metabolism or by changing the effect-concentration relationship.

'You are old, Father William,' the young man said,
'And your hair has become very white;
And yet you incessantly stand on your head –
Do you think, at your age, it is right?"

'In my youth,' Father William replied to his son,
'I feared it might injure the brain;
But now that I'm perfectly sure I have none,
Why I do it again and again.'

excerpted from 'Father William' by Lewis Carroll

Father William demonstrates that spirited independence and sense of humor we all hope to express in our old age. Central to that goal, however, is the preservation of cognition, good mood, personality, and health. This book enhances our understanding of the role hormones play in the geriatric mental disorders that can threaten our relationships and self. The endocrine basis of geriatric psychiatry is a new area of investigation, and our field does not yet have the data to comprehensively review all hormones involved in mental disorders and the aging. As research progresses, our understanding of the pathogenesis of these disorders will increase and lead us to more effective hormonal interventions and, possibly, the ability to prevent some of these debilitating disorders.

Acknowledgments

This book was made possible (developed and completed) through my career development award from the National Institutes of Health. Ira Katz has encouraged and assisted me in my psychiatric research career development and with this book. I am especially grateful to him. Jeane Ann Grisso has been a stimulative and generous mentor, role model and friend. Enid Light and Barry Lebowitz, at the National Institutes of Mental Health, were instrumental in focusing the scientific community on the endocrine aspects of mental disorders and my own career development.

I am indebted to several mentors for their advice and encouragement: James Stinnett, Ellen Freeman, and Dwight Evans, the chair of the Department of Psychiatry at the University of Pennsylvania. Peter Schmidt at the National Institutes of Health has been exceptionally generous in helping me refine my understanding of sex steroids and mental disorders in aging. I would also like to convey my warm appreciation to Edward Schweizer, Gary Gottlieb, and Peter Whybrow.

This book has been enhanced by a generous unrestricted educational grant from Pfizer, which has a demonstrated commitment to women's mental health. Cathryn Clary at Pfizer was invaluable in obtaining this grant which allowed for editorial assistance with this book. Jennifer Fisher Wilson has provided superb editorial assistance. The staff of Cambridge University Press have been important in supporting this project. I would like to acknowledge the important contributions of the chapter authors and their hard work and flexibility.

My family has been crucial in this project. My parents, Helen and Herbert Morrison, and my sister, Margaret Gimmy, have my warmest acknowledgments. My son, Nathaniel Selzer, and my stepchildren, Molly and C. J. Selzer, are a continual source of delight, ideas, and inspiration. And, finally, I am always grateful to my husband, Michael Selzer, for his loving support and the warm, glittering mysteries that we share together.

Mary F. Morrison, editor

Part I

Overview

Summary chapter.
The endocrine basis of geriatric psychiatry:
an integrative approach

John E. Morley

Introduction

Life is becoming less like a short sprint and more like a marathon.
Kofi Anan, UN Secretary General, October 1, 1998

Man is born, grows up and dies according to laws which have never been properly investigated either as a whole or in the mode of their mutual reactions.
Quetelet, 1835

The world is rapidly aging. The concept of a few older persons aging successfully into old age was well established at the time of the ancient Greek philosophers, e.g. Socrates, 98 years; Sophocles, 91 years; and Plato, 81 years. In 1900 the average citizen of the United States lived less than 50 years, whereas at the end of the century life expectancy has reached the late seventies. By the year 2030, the percentage of older individuals in the population of most developed nations will be approaching 20%. However, it is not only in the developed nations that persons are living longer. By the year 2000 approximately two-thirds of older persons will live in developing nations, e.g. 300 million in China and 170 million in India.

It is against the backdrop of this age wave that there has been an increasing interest in understanding the scientific basis of the aging process, both physiological and pathological. In the area of mental disorders and aging there have been tremendous advances in our understanding of the pathophysiology of these disorders and an extraordinary development of new therapeutic agents.

Since the original work by Moos and Solomon (1965) recognizing the important mind–body connections with disease, there has been an explosion in our knowledge of how the mind communicates with the body and the body with the mind. It is now recognized that, in many cases, their communications involve the secretion of the ductless glands, i.e. hormones. It is also clear that many peptide hormones have a second role as neurotransmitters within the central nervous system.

In addition, the immune system releases a series of peptide hormones, better recognized as cytokines, that both modulate the endocrine system and a variety of behaviors. Behavior, in turn, through hormonal release and the autonomic nervous system, can modulate the immune system. These interactions have spawned the field of psychoneuroimmunology. The waning immune system seen with aging creates special challenges for the understanding of how behavior–endocrine interactions modulate the immune system of older persons.

This book is presented to the reader as an overview of the endocrine basis of geriatric psychiatry. It is hoped that, with the material provided in this book, the intrepid researcher will be able to revolutionize this field in the next millennium. This chapter will attempt to integrate some of the more exciting findings in the field of hormones, aging, and mental disorders and provide some signposts for where the future advances may lie.

Endocrine disorders as a cause of mental illness

The concept of endocrine disorders resulting in mental illness is well established. Early reports of hypothyroidism discussed 'myxedema madness.' This is especially important in older persons where atypical presentations are common. Thus, we see apathetic hyperthyroidism, with depression and weight loss being major symptoms. Older hypothyroid patients often present with cognitive abnormalities that are reversed with thyroid hormone replacement (Osterweil et al., 1992). Hypothyroidism can also present as depression. Both an excess and a deficiency of thyroid hormone can present as delirium or as a reversible cause of dementia. Addison's disease (hypoadrenocortisolism) often presents insidiously in older persons with a mild delirium, abdominal pain, hypotension, hyperkalemia, weight loss, and hypoglycemia. Hypercalcemia is not rare in older persons and can present with either depression or cognitive impairment. Pheochromocytoma – the classical medical cause of a panic attack – occurs as commonly in persons over 60 years of age as in younger persons, but the diagnosis is rarely made.

Diabetes mellitus has been shown to be associated with cognitive impairment secondary to hyperglycemia and dementia secondary to vascular infarcts (Morley, 1998). This can lead to major problems with compliance leading to worsening glycemic control. Depression occurs more commonly in older persons with diabetes mellitus, and depression is a major cause of noncompliance leading to increased hospitalizations and mortality in older diabetics (Rosenthal et al., 1998). Both hypoglycemia and hyperglycemia can present with delirium.

Hypopituitarism can present with delirium. Elevated prolactin levels are associated with decreased libido and impotence. Adult growth hormone deficiency has been associated with fatigue.

Table 1.1. Behavioral effects of endocrine disorders

Delirium	Dementia	Depression	Anxiety/panic
Hypoglycemia	Hypothyroidism	Hypothyroid	Pheochromocytoma
Hyperglycemia	Vitamin B_{12} deficiency	Hyperthyroid	Hyperthyroidism
Hyponatremia	Diabetes mellitus	Addison's disease	
(syndrome of			
inappropriate ADH)			
Hypothyroidism	Hyperparathyroidism	Diabetes mellitus	
Hypopituitarism		Hypercalcemia	
Addison's Disease			
Vitamin B deficiency			
Hypercalcemia			

Older persons often have elevated levels of circulating cytokines due to chronic disorders. In addition, acute infections lead to a marked increase in cytokines. Tumor necrosis factor α and interleukin-1 both produce delirium. While this may, in part, be due to small amounts crossing the blood–brain barrier (Banks et al., 1994), the major effect appears to be on ascending vagal fibers through neuronal synapses from the nucleus tractus solitarius to the amygdala to the hippocampus, resulting in release of interleukin-1 from hippocampal microglial cells. This glial interleukin-1, in turn, results in decreased release of acetylcholine and cognitive impairment. Cytokines may also play a role in the pathogenesis of dysphoria associated with physical illness.

Table 1.1 summarizes the endocrine disorders responsible for some major psychiatric symptoms in older persons.

Hormones and aging

As shown in Table 1.2, the majority of hormones show a physiological decline with aging. This has led to an enthusiasm for hormone replacement as a modern-day fountain of youth. Unfortunately, with the exception of the data for estrogen and testosterone replacement, the controlled studies in humans have failed to match the promise of animal studies.

Dehydroepiandrosterone (DHEA) and its sulfate show the largest decline of any of the hormones with aging. The function of this adrenal cortical hormone remains elusive. Replacement studies in middle-aged persons suggested an improved mood (Morales et al., 1994) but this could not be replicated by another group (Wolf et al., 1998). As pointed out by Wolkowitz (Chapter 7), DHEA may have a role to play in

Table 1.2. Hormonal changes with aging

Decrease	No change	Increase
Insulin growth Factor I	Epinephrine	Insulin
Vitamin 25(OH)D	Thyroxine	Vasopressin (basal)
Testosterone (males)	Amylin	Cholecystokinin
Estradiol (females)	Glucagon	Atrial naturetic peptide
DHEA and its sulfate	Glucagon like Peptide I	Norepinephrine
Triiodothyronine	Thyrotropin	Epinephrine (> 80 years)
1,25(OH)$_2$ Vitamin D	Calcitonin	FSH
Inhibin	Activin (females)	LH (women)
Arginine vasopressin (nocturnal	ACTH	Parathormone
increase)		
Pregnenolone	Prolactin (females)	Cortisol
		Activin (males)
		Prolactin (males)

depression, but adequate control trials are not yet available. In men, but not in women, high doses of DHEA (100 mg daily) have increased muscle mass and strength (Morales et al., 1998). In mice, DHEA is a potent enhancer of memory, most probably by a nongenomic effect involving GABA (Flood et al., 1992). However, while some epidemiological studies have suggested that DHEA may be correlated with the decline in functional status with aging (Morrison et al., 1998; Rudman et al., 1990b), there is no clear evidence for DHEA improving cognition in humans (Horani & Morley, 1997).

Pregnenolone is the first steroid hormone formed from cholesterol on the adrenal cortex. It is the true 'mother hormone.' In mice it is the most potent memory enhancer yet to be discovered (Flood et al., 1995).

Unfortunately, our study in humans failed to demonstrate any clear cognitive effects of pregnenolone at a 50 mg dose. Previous studies have suggested that pregnenolone may enhance attention and improve function through this route (Horani & Morley, 1997). Pregnenolone may also have small effects on improving sleep.

Melatonin is produced by the pineal gland. Descartes originally suggested that the pineal was the seat of the soul. At present, the best data for melatonin is an effect on sleep in older persons (Dawson et al., 1998). Continued studies on the potential role of melatonin on mental function are warranted.

In the 1980s, Dan Rudman (1985) suggested that aging was due to a growth hormone 'menopause.' His early study suggested positive effects of growth hormone in older men (Rudman et al., 1990a; Cohn et al., 1993). However, subsequent studies have only been able to demonstrate an increase in muscle mass without an increase in muscle strength and no positive behavioral effects (Papadakis et al., 1996). Overall, side-effects have been extremely rate limiting. This is in contradistinction to growth hormone replacement in growth hormone-deficient younger men where positive effects on mood have been demonstrated (Burman & Deijen, 1998). The recent availability of orally active growth hormone secretagogues may allow replacement with more physiological levels of growth hormone.

Arginine vasopressin (AVP) levels increase during the day but the nocturnal surge is attenuated with aging. This is responsible for the well-known nocturia that occurs with aging. In addition, AVP has been demonstrated in animals to enhance memory. In rodents the decline in AVP that occurs with aging is related to the decline in testosterone (see below) and can be restored with testosterone replacement.

Cortisol levels show no change or a small increase with aging. This is most probably predominantly due to the decrease in cortisol production rate that occurs with aging. Thyroxine levels remain stable throughout the lifespan as the decrease in thyroxine production rate is balanced by a decrease in thyroxine clearance. Triiodothyronine levels decline slightly in persons beyond 80 years of age.

25(OH) vitamin D levels decline with aging resulting in an increase in parathyroid homone levels and an increased loss of calcium from bone, resulting in osteoporosis in the old–old (Type II osteoporosis). This can have an indirect effect on mental function as it can lead to lumbar spinal fractures with severe pain.

Norepinephrine increases in the young old and epinephrine in the old–old. This is due predominantly to a postreceptor defect. This postreceptor defect leads to a decreased catecholamine responsiveness with aging. This may result in altered stress responses in older individuals.

Estrogen and cognitive dysfunction

The rapid fall in estrogen in women at the time of the menopause is the most dramatic hormonal change that occurs with aging. This occurrence is marked by hot flashes. Chapters 8 and 9 discuss the putative effects of estrogen deficiency on cognitive dysfunction and dementia in older persons.

Estrogen has a number of effects on the brain that may improve cognition. These include an increase in choline acetyl transferase, an increase in cholinergic neuron survival and an increase in axonal sprouting and dendrite spine formation. Estrogen stimulates nerve growth factor. Estrogen may also protect against vascular dementia through its positive effects on lipids and vasodilation through the stimulation of endothelial nitric oxide.

A number, but not all, cross-sectional studies have suggested that estrogen use is associated with better cognitive function than non-estrogen use. Estrogen use may also delay the onset of Alzheimer's Disease.

One controlled study in nursing home residents suggested improved function in those residents receiving estrogen (Birge, 1996). Other small controlled trials have found some improvement in cognition with estrogen use in postmenopausal women. Progesterone, which is usually co-administered with estrogen, is amnestic (Farr et al., 1995), and this may make it difficult to interpret the effects of some studies on cognition.

Overall, the possible role of estrogen in enhancing cognitive function is extremely exciting, but final proof must await the results of ongoing controlled trials.

Testosterone and behavior

There are now multiple cross-sectional studies demonstrating that testosterone, free testosterone and bioavailable testosterone (albumin plus free testosterone) decline with aging (Morley et al., 1997d). This has been confirmed in a longitudinal study (Morley et al., 1997b). This decline is due primarily to a failure of the gonadotropin-releasing hormone–pituitary unit, and thus luteinizing hormone fails to rise as testosterone declines.

We have recently defined a testosterone deficiency syndrome called Androgen Deficiency in Aging Males (ADAM) that occurs when bioavailable testosterone levels fall below those seen in young males (Table 1.3). This syndrome identified dysphoria as one of the symptoms of testosterone deficiency, as discussed in Chapter 6.

In the SAMP8 mouse, a spontaneous model of cognitive dysfunction due to overproduction of β-amyloid, testosterone levels fall early in the lifespan (Flood & Morley, 1998). Testosterone replacement reverses the memory and learning defects seen in these mice. Testosterone appears to produce this effect by suppressing amyloid precursor protein production in the limbic system.

Cross-sectional studies have suggested that bioavailable testosterone is a major factor in age-related cognitive decline (Morley et al., 1997c). Two interventional studies in older males have shown that testosterone replacement results in enhanced visual–spatial cognitive function (Janowsky et al., 1994).

Testosterone has also been clearly demonstrated to increase libido (Hajjar et al., 1997). Testosterone replacement results in increased strength (Sih et al., 1997; Urban et al., 1995).

Since the time before Christ, when Areteaus the Cappadocian first demonstrated behavior effects in cocks when they were castrated, our knowledge of the effects of testosterone on behavior has come a long way (Chapter 6). However, it is important to realize that many of these effects are small – although small effects can have dramatic affects on quality of life.

Table 1.3. St Louis University. ADAM: Androgen deficiency in aging males

Questionnaire
1. Do you have a decrease in libido (sex drive)?
2. Do you have a lack of energy?
3. Do you have a decrease in strength and/or endurance?
4. Have you lost weight?
5. Have you noticed a decreased 'enjoyment of life'?
6. Are you sad and/or grumpy?
7. Are your erections less strong?
8. Have you noted a recent deterioration in your ability to play sports?
9. Are you falling asleep after dinner?
10. Has there been a recent deterioration in your work performance?

Positive questionnaire is defined as 'yes' answers to questions 1 or 7 and/or 'yes' answers to any three other questions.

Depression and the hypothalamic–pituitary–adrenal axis

Some of the most important advances on the understanding of hormones and behavior in the last decade have come from the increased recognition of the role of the hypothalamic–pituitary–adrenal axis in depression (Chapter 3). Stress activates this axis through the actuation of hypothalamic corticotropin releasing factor (CRF). CRF levels are elevated in the majority, but not all, persons with depression.

CRF appears to play a particularly important role in the genesis of the vegetative signs of depression. These include sleep disturbance, decreased locomotion, anorexia, and weight loss. Older persons with depression are more likely to have anorexia and weight loss than young depressives (Fitten et al., 1989). In addition, the elevated glucocorticoid levels in depression lead to hippocampal neuronal loss and impaired cognition (the pseudodementia syndrome of depression in older persons). The elevated cortisol levels also increase the likelihood of older depressed women to develop osteoporosis (Michelson et al., 1996).

Alcoholism is associated with direct activation of the hypothalamic–pituitary–adrenal axis (Willenbring et al., 1984). This could, in turn, result in some of the depressive symptoms seen in older alcoholics.

An interesting therapeutic development in the treatment of late life depression has been the use of electromagnetic brain stimulation (EBS). Our unpublished studies have suggested that EBS has direct effects on the hypothalamic–pituitary–adrenal axis.

The potential of the treatment of vegetative symptoms, such as weight loss, in older depressives with CRF antagonists is enormously exciting.

Anorexia of aging and hormones

Food intake declines throughout the lifespan, and beyond the age of 70 years, there is a declining in body mass (Morley, 1997). A part of this decline in food intake is due to overproduction of the gastrointestinal hormone, cholecystokinin, and an enhancement of its satiating effect with aging (Silver et al., 1988; Morley et al., 1997a). In addition to this there is a decrease in the ability of the gastric fundus to relax to accept normal sized meals. This leads to early satiation in older persons and is due to a deficiency in nitric oxide (Morley & Flood, 1994).

Leptin is a peptide hormone produced by fat cells (Morley et al., 1999). It plays a role in decreasing intake through inhibiting neuropeptide Y in the central nervous system. Testosterone deficiency with aging leads to an increase in circulating leptin levels with aging and this is responsible for the greater decrease in food intake that occurs with aging in men. Estradiol has no effect on leptin.

A number of neurotransmitters within the hypothalamus drive food intake. Dynorphin (an opioid peptide) increases fat intake and neuropeptide Y increases carbohydrate intake. Both of these peptides decline with aging. Their effects appears to be mediated by activation of nitric oxide in the hypothalamus. Levels of the mRNA for nitric oxide synthase also decline with aging (Morley et al., 1996).

Depression is the most common cause of anorexia and weight loss in older persons (Wilson et al., 1998). Anorexia nervosa (or tardive) can reoccur in older women and appears for the first time in older men. The potential relationship of this condition to sex hormone changes in the elderly is in need of exploration. Late life paranoia can also be associated with refusal to eat because of fear that the food is poisoned.

Dementia is most often associated with failure to eat, apraxia of swallowing, and weight loss. In the midstages of dementia some patients develop hyperphagia. Ingestion of unpalatable objects, e.g. coprophagia, can also occur in demented persons. While it has been suggested that Alzheimer's disease may be associated with an increased metabolic rate, double labeled water studies have failed to confirm this (Poehlman et al., 1997).

The endocrinology of disturbances of food intake and metabolism associated with aging represents one of the cutting edge issues in geriatric psychiatry.

Conclusions

As illustrated in Fig. 1.1, the interaction of hormones and behavior is inordinately complex. In older persons hormonal alterations can lead to depression, delirium, dementia, and panic attacks. Depression or a decline in food intake can lead to

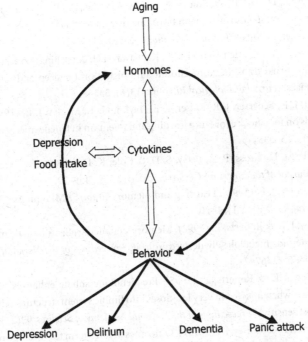

Figure 1.1.   The interaction of hormones and behavior in the aging brain.

marked alterations in hormonal levels. Aging can result in a decline in hormonal levels making the aging brain more vulnerable to developing cognitive defects. Cytokines produced by the immune system can directly alter both hormones and behavior. With the increased computer power in the next millennium, together with full knowledge of the human genome, we should be much more capable of understanding these complex interactions and developing new approaches to the management of mental disorders in older persons. However, it is perhaps best to close with the comment of the English philosopher, Emerson Pugh: 'If the human brain were so simple that we could understand it, we would be so simple that we couldn't.'

REFERENCES

Banks, W. A., Kastin, A. J. & Ehrensing, C. A. (1994). Blood-borne interleukin-1 alpha is transported across the endothelial blood–spinal cord barrier of mice. *Journal of Physiology*, **479** (2), 257–64.

Birge, S.J. (1996). Is there a role for estrogen replacement therapy in the prevention and treatment of dementia? *Journal of the American Geriatric Society*, **44**(7), 865–70.

Burman, P. & Deijen, J.B. (1998). Quality of life and cognitive function in patients with pituitary insufficiency. *Psychotherapy and Psychosomatics*, **67**(3), 154–67.

Cohn, L., Feller, A.G., Draper, M.W., Rudman, I.W. & Rudman, D. (1993). Carpal tunnel syndrome and gynaecomastia during growth hormone treatment of elderly men with low circulating IGF-1 concentrations. *Clinical Endocrinology*, 39(4), 417–25.

Dawson, D., Rogers, N.L., van den Heuvel, C.J., Kennaway, D.J. & Lushington, K. (1998). Effect of sustained nocturnal transbuccal melatonin administration on sleep and temperature in elderly insomniacs. *Journal of Biological Rhythms*, 13(6), 532–8.

Farr, S. A., Flood, J. F., Scherrer, J. F., Kaiser, F. E., Taylor, G. T., Morley, J. E. (1995). Effect of ovarian steroids on footshock avoidance learning and retention in female mice. *Physiology and Behavior*, 58(4), 715–23.

Fitten, L. J., Morley, J. E., Gross, P. L., Petry, S. D. & Cole, K. D. (1989). Depression (Clinical Conference). *Journal of the American Geriatric Society*, 37(5), 459–72.

Flood, J. F. and Morley, J. E. (1998). Learning and memory in the SAMP8 mouse. *Neuroscience and Biobehavioral Review*, 22(1), 1–20.

Flood, J. F., Morley, J. E. & Roberts, E. (1992). Memory-enhancing effects in male mice of pregnenolone and steroids metabolically derived from it. *Proceedings of the National Academy of Sciences*, USA, 89(5), 1567–71.

Flood, J. F., Morley, J. E. & Roberts, E. (1995). Pregnenolone sulfate enhances post-training memory processes when injected in very low doses into limbic system structures: the amygdala is by far the most sensitive. *Proceedings of the National Academy of Sciences*, 92(23), 10806–10.

Hajjar, R. R., Kaiser, F. E. & Morley, J. E. (1997). Outcomes of long-term testosterone replacement in older hypogonadal males: a retrospective analysis. *Journal of Clinical Endocrinology and Metabolism*, 82(11), 3793–6.

Horani, M. H. & Morley, J. E. (1997). The viability of the use of DHEA. *Clinical Geriatrics*, 5(4), 34–51.

Janowsky, J. S., Oviatt, S. K. & Orwoll, E. S. (1994). Testosterone influences spatial cognition in older men. *Behavioral Neuroscience*, 108(2), 325–32.

Michelson, D., Stratakis, C., Hill, L., Reynolds, J., Galliven, E., Chrousos, G. & Gold, P. (1996). Bone mineral density in women with depression. *New England Journal of Medicine*, 335(16), 1176–81.

Moos, R. H. & Solomon, G. F. (1965). Personality correlates of the degree of functional incapacity of patients with physical disease. *Journal of Chronic Diseases*, 18(10), 1019–38.

Morales, A. J., Haubrich, R. H., Hwang, J. Y., Asakura, H. & Yen, S. S. (1998). The effect of six months treatment with a 100 mg daily dose of Dehydroepiandrosterone (DHEA) on circulating sex steroids, body composition and muscle strength in age-advanced men and women. *Clinical Endocrinology*, 49(4), 421–32.

Morales, A. J., Nolan, J. J., Nelson, J. C. & Yen, S. S. (1994). Effects of replacement dose of dehydroepiandrosterone in men and women of advancing age. *Journal of Clinical Endocrinogy and Metabolism*, 78(6), 1360–7.

Morley, J. E. (1997). Anorexia of aging: physiologic and pathologic. *American Journal of Clinical Nutrition*, 66(4), 760–73.

Morley, J. E. (1998). The elderly Type 2 diabetic patient: special considerations. *Diabetic Medicine*, 15(12, 4), S41–6.

Morley, J. E. & Flood, J. F. (1994). Effect of competitive antagonism of NO synthetase on weight and food intake in obese and diabetic mice. *American Journal of Physiology*, 266, R164–8.

Morley, J. E., Flood, J. F., Perry, H. M. III & Kumar, V. B. (1997a). Peptides, memory, food intake and aging. *Aging*, 9(4), 17–18.

Morley, J. E., Kaiser, F. E., Perry, H. M. III, Patrick, P., Morley, P. M., Stauber, P. M., Vellas, B., Baumgartner, R. N. & Garry, P. J. (1997b). Longitudinal changes in testosterone, luteinizing hormone, and follicle-stimulating hormone in healthy older men. *Metabolism: Clinical and Experimental*, 46(4), 410–13.

Morley, J. E., Kaiser, F. E., Raum, W. J., Perry, H. M. III, Flood, J. F., Jensen, J., Silver, A. J. & Roberts, E. (1997c). Potentially predictive and manipulable blood serum correlates of aging in the healthy human male: progressive decreases in bioavailable testosterone, dehydroepiandrosterone sulfate, and the ratio of insulin-like growth factor 1 to growth hormone. *Proceedings of the National Academy of Sciences, USA*, 94(14), 7537–42.

Morley, J. E., Kaiser, F. E., Sih, R., Hajjar, R. & Perry, H. M. III. (1997d). Testosterone and frailty. *Clinical Geriatric Medicine*, 13(4), 685–95.

Morley, J. E., Kumar, V. B., Mattammal, M. B., Farr, S., Morley, P. M. & Flood, J. F. (1996). Inhibition of feeding by a nitric oxide synthase inhibitor: effects of aging. *European Journal of Pharmacology*, 322(1), 15–19.

Morley, J. E., Perry, H. M. III, Baumgartner, R. & Garry, P. J. (1999). Commentary. Leptin, adipose tissue and aging: is there a role for testosterone? *Journal of Gerontology*, B108–9.

Morrison, M. F., Katz, I. R., Parmelee, P., Boyce, A. A. & TenHave, T. (1998). Dehydroepiandrosterone sulfate (DHEA-S) and psychiatric and laboratory measures of frailty in a residential care population. *American Journal of Geriatric Psychiatry*, 6(4), 277–84.

Osterweil, D., Syndulko, K., Cohen, S. N., Pettler-Jennings, P. D., Hershman, J. M., Cummings, J. L., Tourtellotte, W. W. & Solomon, D. H. (1992). Cognitive function in non-demented older adults with hypothyroidism. *Journal of the American Geriatric Society*, 40(4), 325–35.

Papadakis, M. A., Grady, D., Black, D., Tierney, M. J., Gooding, G. A., Schambelan, M. & Grunfeld, C. (1996). Growth hormone replacement in healthy older men improves body composition but not functional ability. *Annals of Internal Medicine*, 124(8), 708–16.

Poehlman, E. T., Toth, M.J., Goran, M. I., Carpenter, W. H., Newhouse, P. & Rosen, C. J. (1997). Daily energy expenditure in free-living non-institutionalized Alzheimer's patients: a doubly labeled water study. *Neurology*, 48(4), 997–1002.

Rosenthal, M. J., Fajardo, M., Gilmore, S., Morley, J. E. & Naliboff, B. D. (1998). Hospitalization and mortality of diabetes in older adults. A 3-year prospective study. *Diabetes Care*, 21(2), 231–5.

Rudman, D. (1985). Growth hormone, body composition, and aging. *Journal of the American Geriatric Society*, 33(11), 800–7.

Rudman, D., Feller, A. G., Nagraj, H. S., Gergans, G. A., Lalitha, P. Y., Goldberg, A. F., Schlenker, R. A., Cohn, L., Rudman, I. W. & Mattson, D. E. (1990a). Effects of human growth hormone in men over 60 years old. *New England Journal of Medicine*, 323(1), 1–6.

Rudman, D., Shetty, K. R., Mattson, D. E. (1990b). Plasma dehydroepiandrosterone sulfate in nursing home men. *Journal of the American Geriatric Society*, 38(4), 421–7.

Sih, R., Morley, J. E., Kaiser, F. E., Perry, H. M. III, Patrick, P. & Ross, C. (1997). Testosterone replacement in older hypogonadal men: a 12-month randomized controlled trial. *Journal of Clinical Endocrinology and Metabolism*, 82(6), 1661–7.

Silver, A. J., Flood, J. F. & Morley, J. E. (1988). Effects of gastrointestinal peptides on ingestion in old and young mice. *Peptides*, 9(2), 221–5.

Urban, R. J., Bodenburg, Y. H., Gilkison, C., Foxworth, J., Coggan, A. R., Wolfe, R. R. & Ferrando, A. (1995). Testosterone administration to elderly men increases skeletal muscle strength and protein synthesis. *American Journal of Physiology*, 269(5, 1), E820–6.

Willenbring, M. L., Morley, J. E., Niewoehner, C. B., Heilman, R. O., Carlson, C. H. & Shafer, R. B. (1984). Adrenocortical hyperactivity in newly admitted alcoholics: prevalence, course and associated variables. *Psychoneuroendocrinology*, 9(4), 415–22.

Wilson, M. M., Vaswani, S., Liu, D., Morley, J. E. & Miller, D. K. (1998). Prevalence and causes of undernutrition in medical outpatients. *American Journal of Medicine*, 104(1), 56–63.

Wolf, O. T., Naumann, E., Hellhammer, D. H. & Kirschbaum, C. (1998). Effects of dehydroepi-androsterone replacement in elderly men on event-related potentials, memory, and well-being. *Journal of Gerontology. Series A, Biological Sciences and Medical Sciences*, 53(5), M385–90.

Overview of steroids in the aging brain

Loretta M. Flanagan-Cato

Introduction

Steroid and thyroid hormones are often considered together because they share a similar cellular mechanism of action in their influence on neural structure and function. The nervous system is particularly sensitive to steroids and thyroid hormone during development, and these hormones also modulate neuronal and glial functions during adulthood. Aging-induced changes in these hormone systems are likely to influence physiological, cognitive, and emotional processes. Previously, it was believed that the effects of gonadal steroids on the adult nervous system were restricted to areas involved in reproduction; however, in recent years it has become evident that sex steroids affect other functions, such as learning and memory.

This chapter provides a review of the current understanding of the basic mechanisms of hormone effects in the brain, with an emphasis on the biosynthesis, the site of action, and the emerging diversity of cellular mechanisms employed by hormones to affect neuronal function.

Biosynthesis, release, and serum transport

Endocrine steroid synthesis

The precursor for all steroid biosynthesis is cholesterol, which can be derived from either animal fats in the diet or from local synthesis depending on the tissue. Specific cell-surface receptors bind circulating low-density lipoproteins that are rich in cholesterol. The protein–cholesterol complex then is transported into the cell by endocytosis, and the cholesterol is split from the lipoprotein, esterified, and stored in cytoplasmic vacuoles. The rate-limiting step in synthesizing all steroid hormones is the first step, accomplished by the action of the cytochrome P450 side chain cleavage enzyme, also known as 20,22-desmolase, which converts cholesterol into pregnenolone. Each steroidogenic endocrine tissue expresses specific enzymes that allow a multistep conversion of pregnenolone to the appropriate steroid hormones. Because of their lipophilic structure, only small amounts of these hormones are stored intracellularly. When more is needed, the biosynthetic pathway must be activated at the rate-limiting 20,22-desmolase reaction. Generally, after secretagogues bind to their plasma membrane receptors, adenylyl cyclase is activated and cyclic AMP levels increase. Cyclic AMP, then, activates protein kinases that convert cholesterol esters to free cholesterol, and, thus, this provides the substrate for steroid synthesis. For adrenal and sex steroids, as well as for thyroid hormone, the major secretagogues are peptide hormones released from the anterior pituitary, which themselves are triggered by hypothalamic releasing hormones. In order to maintain appropriate activity of each of these hormone systems, steroids and thyroid hormone provide negative feedback regulation on either the pituitary or the hypothalamus, or both.

Within the hypothalamic–pituitary–adrenal axis, glucocorticoid secretion is controlled by adrenocorticotropic hormone (ACTH). ACTH increases the interaction of cholesterol with the side chain cleavage enzyme. Once pregnenolone is available in the adrenal cortex, it is rapidly, sequentially modified to form one of the three major types of adrenal hormones, depending on cell type: cortisol, aldosterone, or dehydroepiandrosterone. Plasma levels of cortisol rise within minutes of an intravenous infusion of ACTH. Under ordinary circumstances, the secretion of cortisol is both episodic and variable with a major burst of activity in the early morning hours before awakening. The activity of this axis is set by the negative feedback control that cortisol exerts on both hypothalamic corticotropic hormone (CRH) and pituitary ACTH synthesis and release.

The hypothalamic–pituitary–gonadal axis controls ovarian secretion mainly through the pituitary release of luteinizing hormone (LH) and follicle stimulating hormone (FSH). The major steroids produced by the ovary are progesterone and estradiol, although some androgens are released as well. Prolactin also influences progesterone secretion by modulating the number of LH receptors in the ovary, whereas growth hormone facilitates the actions of FSH through the local production of local insulin-like growth factor I. Both LH and FSH stimulate the production of progesterone and estradiol. Only LH, however, promotes ovarian production of androgens. Estradiol can be synthesized from either estrone or testosterone by an aromatase enzyme. Other estrogens present in the bloodstream, namely estrone and estriol, have little bioactivity relative to estradiol because of their rapid degradation.

In males, LH controls testosterone synthesis, which occurs in Leydig cells in the testes and, to some extent, the adrenal cortex. The first four enzymes in this biosynthetic pathway are present in both the testes and the adrenal cortex, with the final enzymatic step primarily present in the testes. Two types of active metabolites that are formed in peripheral tissues and the brain mediate many androgen effects, and in this regard testosterone can be considered a prohormone. The first category of active metabolites is the 5α-reduced steroids, primarily dihydrotestosterone (5α-DHT), which mediates many androgen actions in target tissues. Approximately 7% of the total testosterone is converted to 5α-DHT by 5α-reductase. Although both testosterone and 5α-DHT bind to a common androgen receptor, 5α-DHT is the main intracellular androgen and is about twice as potent as testosterone in androgen bioassay systems. 5α-reductase has a distinct tissue localization with the most activity found in the reproductive accessory organs, the liver, and the skin. Some activity is also found in the brain. The second category of active testosterone metabolites is estrogen formed by the aromatization of androgens in a number of tissues, including the brain. In males, 85% to 90% of the estrogens are formed outside the testes, and the overall rate of aromatization appears to rise with advancing age. Both the 5α-reduction and the aromatization of testosterone are physiologically irreversible processes. Thus, in males, the physiological actions of testosterone are the result of combined effects of 5α-reduced androgens and estrogens. In women, androgens are produced by both the ovary and adrenal, and while testosterone is the primary active androgen in women, dehydroepiandrosterone and androstenedione are also present.

Once in the circulation, steroid hormones tend to be bound to plasma proteins. For instance, cortisol is largely bound to a specific glucocorticoid binding protein, transcortin, with a small percent bound to albumin. Only about 5% of circulating cortisol is 'free.' Likewise, about 70% of circulating estrogens are bound to plasma proteins, such as albumin and testosterone binding globulin (TeBG). Estrogens have a lower affinity for TeBG than androgens, resulting in a greater availability of estrogens to the tissues. Progesterone also appears to circulate bound to plasma proteins, but the characteristics of this association are not known. Testosterone circulates in the plasma largely bound to plasma proteins, primarily albumin and TeBG. In normal men, only about 2% of testosterone is unbound. However, dissociation of testosterone occurs in the microcirculation in vivo so that tissue availability of steroid hormones is greater than the 'free' concentration measured in vitro. After synthesis and release, most steroids are inactivated in the liver where they are converted to tetrahydro forms, conjugated to glucuronides, and finally, excreted into the urine.

In summary, endocrine release of adrenal and gonadal steroids is controlled by peptide hormones that activate the biosynthesis pathway. Endocrine tissues differ in the expression of receptors for these peptide secretagogues and the enzymatic elements of the steroidogenic pathway. Cholesterol conversion to pregnenolone is the rate-limiting step in biosynthesis for all steroids. Because of limited storage mechanisms, synthesis and release are nearly synonymous for endocrine steroids. Secretion of each of these hormones changes with the aging process (as further discussed in Chapters 3, 5, and 6).

Neurosteroids

The nervous system can be influenced by steroids released from peripheral tissues as well as by locally generated steroids. The term 'neurosteroid' has been used to refer both to steroids that are synthesized in the brain de novo and to those synthesized by in situ metabolism of blood-borne precursors. Pregnenelone and progesterone are considered neurosteroids based on several lines of evidence. First, levels of these steroids remain high in the brain after gonadectomy and adrenalectomy (Baulieu, 1991; Robel & Baulieu, 1994). Second, the CNS oligodendrocytes possess the necessary enzymes to synthesize these steroids from cholesterol, namely, P450 side chain cleavage enzyme, 3β-hydroxysteroid dehydrogenase, and 5α-reductase (Le Goascogne et al., 1987; Celotti et al., 1992; Mellon & Deschepper, 1993; Guennoun et al., 1995; Sanne & Krueger, 1995). Third, studies in cultured oligodendrocytes have shown that these cells produce pregnenelone when given the appropriate precursors (Hu et al., 1987; Jung-Testas et al., 1989). The available evidence indicates that neurosteroids are formed in the mammalian brain during development and adulthood, and it is possible that decreases in their levels contribute to aging in the brain. For instance, in rodents, higher brain levels of progesterone and dehydroepiandrosterone are associated with less decline of cognitive function with aging (Flood & Roberts, 1988; Robel et al., 1995), and preliminary studies have suggested that neurosteroids participate in regeneration, particularly myelin repair (Le Goascogne et al., 1987, 1989; Jung-Testas et al., 1991, 1994; Sanne & Krueger, 1995). Although further research is needed, such results indicate that neurosteroids may be therapeutically useful.

Many steroids, however, cannot be synthesized in the CNS. Cytochrome P450$-_{17\alpha}$ – the enzyme that converts pregnenolone to dehydroepiandrosterone and progesterone to androstenedione, the obligate precursors for androgens – does not seem to be present in the brain. Glucocorticoids also are probably not neurosteroids because their levels in brain become undetectable after removal of steroidogenic endocrine glands (Mellon, 1994). Estrogens, however, can be synthesized in the brain by the aromatization of circulating testosterone.

In summary, brain functions may be modulated by locally synthesized neurosteroids in addition to being influenced by peripherally derived steroid hormones. There is substantial evidence that pregnenolone and progesterone can be synthesized by glia in the nervous system, and particular populations of neurons convert testosterone to estradiol. Neurosteroids may counteract some of the effects of aging in the brain.

Thyroid hormones

The substrates for thyroid hormone biosynthesis are iodide and the amino acid tyrosine. The thyroid gland concentrates inorganic iodide from the extracellular fluid by an active, saturable energy-dependent process. Both thyroid-stimulating hormone (TSH) and a thyroid regulatory mechanism control the iodide transport mechanism. Tyrosine residues are iodinated by thyroid peroxidase, a membrane bound heme-protein enzyme. Within the matrix of the large protein thyroglobulin, the precursor amino acids diiodotyrosine and monoiodotyrosine are converted by a coupling reaction to the two principle thyroid hormones: T4 (3,5,3',5'-tetraiodothyronine) and T3 (3,5,3'-triiodothyronine), respectively. The specific tertiary structure of thyroglobulin is thought to be important for efficient coupling since disruption of its native structure results in very low levels of T4 formation. Within thyroglobulin, the T4 to T3 ratio is ten to one.

Release of thyroid hormone is prompted by circulating TSH, which activates adenylyl cyclase. In contrast to steroid hormones, the thyroid contains a several week supply of thyroid hormones in its thyroglobulin pool. TSH causes digestion of thyroglobulin which liberates T4 and T3. The free T4 and T3, being lipophilic like steroids, diffuse from the cell into the circulation. However, iodotyrosines are largely prevented from being released into the circulation by the action of an intracellular deiodinase, and the free iodide is salvaged for reuse. Thyroglobulin also is not released into the circulation in appreciable amounts unless there is trauma or inflammation of the thyroid. Thyroid hormone in the circulation is largely bound to thyroid hormone-binding globulin (TBG), prealbumin, and albumin, so less than 1% of T4 and T3 are 'free.' T4 binds more tightly to serum binding proteins than T3, resulting in lower metabolic clearance rates and in a longer serum half-life. Specifically, the serum half-life of T4 is about 7 days, whereas for T3 it is less than a day.

In summary, the precursors, the biosynthetic process, and the release mechanisms for thyroid hormones differ from those for steroid hormones. Like steroids, however, thyroid hormones are lipophilic, they are chaperoned in the circulation, and they provide negative feedback regulation on their own secretion. With aging, there are often changes in thyroid hormone secretion (as further discussed in Chapter 4).

Receptors

General principles

Steroid and thyroid hormones enter cells by diffusion and bind to cognate intracellular receptors. These receptor proteins share three properties: they have a nuclear site of action, they bind to specific DNA sequences, and they regulate gene transcription (Evans, 1988). These functional similarities between the steroid and thyroid hormone receptors are consonant with their molecular homologies. In particular, sequence comparisons have revealed that all these receptors have three regions of sequence homology: a region with DNA binding capability that functions as two zinc fingers; a hormone binding domain that consists of a hydrophobic pocket; and a region that allows these receptors to dimerize in solution.

Hormone binding 'activates' or 'transforms' the receptors, which is thought to trigger a conformational change, a dissociation from a complex that includes heat shock proteins, and an increased affinity for regulatory elements of the genome. Steroids alter protein synthesis by regulating the rate of gene transcription and increasing the stability of mRNA. There are relatively few examples where steroids influence protein expression by affecting mRNA translation. Once the hormone–receptor complex has interacted with the DNA, the receptor is recycled to an unoccupied form in a process that may involve dephosphorylation.

Steroid-regulated genes possess steroid receptor binding sites known as hormone response elements (HREs), which consist of imperfect hexanucleotide pallindromic sequences that attract receptor dimers. The association of hormone receptor dimers with these sequences alters the probability of transcription occurring. Given that RNA polymerase II is not in excess in the nucleus, genes are in competition for this enzyme. Thus, regulatory DNA sequences can bind proteins that attract this enzyme to their location, acting as a thermostat to control the basal rate of transcription. While glucocorticoids, mineralocorticoids, androgen, and progesterone activate similar positive HREs, estrogen has a quite different response element which resembles that for thyroid hormone.

The stoichiometry of thyroid hormone receptor (TR) binding to DNA is different than that of steroid receptor binding. In particular, the binding affinity of a TR monomer or homodimer to thyroid responsive elements is relatively weak. Instead, a single TR binds to DNA stably as part of a heterodimer with other proteins, such as with the retinoid X receptor, which is responsive to 9-*cis* retinoic acid. In another deviation from the steroid receptors, the unliganded TR is located in the nucleus bound to thyroid HREs because TR is not anchored to heat shock proteins. For this reason, basal transcription of genes activated by thyroid hormone is repressed by the unliganded TR. This is particularly relevant for a subtype of TR, namely TRα2. Unlike other isoforms of TR, the TRα2 receptors are not regulated by thyroid hormone, and therefore they are not hormone dependent in their DNA binding. As such, TRα2 antagonizes the activity of the ligand-dependent TRs in a dominant-negative fashion. Thus, the expression of TRα2 may be crucial in tissue-specific responses to thyroid hormone for brain development and function.

In summary, activated steroid and thyroid hormone receptors are transcription factors, that, by binding to regulatory DNA sequences, can modulate expression of particular genes. In most, but not all, cases, this regulation occurs in a ligand-dependent fashion. The effect of aging on the levels of receptors for these hormones in the brain has not been well studied.

CNS Localization and subtypes

There are two known subtypes of glucocorticoid receptors. The Type I receptor, which also binds mineralocorticoids, has a high affinity for glucocorticoids (K_D = 0.5 to 1 nM) and is extensively occupied at low, physiological levels of glucocorticoids. The Type II receptor is more selective for glucocorticoids, although with a lower affinity than the Type I receptor (K_D = 5 to 10 nM). The Type II receptor is occupied when glucocorticoids are elevated, such as during stress (Reul & De Kloet, 1985). Both of these receptor subtypes are expressed in the brain, although with somewhat differing distributions, as shown by receptor autoradiography, immunocytochemistry, and in situ hybridization (Warembourg, 1975; Fuxe et al., 1985; Aronsson et al., 1988). The hippocampal formation is one of the prime targets of glucocorticoid action with the greatest levels of receptor binding activity and mRNA for both Type I and Type II receptors, particularly in pyramidal cells of the CA1, CA3, and the granule cells of the dentate gyrus. These glucocorticoid receptors participate in learning and memory functions (Diamond & Rose, 1994; Bodnoff et al., 1995), regulation of the hypothalamic–pituitary–adrenal axis (Jacobson & Sapolsky, 1991), and neuronal viability (Stein-Behrens et al., 1992). The colocalization of both Type I and Type II receptors in these regions implies differential regulation by circadian rhythms and stress. Brain regions that express mainly the Type II receptors include the hypothalamic paraventricular nucleus, the central nucleus of the amygdala, limbic-related areas of thalamus, the neocortex, the locus coeruleus, and the dorsal raphe nucleus. Thus, at higher levels, glucocorticoids influence regions known to participate in endocrine and autonomic responses, arousal, and affect. The distribution of the Type I receptors is more limited, and includes the limbic system, hypothalamus, and the circumventricular organs. These receptors may participate in the behavioral, endocrine, and autonomic activities, as influenced by mineralocorticoids or basal levels of glucocorticoids.

Estrogen receptors were first localized in the brain using receptor autoradiography after in vivo administration of tritiated estradiol (Pfaff & Keiner, 1973; Stumpf et al., 1975). This technique identified estrogen receptors in abundance in hypothalamic and preoptic structures involved in gonadotropin regulation and reproductive behaviors. In addition, estrogen receptors were found in the catecholamine neurons associated with the reticular activating system, the emotional integration systems of the periaqueductal gray and the amygdala, and the limbic system, but very few receptors were found in the hippocampus and neocortex. These findings were later confirmed with immunocytochemistry (Sar & Parikh, 1986; Fuxe et al., 1987; Press & Greene, 1988) and in situ hybridization (Simerly et al., 1990) for the estrogen receptor protein and mRNA, respectively.

Rather recently, it was discovered that more than one form of estrogen receptor exists (Kuiper et al., 1996; Mosselman et al., 1996). The novel subtype, dubbed estrogen receptor-β, has a very similar pharmacological profile to the α form (Kuiper et al., 1997), however, the β form displays a different tissue distribution. For example, estrogen receptor-α is found in abundance in the hypothalamic ventromedial nucleus, whereas estrogen receptor-β is not abundant there (Shughrue et al., 1996). The mRNA for the β form of the receptor was found in several hypothalamic neuroendocrine structures, such as the paraventricular nucleus, as well as limbic areas such as the amygdala, and reticular areas such as the dorsal raphe nucleus. The variant β_2 is also present in the brain, including the frontal cortex, hippocampus, and hypothalamus, but in much less abundance than the originally identified β receptor (Petersen et al., 1998). The behavioral consequences of each of these subtypes are not completely parsed as yet. However, in vitro studies indicate that expression of the α vs. the β receptor has opposite effects on the interactions with transcription factors that bind to the transcription enhancer element known as AP-1, which mediates the effects of immediate early genes on transcriptional activation (Paech et al., 1997).

Progestin receptors were first localized in the brain with receptor autoradiography and microdissection techniques (MacLusky & McEwen, 1978, 1980; Warembourg, 1978), with the highest concentrations found in the preoptic area and mediobasal hypothalamus. These early studies indicated that hypothalamic progestin receptors were up-regulated by estrogen, whereas in other regions such as the cerebral cortex, amygdala, hippocampus, caudate–putamen, cerebellum, and midbrain, progestin binding activity occurred independently of estrogen treatment. Subsequent studies confirmed this localization using immunocytochemistry (Warembourg et al., 1986; Blaustein et al., 1988; Don Carlos et al., 1989). In situ hybridization studies have shown that estrogen regulates the level of progestin receptors in the hypothalamus at a transcriptional level (Romano et al., 1989). More recently, it has become apparent that the progestin receptor is present in both a long and a short form, depending on an alternate translation initiation event (Conneely et al., 1989). These two proteins differ by the presence of a 164 amino acid segment in the amino terminus of the long form, which leads to differential interactions with other transcription factors (McDonnell et al., 1994).

Androgen receptors have been localized in the brain using receptor autoradiography (Sar & Stumpf, 1977) and in situ hybridization (Simerly et al., 1990). In particular, androgen receptors were consistently found in the olfactory cortex, the septum, the preoptic area, the hypothalamus, the extended amygdala, and the hippocampal formation. Many of these areas are known to participate in reproductive behaviors and endocrine function. However, it is noteworthy that regions that regulate stress responses, such as the hypothalamic region that contains CRH neurons and the reticular formation, also express androgen receptors. The brain also expresses 5α-reductase, allowing local conversion of testosterone to its more potent androgen metabolite, 5α-DHT. There are two isoforms of this enzyme expressed in the brain (Melcangi et al., 1998). Type 1 shows no sexual dimorphism and is not regulated by androgens. Type 2, in contrast, is controlled by testosterone and is most abundant at the time of sexual differentiation of the brain. The distribution of 5α-reductase generally overlaps with the distribution of androgen receptors, including the preoptic area and hypothalamus (Selmanoff et al., 1977).

It is important to realize that many effects of testosterone in the brain may actually be mediated by estrogen receptors depending on the presence of the aromatase enzyme. In general, the localization of aromatase in the brain corresponds to the expression of estrogen receptors, based on enzymatic activity and mRNA levels (Roselli et al., 1985, 1998; Roselli & Resko, 1987). In animal models, the most prominent sites of aromatase activity are found in the extended amygdala and hypothalamic areas involved in neuroendocrine control and reproductive behavior. In human brain, aromatase mRNA has been detected in the pons, thalamus, hypothalamus, amygdala, hippocampus, and frontal cortex (Sasano et al., 1998). Androgens and estrogens up-regulate the expression of aromatase in most of these areas in animal studies.

It is now well recognized that thyroid hormone is critical for normal neurological function. Three subtypes of TR, all of which belong to the superfamily of steroid receptors, are particularly prevalent in the brain: TRα1, TRβ1, and TRβ2 (Puymirat, 1992). These receptors have been localized, using in situ hybridization and immunocytochemistry, in various nuclei of the hypothalamus, including the arcuate, paraventricular, and ventromedial, as well as the piriform cortex, CA1 of the hippocampus, caudate putamen, and the Purkinje cells of the cerebellum (Bradley et al., 1992; Lechan et al., 1993). Sites of brain expression for these receptor isoforms suggest that they may be involved in thermoregulation, metabolism, appetite, mood, or cognitive function.

Biological effects of steroids

Classical effects involve changes in neurotransmission

There have been a large number of studies documenting the effects of adrenal or ovarian steroids on the synthesis and release of various neurotransmitters and on the expression of various receptors in discrete brain areas. In many cases, the effects of steroids parallel changes that occur within these neurotransmitter systems during either stress or reproductive cycles. An exhaustive list of such effects is beyond the scope of this chapter. In most examples, such changes occur in a time course that is consistent with a genomic mechanism of action, requiring changes in transcription. As discussed below, however, it has become apparent that the effects of steroids and their receptors cannot be limited to genomic effects on neurochemistry.

Novel effects of steroids

In addition to modulating neurochemistry, steroids cause structural changes in the brain, such as changes in the synaptic organization and electrical coupling of neurons. Thus, steroids can transiently alter the hard wiring of particular circuits in the adult brain. For example, in the ventromedial hypothalamus and the CA1 region of the hippocampus, estrogen increases the density of dendritic spines and synaptic specializations (Frankfurt et al., 1990; Gould et al., 1990; Woolley et al., 1990; Frankfurt & McEwen, 1991; Woolley & McEwen, 1993). At least in the hippocampus, the effect is likely to be secondary to changes in neural input because changes in spine density in hippocampal pyramidal neurons requires NMDA receptor activation (Woolley & McEwen, 1994; Woolley et al., 1996). Importantly, these estrogen-induced morphological changes are correlated with increased postsynaptic sensitivity to NMDA-mediated synaptic input (Woolley et al., 1997). Although these estrogen-induced spines appear to be dependent on synaptic activity (Murphy & Segal, 1996, 1997; Murphy et al., 1998), their time course suggests that they are secondary to genomic effects in other nodes in the neural circuitry.

Recent discoveries have shown that at least some steroid receptors can be activated by mechanisms other than ligand binding. For instance, dopamine receptor agonists mimic the effect of progesterone on female sexual behavior in rats, and this effect is abolished with progestin receptor antagonists or antisense, and in transgenic mice deficient in progestin receptors (Mani et al., 1994, 1996). In addition, progestin receptor antagonists reduce mating-induced expression of immediate early genes in the hypothalamus in the absence of progesterone, suggesting that endogenous neurotransmitters facilitated mating by activating the progestin receptor (Auger et al., 1997). Non-steroid activation of the estrogen receptor also has been documented (Ignar-Trowbridge et al., 1992). Such results indicate that steroid receptors are not necessarily innocent bystanders in neural function in the absence of their steroid ligand.

Another novel effect of steroids involves modulation of membrane-bound receptors. Selye first reported that progesterone and several of its metabolites have anesthetic and sedative effects which occur more rapidly than would be expected of a transcription-mediated event (Selye, 1942). Much later electrophysiological and pharmacological work on the GABA–A receptor demonstrated that such steroids act as allosteric agonists of this receptor to facilitate the actions of GABA (Majewska et al., 1986; Gee et al., 1987; Dayanithi & Tapia-Arancibia, 1996). Behavioral consequences of steroid–GABA interactions include the effect of progestin metabolites, such as allopregnanolone, to rapidly alter reproductive and anxiety-like behaviors (Frye & DeBold, 1993; Frye et al., 1996; Brot et al., 1997). Progesterene and its metabolites also directly modulate oxytocin receptors (Grazzini et al., 1998) and N-methyl-D-aspartate (NMDA) receptors (Park-Chung et al., 1997).

There also are rapid effects of estrogens, such as increased K^+–stimulated dopamine release in the nucleus accumbens (Thompson & Moss, 1994), reduced calcium currents in the neostriatum (Mermelstein et al., 1996), and potentiated kainate-induced depolarization in hippocampal pyramidal cells in a protein kinase A-dependent fashion (Wong & Moss, 1992; Gu & Moss, 1996). Given the lack of evidence for classical estrogen receptors in these regions, non-receptor targets have been proposed (Balthazart & Ball, 1998). For instance, aromatase may act as a bifunctional enzyme to generate locally catechol estrogens, powerful competitive inhibitors of catechol o-methyl transferase. Thus, it has been proposed that, since the mammalian telencephalon generally expresses aromatase but not estrogen receptors, local conversion of estrogen may non-genomically alter neuronal function by altering catecholamine levels.

Sexual dimorphisms

Although there are no gross sexual dimorphisms in the general pattern of expression of androgen and estrogen receptors in the brain (Simerly et al., 1990), the density of estrogen and progesterone receptors in the preoptic area and hypothalamic is higher in female than in male rats (Rainbow et al., 1982; Brown et al., 1988). Conversely, there are higher levels of aromatase activity in these brain regions in male rats compared with females (Roselli et al., 1996; Roselli & Klosterman, 1998). Major sex differences in steroid receptors beyond areas involved in reproduction have not been noted.

Interactions with other steroids

Estrogens and glucocorticoids often act in opposition to regulate physiological responses. For example, estrogen is well known to stimulate uterine and breast growth and bone formation. In contrast, glucocorticoids block uterotrophic effects, inhibit breast cell proliferation, and reduce bone formation (Bigsby, 1993). Estrogen enhances the hypothalamic–pituitary–adrenal response during stress, yet glucocorticoids exert a negative feedback effect (Burgess & Handa, 1992). In the brain, estrogen is associated with neuronal spouting and neurite outgrowth (Toran-Allerand, 1996), whereas glucocorticoids can cause dendritic atrophy and cell death (Sapolsky et al., 1990). There are several possible levels of interaction between glucocorticoids and estrogens. For example, the hepatic synthesis of trans-cortin is increased by estrogen. In addition, it now appears that physiological inter-actions of estrogen and glucocorticoids also may be mediated by interactions of the estrogen and glucocorticoid receptors at AP-1 binding sites (Uht et al., 1997). In particular, estrogen and glucocorticoid receptor activation exert opposing regula-tion on the AP-1 response element. This site mediates regulation by various imme-diate early gene products, such as Fos and Jun. Thus, the antagonistic effects of these steroids on various tissues may be mediated by receptor interactions at par-ticular DNA sites.

As mentioned above, the progestin receptor binds with equal affinity to the same HRE as do the Type I and Type II glucocorticoid receptors. The sharing of a common DNA binding sequence may be responsible for the partial agonist prop-erties of progesterone for glucocorticoid actions. Despite sharing a common HRE, glucocorticoid receptors are much more efficient than progestin receptors in recruiting additional transcription factors that expose the chromatin. Thus, the progestin receptors may only enhance gene expression at sites that are already rel-atively accessible.

Another example of functional antagonism between these receptor systems can be found with estrogen and thyroid hormone. For example, increased levels of thyroid hormone during reduced ambient temperatures seem to mediate the sup-pression of female reproductive behavior during cold stress. The mechanism may involve direct competition of TR and estrogen receptors for consensus sequences given that the half-site consensus sequence for the thyroid hormone response element is identical to that for the estrogen response element. In vitro transfection studies have shown that $TR\alpha1$ inhibited estrogen induction of reporter gene expression. This interaction between estrogen receptors and TR appears to be physiologically relevant. In particular, thyroid hormone is able to inhibit the effects of estrogen on brain expression of specific proteins (Zhu et al., 1996) and on repro-ductive behavior (Dellovade et al., 1996).

Summary and conclusions

Receptors for steroids and thyroid hormones belong to a superfamily of transcrip-tion factors which regulate gene expression and are found in limbic and hypotha-lamic areas of the brain, and to a lesser extent the neocortex and areas that regulate attention and arousal. The behavioral effects of each of these hormones should not be considered in isolation, however, because cooperative or antagonistic effects on gene expression can occur based on receptor-receptor interactions. In addition, some steroids, particularly progesterone and its metabolites, regulate membrane-bound receptors such as the GABA–A and NMDA channels. Furthermore, certain steroid receptors can be activated independently of ligand binding, for example by second messenger cascades initiated by catecholamines or peptides.

Finally, in addition to endocrine sources, the brain generates some steroids. This diversity of regulation and function provides a cellular basis for the integration of interoceptive hormonal cues with other modes of neural processing. At the same time, this complexity of mechanisms makes it especially challenging to study the effects of aging, where parallel changes occur in multiple hormone systems.

REFERENCES

Aronsson, M., Fuxe, K., Dong, Y., Agnati, L. F., Okret, S. & Gustafsson, J-A. (1988). Localization of glucocorticoid receptor mRNA in the male rat brain by in situ hybridization. *Proceedings of the National Academy of Sciences, USA*, 85, 9331–5.

Auger, A. P., Moffatt, C. A. & Blaustein, J. D. (1997). Progesterone-independent activation of rat brain progestin receptors by reproductive stimuli. *Endocrinology*, 138, 511–14.

Balthazart, J. & Ball, G. F. (1998). New insights into the regulation and function of brain estrogen synthase (aromatase). *Trends in Neuroscience*, 21, 243–9.

Baulieu, E-E. (1991). Neurosteroids: A new function in the brain. *Biology of the Cell*, 71, 3–10.

Bigsby, R. M. (1993). Progesterone and dexamethasone inhibition of estrogen-induced synthesis of DNA and complement in rat uterine epithelium: effect of antiprogesterone compounds. *Journal of Steroid Biochemistry and Molecular Biology*, 45, 295–301.

Blaustein, J., King, J. C., Toft, D. O. & Turcotte, J. (1988). Immunocytochemical localization of estrogen-induced progestin receptors in guinea pig brain. *Brain Research*, 474, 1–15.

Bodnoff, S. R., Humphreys, A. G., Lehman, J. C., Diamond, D. M., Rose, G. M. & Meaney, M. J. (1995). Enduring effects of chronic corticosterone treatment on spatial learning, synaptic plasticity, and hippocampal neuropathology in young and mid-aged rats. *Journal of Neuroscience*, 15, 61–9.

Bradley, D. J., Towle, H. C. & Young III, W. S. (1992). Spatial and temporal expression of α- and β-thyroid hormone receptor mRNAs, including the β2-subtype, in the developing mammalian nervous system. *Journal of Neuroscience*, 12, 2288–302.

Brot, M. D., Akwa, Y., Purdy, R. H., Koob, G. F. & Britton, K. T. (1997). The anxiolytic-like effects of the neurosteroid allopregnanolone: interactions with GABA$_A$ receptors. *European Journal of Pharmacology*, 325, 1–7.

Brown, T. J., Hochberg, R. B., Zielinski, J. E. & MacLuskey, N. J. (1988). Regional sex differences in cell nuclear estrogen-binding capacity in the rat hypothalamus and preoptic area. *Endocrinology*, 123, 1761–71.

Burgess, L. H. & Handa, R. J. (1992). Chronic estrogen-induced alterations in adrenocorticotropin and corticosterone secretion, and glucocorticoid receptor-mediated functions in female rats. *Endocrinology*, **131**, 1261–9.

Celotti, F., Melcangi, R. C. & Martini, L. (1992). The 5α-reductase in the brain: molecular aspects and relation to brain function. *Frontiers in Neuroendocrinology*, **13**, 163–215.

Conneely, O. M., Kettelberger, D. M., Tsai, M-J., Schrader, W. T. & O'Malley, B. W. (1989). The chicken progesterone receptor A and B isoforms are products of an alternate translation initiation event. *Journal of Biological Chemisty*, **264**, 14062–4.

Dayanithi, G. & Tapia-Arancibia, L. (1996). Rise in intracellular calcium via a nongenomic effect of allopregnanolone in fetal rat hypothalamic neurons. *Journal of Neuroscience*, **16**, 130–6.

Dellovade, T. L., Zhu, Y-S., Krey, L. & Pfaff, D. W. (1996). Thyroid hormone and estrogen interact to regulate behavior. *Proceedings of the National Academy of Sciences, USA*, **93**, 12581–6.

Diamond, D. M. & Rose, G. M. (1994). Stress impairs LTP and hippocampal-dependent memory. *Annals of the New York Academy of Sciences*, **746**, 411–14.

Don Carlos, L. L., Greene, G. L. & Morrell, J. I. (1989). Estrogen plus progesterone increases progestin receptor immunoreactivity in the brain of ovariectomized guinea pigs. *Neuroendocrinology*, **50**, 613–23.

Evans, R. M. (1988). The steroid and thyroid hormone receptor super-family. *Science*, **240**, 889–95.

Flood, J. F. & Roberts, E. (1988). Dehydroepiandrosterone sulfate improves memory in aging mice. *Brain Research*, **448**, 178–81.

Frankfurt, M. & McEwen, B. S. (1991). Estrogen increases axodendritic synapses in the VMN of rats after ovariectomy. *NeuroReport*, **2**, 380–2.

Frankfurt, M., Gould, E., Woolley, C. S. & McEwen, B. S. (1990). Gonadal steroids modify dentritic spine density in ventromedial hypothalamic neurons: a Golgi study in the adult rat. *Neuroendocrinology*, **51**, 530–5.

Frye, C. A. & DeBold, J. F. (1993). 3α-OH-DHP and 5α-THDOC implants to the ventral tegmental area facilitate sexual receptivity in hamsters after progesterone priming to the ventral medial hypothalamus. *Brain Research*, **612**, 130–7.

Frye, C. A., Van Keuren, K. R., Rao, P. N. & Erskine, M. S. (1996). Analgesic effects of the neurosteroid 3α-androstanediol. *Brain Research*, **709**, 1–9.

Fuxe, K., Cintra, A., Agnati, L. F., Harfstrand, A., Wikstrom, A. C., Okret, S., Zoli, M., Miller, L. S., Greene, J. L. & Gustafsson, J. A. (1987). Studies on the cellular localization and distribution of glucocorticoid receptor and estrogen receptor immunoreactivity in the central nervous system of the rat and their relationship to the monoaminergic and peptidergic neurons. *Journal of Steroid Biochemistry*, **27**, 159–70.

Fuxe, K., Wikstrom, A. C., Okret, S., Agnati, L. F., Harfstrand, A., Yu, Z, Y., Granholm, L., Zoli, M., Vale, W. & Gustafsson, J. A. (1985). Mapping of glucocorticoid receptor immunoreactive neurons in the rat tel- and diencephalon using a monoclonal antibody against rat liver glucocorticoid receptor. *Endocrinology*, **117**, 1803–12.

Gee, K. W., Chang, W-C., Brinton, R. E. & McEwen, B. S. (1987). GABA-dependent modulation of the Cl$^-$ ionophore by steroids in the rat brain. *European Journal of Pharmacology*, **136**, 419–23.

Gould, E., Woolley, C. S., Frankfurt, M. & McEwen, B. S. (1990). Gonadal steroids regulate dendritic spine density in hippocampal pyramidal cells in adulthood. *Journal of Neuroscience,* **10**, 1286–91.

Grazzini, E., Guillon, G., Mouillac, B. & Zingg, H. H. (1998). Inhibition of oxytocin receptor function by direct binding of progesterone. *Nature,* **392**, 509–12.

Gu, Q. & Moss, R. L. (1996). 17β-estradiol potentiates kainate-induced currents via activation of the cAMP cascade. *Journal of Neuroscience,* **16**, 3620–9.

Guennoun, R., Fiddes, R. J., Gouezou, M., Lombes, M. & Baulieu, E-E. (1995). A key enzyme in the biosynthesis of neurosteroids, 3β-hydroxysteroid dehydrogenas (3β-HSD), is expressed in rat brain. *Molecular Brain Research,* **30**, 287–300.

Hu, Z. Y., Bourreau, E., Jung-Testas, I., Robel, P. & Baulieu, E-E. (1987). Oligodendrocyte mitochondria convert cholesterol to pregnenolone. *Proceedings of the National Academy of Sciences, USA,* **84**, 8215–29.

Ignar-Trowbridge, D. M., Nelson, K. G., Bidwell, M. C., Curtis, S. W., Washburn, T. F., McLachlan, J. A. & Korach, K. S. (1992). Coupling of dual signalling pathways: EGF action involves the estrogen receptor. *Proceedings of the National Academy of Sciences, USA,* **89**, 4658–62.

Jacobson, L. & Sapolsky, R. M. (1991). The role of the hippocampus in feedback regulation of the hypothalamo-pituitary-adrenocortical axis. *Endocrine Reviews,* **12**, 118–34.

Jung-Testas, I., Hu, Z. Y., Robel, P. & Baulieu, E-E. (1989). Biosynthesis of pregnenolone and progesterone in primary cultures of rat glial cells. *Endocrinology,* **125**, 2083–91.

Jung-Testas, I., Renoir, J. M., J.M., G. & Baulieu, E.-E. (1991). Estrogen-inducible progesterone receptors in primary cultures of rat glial cells. *Experimental Cellular Research,* **193**, 12–19.

Jung-Testas, I., Schumacher, M., Robel, P. & Baulieu, E-E. (1994). Actions of steroid hormones and growth factors on glial cells of the central and peripheral nervous system. *Journal of Steroid Biochemistry and Molecular Biology,* **48**, 145–54.

Kuiper, G. G. J. M., Carlsson, B., Grandien, K., Enmark, E., Haggblad, J., Nilsson, S. & Gustafsson, J-A. (1997). Comparison of the ligand binding specificity and transcript tissue distribution of estrogen receptors α and β. *Endocrinology,* **138**, 863–70.

Kuiper, G. G. J. M., Enmark, E., Pelto-Huikko, M., Nilsson, S. & Gustafsson, J.-A. (1996). Cloning of a novel estrogen receptor expressed in rat prostate and ovary. *Proceedings of the National Academy of Sciences, USA,* **93**, 5925–30.

Le Goascogne, C., Gouezou, M., Robel, P., Defaye, G., Chambaz, E., Waterman, M. R. & Baulieu, E-E. (1989). The cholesterol side chain cleavage complex in human brain white matter. *Journal of Neuroendocrinology,* **1**, 153–6.

Le Goascogne, C., Robel, P., Gouezou, M., Sananes, N., Baulieu, E-E. & Waterman, M. (1987). Neurosteroids: cytochrome P450scc in rat brain. *Science,* **237**, 1212–15.

Lechan, R. M., Qi, Y., Berrodin, T. J., Davis, K. D., Schwartz, H. L., Strait, K. A., Oppenheimer, J. H. & Lazar, M. A. (1993). Immunocytochemical delineation of thyroid hormone receptor β2-like immunoreactivity in the rat central nervous system. *Endocrinology,* **132**, 2461–9.

MacLusky, N. J. & McEwen, B. S. (1978). Oestrogen modulates progestin receptor concentrations in some brain regions but not in others. *Nature,* **274**, 276–7.

MacLusky, N. J. & McEwen, B. S. (1980). Progestin receptor in rat brain: distribution and properties of cytoplasmic progestin-binding sites. *Endocrinology,* **106**, 192–202.

Majewska, M. D., Harrison, N. L., Schwartz, R. D., Barker, J. L. & Paul, S. M. (1986). Steroid hormone metabolites are barbiturate-like modulators of the GABA receptor. *Science*, 232, 1004–7.

Mani, S. K., Allen, J. M. C., Clark, J. H., Blaustein, J. D. & O'Malley, B. W. (1994). Convergent pathways for steroid hormone- and neurotransmitter-induced rat sexual behavior. *Science*, 265, 1246–9.

Mani, S. K., Allen, J. M. C., Lydon, J. P., Mulac-Jericevic, B., Blaustein, J. D., DeMayo, F. J., Conneely, O. & O'Malley, B. W. (1996). Dopamine requires the unoccupied progesterone receptor to induce sexual behavior in mice. *Molecular Endocrinology*, 10, 1728–37.

McDonnell, D. P., Shahbaz, M. M., Vegeto, E. & Goldman, M. E. (1994). The human progesterone receptor A-form functions as a transcriptional modulator of mineralocorticoid receptor transcriptional activity. *Journal of Steroid Biochemistry and Molecular Biology*, 48, 425–32.

Melcangi, R. C., Poletti, A., Cavarretta, I., Celotti, F., Colciago, A., Magnaghi, V., Motta, M., Negri-Cesi, P. & Martini, L. (1998). The 5α-reductase in the central nervous system: expression and modes of control. *Journal of Steroid Biochemistry and Molecular Biology*, 65, 295–9.

Mellon, S. H. (1994). Neurosteroids: biochemistry, modes of action, and clinical relevance. *Journal of Clinical Endocrinology and Metabolism*, 78, 1003–8.

Mellon, S. H. & Deschepper, C. F. (1993). Neurosteroid biosynthesis: genes for adrenal steroidogenic enzymes are expressed in brain. *Brain Research*, 629, 283–92.

Mermelstein, P. G., Becker, J. B. & Surmeier, D. J. (1996). Estradiol reduces calcium currents in rat neostriatal neurons via a membrane receptor. *Journal of Neuroscience*, 16, 595–604.

Mosselman, S., Polman, J. & Dijkema, R. (1996). ER β: identification and characterization of a novel human estrogen receptor. *FEBS Letters*, 392, 49–53.

Murphy, D. D. & Segal, M. (1996). Regulation of dendritic spine density in cultured rat hippocampal neurons by steroid hormones. *Journal of Neuroscience*, 16, 4059–68.

Murphy, D. D. & Segal, M. (1997). Morphological plasticity of dendritic spines in central neurons is mediated by activation of cAMP response element binding protein. *Proceedings of the National Academy of Sciences, USA*, 94, 1482–7.

Murphy, D. D., Cole, N. B., Greenberger, V. & Segal, M. (1998). Estradiol increases dendritic spine density by reducing GABA neurotransmission in hippocampal neurons. *Journal of Neuroscience*, 18, 2550–9.

Paech, K., Webb, P., Kuiper, G. G. J. M., Nilsson, S., Gustafsson, J-A., Kushner, P. J. & Scanlan, T. S. (1997). Differential ligand activation of estrogen receptors ERα and ERβ at AP1 sites. *Science*, 277, 1508–10.

Park-Chung, M., Wu, F.-S., Purdy, R. H., Malayev, A. A., Gibbs, T. T. & Farb, D. H. (1997). Distinct sites for inverse modulation of N-methyl-D-aspartate receptors by sulfated steroids. *Molecular Pharmacology*, 52, 1113–23.

Petersen, D. N., Tkalcevic, G. T., Koza-Taylor, P. H., Turi, T. G. & Brown, T. A. (1998). Identification of estrogen receptor β₂, a functional variant of estrogen receptor β expressed in normal rat tissues. *Endocrinology*, 139, 1082–92.

Pfaff, D. W. & Keiner, M. (1973). Atlas of estradiol-concentrating cells in the central nervous system of the female rat. *Journal of Comparative Neurology*, 151, 121–58.

Press, M. F. & Greene, G. L. (ed.) (1988). Immunocytochemical localization of estrogen and progesterone receptors. *Advances in Immunohistochemistry.* New York: Raven Press.

Puymirat, J. (1992). Thyroid receptors in the rat brain. *Progress in Neurobiology,* 39, 281–94.

Rainbow, T. C., Parsons, B. & McEwen, B. S. (1982). Sex differences in rat brain oestrogen and progestin receptors. *Nature,* 300, 648–9.

Reul, J. M. H. M. & De Kloet, E. R. (1985). Two receptor systems for corticosterone in rat brain: microdistribution and differential occupation. *Endocrinology,* 117, 2505–11.

Robel, P. & Baulieu, E-E. (1994). Neurosteroids. Biosynthesis and function. *Trends in Endocrinology and Metabolism,* 5, 1–8.

Robel, P., Young, J., Corpechot, C., Mayo, W., Perche, F., Haug, M., Simon, H. & Baulieu, E-E. (1995). Biosynthesis and assay of neurosteroids in rats and mice: functional correlates. *Journal of Steroid Biochemistry and Molecular Biology,* 53, 335–60.

Romano, G. J., Krust, A. & Pfaff, D. W. (1989). Expression and estrogen regulation of progesterone receptor mRNA in neurons of the mediobasal hypothalamus: an *in situ* hybridization study. *Molecular Endocrinology,* 3, 1295–300.

Roselli, C. E. & Klosterman, S. A. (1998). Sexual differentiation of aromatase activity in the rat brain: effects of perinatal steroid exposure. *Endocrinology,* 139, 3193–201.

Roselli, C. E. & Resko, J. A. (1987). The distribution and regulation of aromatase activity in the central nervous system. *Steroids,* 50, 495–508.

Roselli, C. E., Abdelgadir, S. E., Ronnekleiv, O. K. & Klosterman, S. A. (1998). Anatomic distribution and regulation of aromatase gene expression in the rat brain. *Biology of Reproduction,* 58, 79–87.

Roselli, C. E., Horton, L. E. & Resko, J. A. (1985). Distribution and regulation of aromatase activity in the rat hypothalamus and limbic system. *Endocrinology,* 117, 2471–7.

Roselli, C. E., Klosterman, S. A. & Fasasi, T. A. (1996). Sex differences in androgen responsiveness in the rat brain: regional differences in the induction of aromatase activity. *Neuroendocrinology,* 64, 139–45.

Sanne, J. L. & Krueger, K. E. (1995). Expression of cytochrome P450 side-chain cleavage enzyme and 3β-hydroxysteroid dehydrogenase in the rat central nervous system: a study by polymerase chain reaction and in situ hybridization. *Journal of Neurochemistry,* 65, 528–36.

Sapolsky, R. M., Uno, H., Rebert, C. S. & Finch, C. E. (1990). Hippocampal damage associated with prolonged glucocorticoid exposure in primates. *Journal of Neuroscience,* 10, 2897–902.

Sar, M. & Parikh, I. (1986). Immunohistochemical localization of estrogen receptor in rat brain, pituitary and uterus with monoclonal antibodies. *Journal of Steroid Biochemistry,* 24, 497–503.

Sar, M. & Stumpf, W. E. (1977). Distribution of androgen target cell in rat forebrain and pituitary after [³H]-dihydrotestosterone administration. *Journal of Steroid Biochemistry,* 8, 1131–5.

Sasano, H., Takahashi, K., Satoh, F., Nagura, H. & Harada, N. (1998). Aromatase in the human central nervous system. *Clinical Endocrinology,* 48, 325–9.

Selmanoff, M. K., Brodkin, L. D., Weiner, R. I. & Siiteri, P. K. (1977). Aromatization and 5α-reduction of androgens in discrete hypothalamic and limbic regions of the male and female brain. *Endocrinology,* 101, 841–8.

Selye, H. (1942). Correlations between the chemical structure and the pharmacological actions of the steroids. *Endocrinology*, 30, 437–53.

Shughrue, P. J., Komm, B. & Merchenthaler, I. (1996). The distribution of estrogen receptor-β mRNA in the rat hypothalamus. *Steroids*, 61, 678–81.

Simerly, R. B., Chang, C., Muramatsu, M. & Swanson, L. W. (1990). Distribution of androgen and estrogen receptor mRNA-containing cells in the rat brain: an in situ hybridization study. *Journal of Comparative Neurology*, 294, 76–95.

Stein-Behrens, B., Elliot, E. M., Miller, C. A., Schilling, J. W., Newcombe, R. & Sapolsky, R. M. (1992). Glucocorticoids exacerbate kainic acid-induced extracellular accumulation of excitatory amino acids in the rat hippocampus. *Journal of Neurochemistry*, 58, 1730–5.

Stumpf, W. E., Sar, M. & Keefer, D. A. (1975). Atlas of estrogen target cells in rat brain. *Anatomical Neuroendocrinology*, pp. 104–19. Basel: Karger.

Thompson, T. L. & Moss, R. L. (1994). Estrogen regulation of dopamine release in the nucleus accumbens: genomic- and nongenomic-mediated effects. *Journal of Neurochemistry*, 62, 1750–6.

Toran-Allerand, C. D. (1996). Mechanisms of estrogen action during neural development: mediation by interactions with neurotrophins and their receptors? *Journal of Steroid Biochemistry and Molecular Biology*, 56, 169–178.

Uht, R. M., Anderson, C. M., Webb, P. & Kushner, P. J. (1997). Transcriptional activities of estrogen and glucocorticoid receptors are functionally integrated at the AP-1 response element. *Endocrinology*, 138, 2900–8.

Warembourg, M. (1975). Radioautographic study of the rat brain after injection of $(1,2,^3H)$corticosterone. *Brain Research*, 89, 61.

Warembourg, M. (1978). Radioautographic study of the rat brain, uterus and vagina after [^3H]R-5020 injection. *Molecular and Cellular Endocrinology*, 12, 67–79.

Warembourg, M., Logeat, F. & Milgrom, E. (1986). Immunocytochemical evidence of progesterone receptor in guinea pig central nervous system. *Brain Research*, 384, 121–31.

Wong, M. & Moss, R. L. (1992). Long-term and short-term electrophysiological effects of estrogen on the synaptic properties of hippocampal CA1 neurons. *Journal of Neuroscience*, 12, 3217–25.

Woolley, C. S. & McEwen, B. S. (1993). Roles of estradiol and progesterone in regulation of hippocampal dendritic spine density during the estrous cycle in the rat. *Journal of Comparative Neurology*, 336, 293–306.

Woolley, C. S. & McEwen, B. S. (1994). Estradiol regulates hippocampal dendritic spine density via an N-methyl-D-aspartate receptor-dependent mechanism. *Journal of Neuroscience*, 14, 7680–7.

Woolley, C. S., Gould, E., Frankfurt, M. & McEwen, B. S. (1990). Naturally occurring fluctuation in dendritic spine density on adult hippocampal pyramidal neurons. *Journal of Neuroscience*, 10, 4035–9.

Woolley, C. S., Weiland, N. G., McEwen, B. S. & Schwartzkroin, P. A. (1997). Estradiol increases the sensitivity of hippocampal CA1 pyramidal cells to NMDA receptor-mediated synaptic input: correlation with dendritic spine density. *Journal of Neuroscience*, 17, 1848–59.

Woolley, C. S., Wenzel, H. J. & Schwartzkroin, P. A. (1996). Estradiol increases the frequency of multiple synapse boutons in the hippocampal CA1 region of the adult female rat. *Journal of Comparative Neurology*, 373, 108–17.

Zhu, Y-S., Yen, P. M., Chin, W. W. & Pfaff, D. W. (1996). Estrogen and thyroid hormone interaction on regulation of gene expression. *Proceedings of the National Academy of Sciences, USA*, 93, 12587–92.

Part II

Hormones and mental health in the elderly

3

The hypothalamic–pituitary–adrenal axis in aging: preclinical and clinical studies

John W. Kasckow, Thomas D. Geracioti Jr, Marta Pisarska, Ajit Regmi, Dewleen G. Baker, and James J. Mulchahey

Introduction

All organisms are exposed to stimuli construed as stressors and all organisms mount a characteristic physiologic response to stress to maintain homeostasis (Herman et al., 1996). Many physical illnesses can be linked to life stress, particularly in aged individuals (McEwen & Stellar, 1993; Clauw & Chrousos, 1997; Katz, 1996). Impairments in the physiological responses to stress have particularly been associated with immune, endocrine, neurological, and psychiatric disorders. Examples of neuropsychiatric disorders, which are associated with dysregulation of the stress response, include depression, post-traumatic stress disorder, and neuro-degenerative disorders (Kathol et al., 1989; Charney et al., 1993; McEwen, 1992; Landfield & Eldridge, 1991; Sapolsky et al., 1986; Landfield et al., 1992).

Activation of physiologic stress responses involve the sympathetic nervous system and the hypothalamic–pituitary–adrenal (HPA) axis. The HPA axis is the best characterized component of the physiologic stress response. In aging, this stress component undergoes significant changes. As mentioned, changes are associated with neurologic and psychiatric disorders in late life, and it has been hypothesized that these changes are related to the pathogenesis of some of these disorders. The purpose of this chapter is to discuss the alterations in the HPA axis which occur with normal aging and also to relate these changes within the context of disorders of aging. We will initially discuss the physiology of the HPA axis. This discussion will be followed by a discussion of animal and human studies which have examined the HPA axis in normal aging and disease states in late life.

The physiology of the HPA axis

The HPA axis is responsible for the release of glucocorticoids into the circulation. Hypothalamic releasing factors, which include corticotropin-releasing factor (CRF) and vasopressin (VP) are released into the portal circulation to stimulate

ACTH secretion from the pituitary. CRF is the main secretagogue for ACTH while vasopressin and oxytocin are co-stored and co-released with CRF in the parvocellular paraventricular nucleus of the hypothalamus. The action of vasopressin is to synergize with the actions of CRF in stimulating ACTH release from the corticotropic cells of the anterior pituitary. ACTH, in turn, travels via the circulatory system to the adrenal cortex to stimulate glucocorticoid production: cortisol in humans or corticosterone in rats (Whitnall, 1993). Glucocorticoids have as targets virtually every cell of the body, where they bind to high-affinity receptors in the cytoplasm. They are then translocated to the nucleus where they dimerize and bind to regulatory regions on DNA to alter gene expresssion (Yamamoto, 1985; Drouin et al., 1992). In this way they can interact with a multitude of tissue systems at once. For instance, they can simultaneously increase cardiovascular tone, mobilize glucose from the liver, inhibit nonessential endocrine systems, and affect the immune system. At this point, it is not clear whether glucocorticoids act as a primary defense mechanism for immediate survival or whether they simply reinstate homeostasis following stressful events (Munck et al., 1984; Herman et al., 1996).

The actions of glucocorticoids are generally catabolic and are needed for short term actions. There are several feedback systems which have evolved to inhibit their release. Negative feedback can occur at multiple levels of the stress axis such as at the brain and pituitary. The types of feedback include 'fast' which takes minutes, 'intermediate' which occurs within hours and 'delayed' which occurs within days (Jones & Gillham, 1988; Keller-Wood & Dallman, 1984). There are numerous other inputs which regulate the HPA axis. The noradrenergic neurons from the locus ceruleus as well as the noradrenergic sympathetic neurons originating in the brainstem lateral tegmentum exert modulatory influences on the HPA axis through their synaptic contacts on hypothalamic CRF cells (Holets, 1990). The same is true of serotonin neurons, which arise in the raphe and ascend to synapse on the CRF cells of the hypothalamus (Fuller, 1992).

In the brain, glucocorticoids negatively regulate this system through the hippocampus and hypothalamus and possibly other limbic sites. The type I 'high affinity' or mineralocorticoid (MR) receptors mediate tonic inhibition of the HPA axis through basal glucocorticoid blood levels while the type II 'low affinity' or glucocorticoid (GR) receptors are active during stress or during the peak of the diurnal rhythm when glucocorticoid blood levels are elevated (deKloet & Sutano, 1989; deKloet et al., 1998). Glucocorticoids can also inhibit release of CRF quickly by acting on the cells of the ACTH secretagogues, and it is thought that this is mediated most likely by cell surface receptors (Whitnall, 1993). At this time it is not entirely clear how and where all of the receptor subtypes interact to regulate the system.

Another important aspect of the HPA axis is its rhythmicity. Glucocorticoids have circadian rhythms such that up to 40-fold differences in levels can occur within 24-hour periods in a consistent pattern. The highest levels of secretion occur with the onset of an organism's active period of the 24-hour day. In humans this is the morning while in rats it is the evening. Furthermore, recent research has also revealed that the immune system exhibits close interactions with the HPA axis. There is evidence supporting the ability of immune stressors such as tissue injury, inflammation, and infection (Mobbs, 1996) to activate hypothalamic neuronal circuits. Immune activation stimulates brain stress systems as part of an organism's acute phase response. Part of this initial response includes the production of cytokines, such as interleukin-1 (IL1), interleukin-6, and tumor necrosis factor, which orchestrate elements of the acute phase response to defend the host. Energy demands are similarly increased through cytokine-mediated activation of CNS stress systems, and it is hypothesized that the concomitant induction of sickness behavior ensues so that energy stores are available to fight infection or injury. Much of the sickness behavior that occurs appears to be accounted for by the actions of IL1. IL1 produces a physiologic stress response by directly activating both CRF and VP cells of the hypothalamus (Sapolsky et al., 1987; Berkenbosch et al., 1987; Whitnall, 1993) through various mechanisms. In addition, IL1 can also regulate the HPA axis at other levels including the pituitary and hippocampus (Besedovsky & Del Rey, 1996).

The HPA axis in aging

Animal studies

In rats, the majority of studies examining adrenocortical sensitivity to ACTH in aging have revealed that this arm of the HPA response is overactive (Lorens et al., 1990; Meaney et al., 1992), although there are studies that support the opposite (Cizza et al., 1994). In addition, many aging rats exhibit a delay in the ability of glucocorticoids to return to baseline after stressors (Sapolsky et al., 1986). In this subset of rats, elevated levels of corticosterone are associated with a decline in hippocampal functioning, impaired glucocorticoid negative feedback, significant reductions in corticosteroid receptors, and damage to hippocampal structures (McEwen, 1992). There is evidence that this decrease in hippocampal receptors removes the inhibition that the hippocampus normally exerts on the HPA axis, leading to persistently elevated corticosterone levels (Sapolsky et al., 1983; Meaney et al., 1992; Peiffer et al., 1991). Also, aged rats with elevated corticosterone levels have impairments in cognition, while aged rats without cognitive impairments exhibit basal glucocorticoid levels similar to those observed in young rats (Issa et al., 1990; Sarrieau et al., 1992). Corticosteroids have been reported to impair neuronal electrophysiology and hippocampal long-term potentiation (Joels & DeKloet, 1989; Diamond et al., 1992; Norris et al., 1998). Furthermore, neuronal damage in the hippocampus observed during aging in rats can be accentuauted by stress or glucocorticoid exposure (Kerr et al., 1991). Adrenalectomy in older male rats can reduce Ca^{2+} dependence after hyperpolarization in hippocampal neurons, suggesting one potential mechanism by which corticosteroids can induce damage (Kerr et al., 1989). In addition, immobilization stress in rats will decrease mRNA levels of neurotrophic factors in the hippocampus, specifically that of brain-derived neurotrophic factor (BDNF). Furthermore, corticosterone administration to rats will decrease BNDF levels in the hippocampal dentate gyrus (Smith et al., 1995).

It is not clear exactly how genetic and environmental influences interplay with the HPA axis and the hippocampus with aging. It is known, however, that rats that were handled neonatally have lower basal blood corticosterone levels and higher cognitive functioning once they reach old age as compared with non-handled rats (Meaney et al., 1991). Antidepressant administration can alter this phenomenon. Rowe et al. (1997) have recently demonstrated that the differences in basal HPA activity that are normally observed between cognitively impaired and cognitively intact rats were reduced when the cognitively impaired rats were administered antidepressants. The precise neural mechanisms responsible for these effects are presently unknown, although it has been demonstrated that antidepressants can increase corticosteroid receptor gene expression in the hippocampus, cortex, and other brain areas (Brady et al., 1992; Pepin & Barden, 1992; Seckl & Fink, 1992; Vedder et al., 1993). It is thus hypothesized that the increased levels in glucocorticoids in older cognitively impaired rats are due to increased ACTH release which is, in turn, a result of decreased tonic glucocorticoid negative feedback; antidepressant treatment reverses this. The contribution of serotonergic or noradrenergic systems to this response is an area of active scientific inquiry. Serotonin is known to increase glucocorticoid receptor mRNA expression and receptor binding levels in primary hippocampal cell cultures, although it is not known whether these effects occur in vivo (Mitchell et al., 1990; 1992; Vedder et al., 1993).

The expression of CRF levels in aging rats has been evaluated by various groups. Both increases and decreases in levels of basal hypothalamic CRF peptide in the aging rat have been observed (Cizza et al., 1994; Hauger et al., 1994). In addition, two groups have reported decreases in basal CRF mRNA levels with aging (Kasckow et al., 1999; Givalois et al., 1997), whereas one group failed to detect changes (Hauger et al., 1994). The discrepancies in basal CRF mRNA expression that have been observed in human and rat studies are not well understood. The RNA levels examined in both species were steady state measures of RNA and were measured by exonic probes. Perhaps the use of intronic probes or other functional measures will allow us to reconcile the differences. The use of intronic probes, which measures mRNA levels of recently transcribed RNA prior to processing is known to be a more sensitive measure of gene expression. On the other hand, the use of exonic probes, which has been utilized in the studies cited above, lead to less sensitive measures of gene expression. Exonic probes detect steady state levels of mRNA in addition to recently transcribed mRNA. As a result, quantitation of recently expressed mRNA by exonic probes could be masked by a high level of steady state mRNA which could have accumulated at baseline prior to gene activation.

The majority of studies addressing the effects of stimuli on the CRF system in aging rats have suggested that the CRF system at the hypothalamic level is hyper-responsive (Hauger et al., 1994) although some studies support the opposite (Cizza et al., 1994). The CRF mRNA decreases noted at baseline could be consistent with such a hypothesis of overactivation. There are other neurochemical CNS systems which exhibit lower basal levels of expression in aging, yet respond in an overactivated manner following physiologic stimulation. This has been demonstrated with locus coeruleus noradrenergic neurons (Bondareff et al., 1982; Peskind et al., 1995).

Fewer investigators have examined the hypothalamic vasopressin system and its role in aging. Our group revealed that older rats with higher basal levels of corticosterone in aging exhibit lower basal levels of vasopressin in portal blood (Mulchahey et al., 1999). In those rats, adrenalectomy restored portal vasopressin levels to those observed in young rats. In addition, other investigators have measured absolute numbers of hypothalamic vasopressin neurons. The results have been inconsistent, in that either decreases or increases in aging rats have been noted (Dorsa & Bottemiller, 1982; Calza et al., 1990; Cizza et al., 1994). Another report suggested that the responsiveness of hypothalamic vasopressin neurons may decrease with aging (Hauger et al., 1994). The discrepancies in these results suggest that dynamic measures of CRF or AVP release or production will yield more meaningful results than do static measures of peptide or gene expression.

There are also very few studies that have examined the interaction of cytokines or biogenic amines with the hypothalamic CRF system in aging. Weidenfeld et al. (1989) noted in young rats that IL1 activates the HPA axis by inhibiting hippocampal corticosterone binding, thereby removing negative feedback. One might predict that IL1 would overactivate the HPA axis more robustly in certain subpopulations of aged rats which have higher basal corticosterone levels and lower corticosteroid receptor numbers. Bernardini et al. (1992) injected IL1 centrally into aged rats and noted a prolonged ACTH and corticosterone secretory response compared with young rats. More studies are needed to better understand how cytokines and other neurotransmitter systems interact with the HPA axis in aging.

Human studies

Aging in humans is an inevitable and highly individual process. Both genetic and environmental factors contribute to this process. The speed and degree of aging varies widely among individuals. These principles also apply to the aging HPA axis

(Bjorntorp, 1995). Reports on age-associated changes in the basal activity of the HPA axis in humans are not consistent. There are investigators who have found that cortisol levels in young and elderly humans are not different (Born et al., 1995; Gotthardt et al., 1995; Jensen & Blichert-Toft, 1971; Lakatua et al., 1987; Touitou et al., 1982; Waltman et al., 1991; Halbreich et al., 1984). On the other hand, age-associated increases in basal plasma cortisol levels have been reported (Halbreich et al., 1984; Lupien et al., 1994; Pfohl et al., 1985; Touitou et al., 1983; Ferrari et al., 1985) as well as age-associated decreases (Drafta et al., 1982; Maes et al., 1994; Sherman et al., 1985; Sharma et al., 1989). The differences in these findings can be attributed to the heterogeneity of the aging process, differences and alterations in circadian rhythm, and possibly also to the differences in methodologies employed by the various investigators.

There are studies supporting impaired glucocorticoid feedback regulation in aged humans (Born et al., 1995, Heuser et al., 1994; O'Brien et al., 1994; Seeman & Robbins, 1994), although earlier studies utilizing dexamethasone suppression tests (DST) have been inconsistent (Ansseau et al., 1986; Odio & Brodish, 1989, Rolandi et al., 1987; Waltman et al., 1991; Zimmerman et al., 1987; Burns & Abou-Saleh, 1994). There are also investigators who have reported significant correlations between age and post-dexamethasone cortisol (Asnis et al., 1981; Sharma et al., 1988) but not all findings have been supportive of this relationship (Carroll et al., 1981; Ansseau et al., 1987). Other approaches have supported the hypothesis that healthy elderly individuals exhibit decreased negative cortisol feedback. Wilkinson et al. (1997) demonstrated that ACTH responses following cortisol infusions in elderly humans, who had been treated with the cortisol synthesis inhibitor metyrapone, were delayed relative to younger humans. Furthermore, Heuser et al. (1994) found using the dexamethasone/CRF stimulation test that there is greater cortisol stimulation in older individuals than that observed in their younger counterparts. This latter test involves challenging patients with CRF following dexamethasone pretreatment and is considered to be a more reliable and sensitive test for detecting HPA abnormalities (Holsboer et al., 1992).

Heuser et al. (1994) also demonstrated gender differences in elderly individuals administered the dexamethasone/CRF stimulation test. They revealed that elderly females had higher ACTH responses than elderly males. Deuschle et al. (1997) characterized pulsatile features of the HPA axis with aging. They demonstrated that the diurnal amplitude of the HPA axis flattens in aging (i.e. the diurnal amplitude of cortisol and ACTH relative to the 24-hour mean of these hormones shows an age-associated decline). Based on their studies, the evening cortisol quiescent period is also shortened in the elderly. Compared to males, the mean cortisol in females was significantly increased while the duration of the quiescent period was even more markedly shortened.

It has been hypothesized that the deficits in HPA axis regulation in aging humans may be attributed to dysregulation of the CRF cells of the hypothalamus. Post-mortem studies performed by Raadsheer et al. (1993, 1994) suggest that the number of CRF immunoreactive cells in the hypothalamus increases with aging. Furthermore, the same group reported in elderly humans that there is greater co-localization of vasopressin with CRF cells (Raadsheer et al., 1993). As mentioned above, vasopressin is also a secretagogue of ACTH and often augments the CRF effects on ACTH release. Co-localization of vasopressin in CRF neurons serves as another index of increased secretory activity of CRF neurons. Chronic hyperactivity of CRF neurons in rats induces coproduction of vasopressin in these neurons following repeated hypoglycemia, immobilization, psychosocial stress, and adrenalectomy (Raadsheer et al., 1994; Bartanusz et al., 1993; deGoeij et al., 1991, 1992; Tilders et al., 1993; Whitnall et al., 1993). In addition to HPA-related dysregulation linked to the CRF cells of the hypothalamus, there may also be a pituitary component contributing to the dysregulation. Studies of Dodt et al. (1991) revealed that there are increases in ACTH and cortisol levels in mentally healthy elderly adults following CRF stimulation tests.

The HPA axis in human disease states associated with aging

Several investigators have reported a higher frequency of DST non-suppressors among elderly patients with depression compared with younger depressed patients (Alexopoulos et al., 1984; Keitner et al., 1992). In addition, the HPA axis also appears to be overactivated in Alzheimer's disease. Early Alzheimer's disease is associated with dexamethasone non-suppression, relative to controls when low doses (i.e. 0.5 mg) of dexamethasone are used (Nasman et al., 1995). Based on post-mortem studies, Raadsheer et al. (1995) reported that CRF mRNA levels in the paraventricular nucleus of brains of Alzheimer's disease patients are elevated above those of controls.

There is also evidence supporting HPA axis dysregulation of Alzheimer's patients at the pituitary and adrenal level. Nasman et al. (1996) indicated in Alzheimer's disease patients that ACTH levels resulting from the CRF challenge test are lower than those seen in controls; in the same patients, however, the ratio of cortisol released relative to ACTH was also higher in Alzheimer's disease patients. Dodt et al. (1991) could not replicate this finding although other studies by O'Brien et al. (1994) also suggested that Alzheimer's disease patients exhibit enhanced adrenal responsitivity to ACTH.

Like the animal studies reported above, studies of subgroups of elderly humans with higher cortisol levels have indicated that these individuals are at risk for developing cognitive deficits. Deficits in cognition have been observed in patients with steroid psychosis following treatment with corticosteroids (Hall et al., 1979; Ling et al., 1981; Wolkowitz & Rapaport, 1989). Neuropathologic changes in aged humans are associated with increased basal glucocorticoid levels (Davis et al., 1986; DeLeon et al., 1988; Dodt et al., 1991). Furthermore, patients with Cushing's syndrome, exhibited by overactivity of the HPA axis, have been noted to exhibit significant postive correlations between hippocampal formation volume and scores on verbal memory tests; in addition, there have been significant negative correlations between hippocampal formation volume and plasma cortisol levels in these patients (Starkman et al., 1992). Inverse relationships have also been reported between 24-hour cortisol levels and severity of cognitive decline in Alzheimer's patients (DeLeon et al., 1988; Oxenkrug et al., 1989; Martignoni et al., 1992).

Hippocampal functioning in humans is known to be essential for explicit memory, i.e. memory for conscious or voluntary recollection of previous information (Cohen & Squire, 1980; Graf & Schachter, 1985). It has been speculated that this role of the hippocampus in human memory formation could be impaired as a result of long-term corticosteroid exposure (Lupien et al., 1994). Degeneration of corticosteroid receptors in a subgroup of humans could lead to increased cortisol levels and further degeneration of the hippocampus, consistent with the glucocorticoid cascade hypothesis of aging (McEwen, 1992; Sapolsky et al., 1986). Lupien et al. (1994, 1998) examined healthy elderly subjects who differed in basal cortisol levels. Correlational analyses revealed that the slope of change in cortisol levels over time predicted cognitive deficits in this population. Aged subjects with significant increases in cortisol levels over many years were impaired on tasks measuring selective attention and explicit memory. Thus, impaired performance on cognitive tests in elderly individuals was associated with HPA axis dysregulation and elevated basal cortisol levels.

Conclusions and future directions

Aging is characterized by an overall reduced ability to maintain homeostasis. The development of molecular and cellular approaches coupled with behavioral studies and improved assessment of human physiology have advanced our understanding of how the aging brain handles stress (Holsboer et al., 1992; McEwen, 1999). Aging in humans appears to be associated with glucocorticoid resistance. In addition, there are gender associated differences in human HPA reactivity with aging as well as changes associated with the diurnal rhythm. The preclinical literature suggests that the reactivity of the CRF component of the HPA system may be increased with aging, although not all studies uniformly support this. It also appears that some aging animals develop HPA axis dysregulation characterized by glucocorticoid insensitivity. In these individuals, basal corticosterone levels are elevated and are associated with cognitive decline. A reduction in hippocampal corticosteroid receptors with aging may be one major factor accounting for these changes. The same processes appear also to apply to some aging humans.

In the future, more detailed longitudinal studies in humans are required to assess more precisely the cognitive deficits associated with hypercortisolemic states. In addition, more preclinical studies are needed to better understand the physiologic and molecular mechanisms accounting for changes in the HPA axis with aging. This applies particularly to other systems that interface with the HPA axis. The manner in which age-associated changes in the HPA axis are linked to biogenic amine systems, as well as immune mediators such as cytokines, is not known. Furthermore, the relationship of the aging HPA axis to other limbic neuroendocrine stress circuits have not yet been explored beyond what we know of hippocampal–HPA axis interactions. Investigators have also not yet examined the manner in which the central nucleus of the amygdala or the bed nucleus of the stria terminalis communicate with the HPA axis in the aged animal.

In the upcoming decades, technologic advances in molecular neurobiology, neuroendocrinology, and neuroimaging will allow us to improve assessment of the aging HPA axis at the preclinical and clinical level. It is hoped that this approach will enable investigators to better understand the manner in which the aging brain responds to stress. Knowledge derived from such studies is likely to help investigators develop new diagnostic methods for detecting neuropsychiatric conditions in aged humans. More importantly, it is hoped that developing a concerted and integrated approach toward researching the HPA axis in aging will help investigators develop new therapeutic targets to treat these age related neuropsychiatric diseases.

ACKNOWLEDGMENT

This work was supported by an NIMH Research Career Award (K01-MH01545–01; JWK), a VA Merit Review Entry Program Award (Merit review 2; JWK) and a Merit Review 1 Award (TDG, DGB, JWK, JJM).

REFERENCES

Alexopoulos, G. S., Young, R. C., Kocsis, J. H., Stokes, P. E., Brockner, N. & Butler, T. A. (1984). The dexamethasone-suppression test in geriatric depression. *Biological Psychiatry*, **19**, 1567–71.

Ansseau, M., Depauw, Y., Charles, G., Castro, P., D'Haenen, H., De Vigne, J. P., Hubain, P., Legros, J. J., Pelc, I., Toscano, A., Wilmotte, J. & Mendlewicz, J. (1987). Age and gender effects on the diagnostic power of the DST. *Journal of Affective Disorders*, **12**, 185–91.

Ansseau, M., von Frenckell, R., Simon, C., Sulon, J., Demey-Ponsart, E. & Franck, G. (1986). Prediction of cortisol responses to dexamethasone from age and basal cortisol in normal volunteers: a negative study. *Psychopharmacology*, **90**, 276–7.

Asnis, G. M., Sachar, E., Halbrech, V., Nathan, R. S., Novacenko, H. & Ostrow, L. C. (1981). Cortisol secretion in relation to age in major depression. *Psychosomatic Medicine*, **43**, 235–42.

Bartanusz, V., Jerzova, D., Bertini, L. T., Tilders, F. J. H., Aubry, J. M. & Kiss, J. Z. (1993). Stress-induced increase in vasopressin and corticotropin-releasing factor expression in hypophysiotropic paraventricular neurons. *Endocrinology*, **132**, 895–902.

Berkenbosch, F., van Oers, J., del Rey, A., Tildens, F. & Besedovsky, H. O. (1987). Corticotropin-releasing factor-producing neurons in the rat activated by interleukin-1. *Science*, **238**, 524–6.

Bernadini, R., Mauceri, G., Iurato, M. P., Chiatenza, A., Lempereur, L. & Scapagnini, U. (1992). Response of the hypothalamic–pituitary–adrenal axis to interleukin-1 in the aging rat. *Progress in Neuroendocrinimmunology*, **5**, 166–71.

Besedovsky, H. O. & Del Rey, A. (1996). Immune-neuro-endocrine interactions: facts and hypotheses. *Endocrine Reviews*, **17**, 64–102.

Bjorntorp, P. (1995). Neuroendocrine aging. *Journal of Internal Medicine*, **238**, 401–4.

Bondareff, W., Mountjoy, C. & Roth, M. (1982). Loss of neurons of origin of the adrenergic projection to cerebral cortex (nucleus locus coeruleus) in senile dementia. *Neurology*, **32**, 4–168.

Born, J., Ditschuneit, I., Schreiber, M., Dodt, C. & Fehm, H. L. (1995). Effects of age and gender on pituitary–adrenocoritical responsiveness in humans. *European Journal of Endocrinology*, **132**, 705–11.

Brady, L. S., Gold, P. W., Herkenham, M., Lynn, A. B. & Whitfield, H. J. Sr. (1992). The antidepressants fluoxetine, idazoxan and phenelzine alter corticotropin-releasing factor hormone and tyrosine hydroxylase mRNA levels in rat brain; therapeutic implications. *Brain Research*, **572**, 117–25.

Burns, R. A. & Abou-Saleh, M. T. (1994). Neuroendocrinology of aging. In *Principles and Practice of Geriatric Psychiatry*, ed. J. R. M. Copeland, M. T. Abou-Saleh & D. G. Blazer, pp. 65–71. Chichester, UK: John Wiley.

Calza, L., Giardino, L., Velardo, A., Battistini, N. & Marrama, P. (1990). Influence of aging on the neurochemical organization of the rat paraventricular nucleus. *Journal of Chemical Neuroanatomy*, **3**, 215–31.

Carroll, B. J., Feinberg, M., Grenden, J. F., Tarika, J., Albala, A. A., Haskett, R. F., James, N. M., Kronfol, Z., Lohr, N., Steiner, M., de Vigne, J. P. & Young, E. (1981). A specific laboratory test for the diagnosis of melancholia. *Archives of General Psychiatry*, **38**, 15–22.

Charney, D., Deutch, A. Y., Krystal, J. H., Southwick, S. M. & Davis, M. (1993). Psychobiologic mechanisms of posttraumatic stress disorder. *Archives of General Psychiatry*, **50**, 295–305.

Cizza, G. Calogero, L. S. Brady, G, Bagdy, E. Bergamini, M. R., Blackman, G. P., Chrousos, G. & Gold, P. W. (1994). Male Fischer-344/N rats show a progressive central impairment of the hypothalamic–pituitary–adrenal axis with advancing age. *Endocrinology*, **134**, 1611–20.

Clauw, D. J. & Chrousos, G. P. (1997). Chronic pain and fatigue syndromes: overlapping clinical and neuroendocrine features and potential pathogenic mechanisms. *Neuroimmunomodulation*, **4**, 134–53.

Cohen, N. J. & Squire, L. R. (1980). Preserved learning and retention of pattern analyzing skill in amnesia: dissociation of knowing how and knowing that. *Science*, **210**, 207–10.

Davis, K. L., Davis, B. M., Greenwald, B. S., Mohs, R. C., Mathe, A. A., Johns, C. A. & Horvath, T. B. (1986). Cortisol and Alzheimer's disease. I Basal studies. *American Journal of Psychiatry*, **143**, 300–5.

DeGoeij, D. C. E., Jezova, D. & Tilders, F. J. H. (1992). Repeated stress enhances vasopressin synthesis in corticotropin-releasing factor neurons in the paraventricular nucleus. *Brain Research*, **577**, 165–8.

DeGoeij, D. C. E., Kvetnansky, R., Whitnall, M. H., Jesova, D., Berkenbosch, F. & Tilders, F. J. H. (1991). Repeated stress induces activation of corticotropin-releasing factor (CRF) neurons enhances vasopressin stores and colocalization with CRF in the median eminence of rats. *Neuroendocrinology*, **53**, 150–9.

DeKloet, E. R. & Sutano, W. (1989). Role of corticosteroid receptors in central regulation of the stress response. In *The Control of the Hypothalamo-Pituitary Adrenocortical Axis*, ed. F. C. Rose, pp. 52–82. Madison, CT: International University Press.

DeKloet, E. R., Vreugdenhil, E., Oitzl, M. S. & Joels, M. (1998). Brain corticosteroid receptor balance in health and disease. *Endocrine Reviews*, **19**, 269–301.

DeLeon, M., McRae, T., Tsai, J., George, A., Marcus, D., Freeman, M., Wolf, A. & McEwen, B. (1988). Abnormal cortisol response in Alzheimer's disease linked to hippocampal atrophy. *Lancet*, **ii**, 391–2.

Deuschle, M., Gotthardt, U., Schweiger, U., Weber, B., Korner, A., Schmider, J., Standhardt, H., Lammers, C-H. & Heuser, I. (1997). With aging in humans, the activity of the hypothalamus–pituitary–adrenal system increases and its diurnal amplitude flattens. *Life Sciences*, **61**, 2239–46.

Diamond, D. M., Bennett, M. C., Fleshner, M. & Rose, G. M. (1992). Inverted-U relationship between the level of peripheral and the magnitude of hippocampal primed burst potentiation. *Hippocampus*, **2**, 421–30.

Dodt, C., Dittmann, J., Hruby, J., Spath-Schwalbe, E., Born, J., Schuttler, R. & Fehm, H. L. (1991). Different regulation of adrenocorticotropin and cortisol secretion in young, mentally healthy elderly and patients with senile dementia of the Alzheimer's type. *Journal of Clinical Endocrinology and Metabolism*, **72**, 272–6.

Dorsa, D. & Bottemiller, L. (1982). Age-related changes of vasopressin content of microdissected areas of the rat brain. *Brain Research*, **242**, 151–6.

Drafta, D., Schindler, A. E., Stroe, E. & Neascu, E. (1982). Age related changes of plasma steroids in normal adult males. *Journal of Steroid Biochemistry*, **17**, 683–7.

Drouin, J., Sun, Y. L., Tremblay, S., Lavender, P., Schmidt, T. J., deLean, A. & Nemer, M. (1992). Homodimer formation is rate limiting for high affinity binding by the glucocorticoid receptor. *Molecular Endocrinology*, **6**, 1299–309.

Ferrari, E., Magru, F., Dori, G., Migliorati, G., Nescis, T., Molla, G., Fioravanti, M. & Solerte, S. (1985). Neuroendocrine correlates of the aging brain in humans. *Neuroendocrinology*, **61**, 464–70.

Fuller, R. W. (1992). The involvement of serotonin in regulation of pituitary–adrenocortical function. *Frontiers in Neuroendocrinology*, **13**, 250–70.

Givalois, L., Li, S. & Pelletier, G. (1997). Age-related decrease in the hypothalamic CRH mRNA expression is reduced by dehydroepiandrosterone (DHEA) treatment in male and female rats. *Molecular Brain Research*, **48**, 107–14.

Gotthardt, U., Schweigger, U., Fahrenberg, J., Lauer, C. J., Holsboer, F. & Heuser, I. (1995). Cortisol, ACTH and cardiovascular response to a cognitive challenge paradigm in aging and depression. *American Journal of Physiology*, 268, R865–73.

Graf, P. & Schacter, D. L. (1985). Implicit and explicit memory for new associations in normal and amnesic subjects. *Journal of Experimental Psychology [Human Learning]*, 13, 45–53.

Halbreich, U., Asnis, G. M., Shindledecker, R., Zumoff, B. & Nathan, S. (1985). Cortisol secretion in endogenous depressives. I Basal plasma levels. *Archives of General Psychiatry*, 42, 904–8.

Hall, R. C., Popkin, M. K., Stickney, S. K. & Gardner, E. R. (1979). Presentation of the steroid psychoses. *Journal of Nervous and Mental Disorders*, 167, 229–36.

Hauger, R. L., Thrivikraman, K. V. & Plotsky, P. M. (1994). Age-related alterations of hypothalamic–pituitary–adrenal axis function in male Fischer 344 rats. *Endocrinology*, 134, 1528–36.

Herman, J. P., Prewitt, C. M. F. & Cullinan, W. E. (1996). Neuronal circuit regulation of the hypothalamo-pituitary-adrenocortical stress axis. *Critical Reviews in Neurobiology*, 10(3, 4), 371–94.

Heuser, I., Gotthardt, U., Schweigger, J., Schmider, J., Lammers, C. H., Dettling, M. & Holsboer, F. (1994). Age-associated changes of pituitary–adrenocortical hormone regulation in humans: importance of gender. *Neurobiology of Aging*, 15, 227–31.

Holets, V. R. (1990). The anatomy and function of noradrenaline in the mammalian brain. In *The Pharmacology of Noradrenaline in the Central Nervous System*, ed. D. J. Heal & C. A. Marsden, pp. 1–40. New York: Oxford University Press.

Holsboer, F., Spengler, D. & Heuser, I. (1992). The role of corticotropin-releasing hormone in the pathogenesis of Cushing's disease, anorexia nervosa, alcoholism, affective disorders and dementia. *Progress in Brain Research*, 93, 385–417.

Issa, A. M., Rowe, W., Gauthier, S. & Meant, M. J. (1990). Hypothalamic–pituitary–adrenal activity in aged, cognitively impaired and cognitively unimpaired rats. *Journal of Neuroscience*, 10, 3247–54.

Jensen, M. & Blichert-Toft, M. (1971). Serum corticotrophin, plasma cortisol, and urinary excretion of 17-ketogenic steroids in the elderly (age group: 66–94 years). *Acta Endocrinologica*, 66, 25–34.

Joels, M. & DeKloet, E. R. (1989). Effects of glucocorticoids and norepinephrine on the excitability in the hippocampus. *Science*, 245, 1502–5.

Jones, M. T. & Gillham, B. (1988). Factors involved in the regulation of adrenocorticotropic hormone/β-lipotropic hormones. *Physiologic Reviews*, 68, 743–818.

Kasckow, J. W., Regmi, A., Mulchahey, J. J., Plotsky, P. M. & Hauger, R. L. (1999). Changes in brain corticotropin-releasing factor messenger RNA expression in aged Fischer 344 rats. *Brain Research*, 822, 228–30.

Kathol, R. G., Jaeckle, R. S. & Lopez, J. F. (1989). Pathophysiology of HPA axis: abnormalities in patients with major depression: an update. *American Journal of Psychiatry*, 146, 311.

Katz, I. R. (1996). On the inseparability of mental and physical health in aged persons. Lessons from depression and medical comorbidity. *American Journal of Geriatric Psychiatry*, 4, 1–16.

Keitner, G. I., Ryan, C. E., Kohn, R., Miller, I., Norman, W. H. & Brown, W. A. (1992). Age and the dexamethasone suppression test: results from a broad unselected patient population. *Psychiatry Research*, 44, 9–20.

Keller-Wood, M. & Dallman, M. (1984). Corticosteroid inhibition of ACTH secretion. *Endocrine*

Reviews, 5, 1–24.

Kerr, D. S., Campbell, L. W., Applegate, M. D., Brodish, A. & Landfied, P. W. (1991). Chronic stress-induced acceleration of electrophysiologic and morphometric biomarkers of hippocampal aging. *Journal of Neuroscience*, 11, 1316–24.

Kerr, D. S., Campbell, L. W., Hao, S-Y. & Landfied, P. W. (1989). Corticosteroid modulation of hippocampal potentials: increased effect during aging. *Science*, 245, 1502–5.

Lakatua, D. J., Nicolau, G. Y., Bogdan, C., Plinga, L., Jachimowicz, A., Sackett-Lundeen, L., Petrescu, E., Ungureanu, E. & Haus, E. (1987). Chronobiology of catecholamine excretion in different age groups. *Progress in Clinical and Biological Research*, 227B, 31–50.

Landfield, P. W. & Eldridge, J. C. (1991). The glucocorticoid hypothesis of brain aging and neurodegeneration: recent modifications. *Acta Endocrinologica*, 125, 54–64.

Landfield, P. W., Thibault, O., Mazzanti, M. L., Porter, N. M. & Kerr, D. S. (1992). Mechanisms of neuronal death in brain aging and Alzheimer's disease: role of endocrine-mediated calcium dyshomostasis. *Journal of Neurobiology*, 23, 1247–60.

Ling, M., Perry, P. & Tsuang, M. (1981). Side effects of corticosteroid therapy. *Archives of General Psychiatry*, 38, 471–7.

Lorens, S. A., Hata, N., Handa, R. J., Van deKar, L. D., Guschwan, M., Goral, J., Lee, J. M., Hamilton, M. E., Bethea, C. L. & Clancy Jr., J. (1990). Neurochemical, endocrine and immunologic responses to stress in young and old Fischer 344 rats. *Neurobiology of Aging*, 11, 139–50.

Lupien, S. J., de Leon, M., de Santi, S., Convit, A., Tarshish, C., Nair, N. P. V., Thakur, M., McEwen, B., Hauger, R. L. & Meaney, M. J. (1998). Cortisol levels during human aging predict hippocampal atrophy and memory deficits. *Nature Neuroscience*, 1, 69–73.

Lupien, S., Lecours, A. R., Lussier, I., Schwartz, G., Nair, N. P. Y. & Meaney, M. J. (1994). Basal cortisol levels and cognitive deficits in human aging. *Journal of Neuroscience*, 14, 2893–903.

Maes, M., Calabrese, J., Lee, M. & Meltzer, H. Y. (1994). Effects of age on spontaneous cortisolaemia of normal volunteers and depressed patients. *Psychoneuroendocrinology*, 19, 79–84.

Martignoni, E., Costa, A., Sinforiani, E., Liuzzi, A., Chiodini, P., Mauri, M., Bono, G. & Nappi, G. (1992). The brain as a target for adrenocortical steroids: cognitive implications. *Psychoneuroendocrinology*, 17, 343–54.

McEwen, B. (1992). Re-examination of the glucocorticoid hypothesis of stress and aging. *Progress in Brain Research*, 93, 365–81.

McEwen, B. S. (1999). Stress and the aging hippocampus. *Frontiers in Neuroendocrinology*, 20, 49–70.

McEwen, B. S. & Stellar, E. (1993). Stress and the individual. Mechanisms leading to disease. *Archives of Internal Medicine*, 153, 2093.

Meaney, M. J., Aitken, D. H., Bhatnagar, S. & Sapolsky, R. M. (1991). Postnatal handling attenuates certain neuroendocrine, anatomical, and cognitive dysfunctions associated with aging in female rats. *Neurobiology of Aging*, 12, 31–8.

Meaney, M. J., Aitken, D. H., Sharma, S. & Viau, V. (1992). Basal ACTH, corticosterone and corticosterone-binding globulin levels over the diurnal cycle, and age related changes in hippocampal type I and type II corticosteroid binding capacity in young and aged, handled and non-handled rats. *Neuroendocrinology*, 55, 204–13.

Mitchell, J. B., Betito, K., Rowe, W., Boksa, P. & Meaney, M. J. (1992). Serotonergic regulation of type II corticosteroid receptor in cultured hippocampal cells: the role of serotonin-induced increases in cAMP levels. *Neuroscience*, 48, 631–9.

Mitchell, J. B., Rowe, W., Boksa, P. & Meaney, M. J. (1990). Serotonin regulates type II corticosteroid receptor binding in hippocampal cell cultures. *Journal of Neuroscience*, 10, 1524–33.

Mobbs, C. V. (1996). Neuroendocrinology of aging. In *Handbook of the Biology of Aging*, ed. E. L. Schneider & J. W. Rowe, pp. 234–82. San Diego, CA: Academic Press.

Mulchahey, J. J., Kasckow, J. W., Plotsky, P. M. & Hauger, R. L. (1999). Steroidal regulation of portal arginine–vasopresin levels in aged Fischer 344 rats. *Brain Research*, 822, 243–5.

Munck, A., Guyre, P. M. & Holbrook, N. J. (1984). Physiological functions of glucocorticoids in stress and their relations to pharmacological actions. *Endocrine Reviews*, 5, 25–44.

Nasman, B., Olsson, T., Fagerlund, M., Eriksson, S., Viitanen, M., Carlstrom, K. (1996). Blunted adrenocorticotropin and increased adrenal steroid response to human corticotropin-releasing hormone in Alzheimer's disease. *Biological Psychiatry*, 39, 311–18.

Nasman, B., Olsson, T., Viitanen, M. & Carlstrom, K. (1995). A subtle disturbance in the feedback regulation of the hypothalamic–pituitary–adrenal axis in the early phase of Alzheimer's disease. *Psychoneuroendocrinology*, 20, 211–20.

Norris, C. M., Halpain, S. & Foster, T. C. (1998). Reversal of age-related alterations in synaptic plasticity by blockade of L-type Ca^{2+} channels. *Journal of Neuroscience*, 18, 3171–9.

O'Brien, J. T., Schweitzer, I., Ames, D., Tuckwell, V. & Mastwyk, M. (1994). Cortisol suppression by dexamethasone in the healthy elderly: effects of age, dexamethasone levels, and cognitive function. *Biological Psychiatry*, 36, 389–94.

Odio, M. & Brodish, A. (1989). Age related adaptation of pituitary–adrenocortical responses to stress. *Neuroendocrinology*, 49, 382–8.

Oxenkrug, G. F., Gurevich, D., Siegel, B., Dumaiao, M. S. & Gershon, S. (1989). Correlation between brain–adrenal axis activation and cognitive impairment in Alzheimer's disease: is there a gender effect? *Psychiatry Research*, 29, 169–75.

Peiffer, A., Barden, N. & Meaney, M. J. (1991). Age-related changes in glucocorticoid receptor binding and mRNA levels in the rat brain and pituitary. *Neurobiology of Aging*, 12, 475–9.

Pepin, M. C. & Barden, N. (1992). Decreased glucocorticoid receptor gene promoter activity after antidepressant treatment. *Molecular Pharmacology*, 41, 1016–22.

Peskind, E. R., Wingerson, D., Murray, S., Pascualy, M., Dobie, D. J., Corre, P. L., LeVerge, R., Weith, R. C. & Raskind, M. A. (1995). Effects of Alzheimer's disease and normal aging on cerebrospinal fluid norepinephrine responses to yohimbine and clonidine. *Archives of General Psychiatry*, 52, 774–82.

Pfohl, B., Sherman, B., Schlechte, J. & Stone, R. (1985). Pituitary–adrenal axis rhythm disturbances in psychiatric depression. *Archives of General Psychiatry*, 42, 897–903.

Raadsheer, F. C., Sluiter, A. A., Ravid, R., Tilders, F. J. & Swaab, D. F. (1993). Localization of corticotropin-releasing hormone (CRH) neurons in the paraventricular nucleus of the human hypothalamus; age-dependent colocalization with vasopressin. *Brain Research*, 615, 50–62.

Raadsheer, F. C., Tilders, F. J. & Swaab, D. F. (1994). Similar age related increase of vasopressin colocalization in paraventricular corticotropin-releasing hormone neurons in controls and Alzheimer's patients. Journal of *Neuroendocrinology*, 6, 131–3.

Raadsheer, F. C., van Heerikhuize, J. J., Lucassen, P. J., Hoogendijk, W. J. G., Tilders, F. J. H. &

Swaab, D. F. (1995). Corticotropin-releasing hormone mRNA levels in the paraventricular nucleus of patients with Alzheimer's disease and depression. *American Journal of Psychiatry*, 152, 1372–6.

Rolandi, E., Franceschini, R., Marabini, A., Messina, V., Cataldi, A., Salvemini, M. & Barreca, T. (1987). Twenty four hour beta endorphin secretion pattern in the elderly. *Acta Endocrinologica*, 115, 441–6.

Rowe, W., Steverman, A., Walker, M., Sharma, S., Barden, N., Seckl, J. R. & Meaney, M. J. (1997). Antidepressants restore hypothalamic–pituitary–adrenal feedback function in aged, cognitively impaired rats. *Neurobiology of Aging*, 18, 527–33.

Sapolsky, R. M., Krey, L. C. & McEwen, B. S. (1983). The adrenocortical stress response in the aged male rat: impairment of recovery from stress. *Experimental Gerontology*, 18, 55–64.

Sapolsky, R. M., Krey, L. C. & McEwen, B. S. (1986). The neuroendocrinology of stress and aging: the glucocorticoid cascade hypothesis. *Endocrine Reviews*, 7, 284–301.

Sapolsky, R., Rivier, C., Yamamoto, G., Plotsky, P. & Vale, W. (1987). Interleukin 1 stimulates the secretion of hypothalamic corticotropin-releasing factor. *Science*, 238, 522–4.

Sarrieau, A., Rowe, W., O'Donnell, D., LaRocque, S., Nair, N. P. V., Levin, N., Seckl, J. R. & Meaney, M. J. (1992). hypothalamic–pituitary–adrenal activity and corticosteroid receptor expression in aged, cognitively impaired and cognitively unimpaired rats. *Society for Neuroscience Abstracts*, 18, 669.

Seckl, J. R. & Fink, G. (1992). Antidepressants increase glucocorticoid and mineralocorticoid receptor mRNA expression in rat hippocampus in vivo. *Neuroendocrinology*, 55, 621–6.

Seeman, T. E. & Robbins, R. J. (1994). Aging and hypothalamic–pituitary–adrenal response to challenge in humans. *Endocrine Reviews*, 15, 233–60.

Sharma, M., Palacios-Bois, J., Schwartz, G., Iskandar, H., Thakur, M., Quirion, R., Nair & N. P. Y. (1989). Circadian rhythms of melatonin and cortisol in aging. *Biological Psychiatry*, 25, 305–19.

Sharma, R. P., Pandey, G. N., Janicak, P. G., Peterson, J., Comaty, J. E. & Davis, J. M. (1988). The effect of diagnosis and age on the DST: a metaanalytic approach. *Biolgical Psychiatry*, 24, 555–68.

Sherman, B., Wysham, C. & Pfohl, B. (1985). Age-related changes in the circadian rhythm of plasma cortisol in man. *Journal of Clinical Endocrinology and Metabolism*, 61, 439–43.

Smith, M. A., Makino, S., Kim, S-Y. & Kvetnansky, R. (1995). Stress increases brain-derived neurotropic factor messenger ribonucleic acid in the hypothalamus and pituitary. *Endocrinology*, 136, 3743–50.

Starkman, M. N., Gebarski, S. S., Berent, S. & Schteingart, D. E. (1992). Hippocampal formation volume, memory dysfunction, and cortisol levels in patients with Cushing's syndrome. *Biological Psychiatry*, 32, 756–65.

Tilders, F. J. H., Schmidt, E. D. & deGoeij, D. C. E. (1993). Phenotypic plasticity of CRH neurons during stress. *Annals of the New York Academy of Sciences*, 697, 39–52.

Touitou, Y., Sulon, J., Bogdan, A., Touitou, C., Reinberg, A., Beck, H., Sodoyez, J. C., Demey-Ponsart, E. & Van Cauwenberge, H. (1982). Adrenal circadian system in young and elderly human subjects: a comparative study. *Journal of Endocrinology*, 93, 201–10.

Touitou, Y., Sulon, J., Bogdan, A., Reinberg, A., Sodoyez, J. C. & Demey-Ponsart, E. (1983).

Adrenocortical hormones, ageing and mental conditions: seasonal and circadian rhythms of plasma 18-hydroxy-11-deoxycorticosterone, total and free cortisol and urinary corticosteroids. *Journal of Endocrinology*, **96**, 53–64.

Vedder, H., Weiss, I., Holsboer, F. & Reul, J. M. H. M. (1993). Glucocorticoid and mineralocorticoid receptors in rat neocortical and hippocampal brain cells in culture. Characterization and regulatory studies. *Brain Research*, **605**, 18–24.

Waltman, C., Blackman, M. R., Chrousos, G. P., Riemann, C. & Harman, S. M. (1991). Spontaneous and glucocorticoid inhibited adrenocorticotropin hormone and cortisol secretion are similar in healthy young and old men. *Journal of Clinical Endocrinology and Metabolism*, **73**, 495–502.

Weidenfeld, J., Abramsky, O. & Ovadia, H. (1989). Effect of intereukin-1 on ACTH and corticosterone secretion in dexamethasone and adrenalectomized pretreated male rats. *Neuroendocrinology*, **50**, 650–4.

Whitnall, M. H. (1993). Regulation of the hypothalamic corticotropin-releasing hormone neurosecretory system. *Progress in Neurobiology*, **40**, 573–629.

Whitnall, M. H., Kiss, A. & Aguilera, G. (1993). Contrasting effects of central alpha-1-adrenoreceptor activation on stress-responsive and stress-nonresponsiveness subpopulations of corticotropin-releasing hormone neurosecretory cells in the rat. *Neuroendocrinology*, **58**, 42–8.

Wilkinson, C. W., Peskind, E. R. & Raskind, M. A. (1997). Decreased hypothalamic–pituitary–adrenal axis sensitivity to cortisol feedback inhibition in human aging. *Neuroendocrinology*, **65**, 79–90.

Wolkowitz, O. M. & Rapaport, M. (1989). Long-lasting behavioral changes following prednisone withdrawal. *Journal of the American Medical Association*, **261**, 1731–2.

Yamamoto, K. R. (1985). Steroid receptor regulated transcription of specific genes and gene networks. *Annual Review of Genetics*, **19**, 205–52.

Zimmerman, M., Coryell, W. & Pfohl, B. (1987). The dexamethasone suppresion test in healthy controls. *Psychoneuroendocrinology*, **12**, 245–51.

4

The hypothalamic–pituitary–thyroid axis

Gabriel K. Tsuboyama

Introduction

Aging appears to affect the hypothalamic–pituitary–thyroid (HPT) axis. Between the sixth and eighth decades, serum levels of free tri-iodothyronine (T3) and thyroid-stimulating hormone (TSH) gradually decline while serum thyroxine (T4) remains the same (Mariotti et al., 1993; Muller, 1994; Erfurth & Hagmer, 1995; Monzani et al., 1996). These findings, coupled with decrements in the response of TSH to thyrotropin releasing hormone (TRH), suggest a decrease in responsiveness of the HPT axis with aging. Thyroid function has been known to affect mood and cognition in younger populations, but the impact of these age-related changes, which are not associated with clinical hypothyroidism or hyperthyroidism, on the central nervous system have not been well characterized.

Disorders of thyroid axis function are likely to affect mental function, especially in the elderly (Esposito et al., 1997). The interaction between brain and thyroid hormones starts in utero and continues throughout life, with psychiatric symptoms present in patients with thyroid dysfunction. Depressed mood and psychomotor retardation occur in hypothyroid patients. Anxiety, fatigue, and irritability are observed in hyperthyroidism (Whybrow & Ferrell, 1974; Kathol & Delahunt, 1986). Depression can be a manifestation of unsuspected hypothyroidism (Gold, 1983).

In hypothyroid patients, withdrawal of thyroid replacement may cause increased sadness and anxiety, in particular in those with a prior history of affective illness or mood lability (Denicoff et al., 1990). Patients with severe hypothyroidism may develop a syndrome of marked psychosis (myxedema madness; Asher, 1949).

No simple relationship between the direction of mood changes and the type of thyroid dysfunction has been demonstrated. Depression, for example, has also been associated with hyperthyroidism (Kathol & Delahunt, 1986), and apathy is a striking feature of some patients with thyrotoxicosis (Kleinschmidt & Waxenberg, 1956; Artunkal & Togrol, 1964; Cohen & Swigar, 1979). Hypothyroid patients may develop mania at the onset of thyroid hormone replacement (Josephson &

Mackenzie, 1980). Cognitive impairment, pseudodementia, and irreversible dementia may also occur in severe cases of hypothyroidism (Whybrow et al., 1969; Clarfield, 1988; Nemeroff, 1989; Haupt & Kurz, 1993).

This chapter will review the regulation of the thyroid axis, including the deiod- ination of T4 to T3 and reverse T3 (rT3), and the localization and regulation of TRH. Characteristics of the aging thyroid axis will be reviewed. Characteristics of the thyroid axis in geriatric major depression will be contrasted with that in younger depressed populations. This will include the following: thyroid axis char- acteristics in major depression, depressive syndromes in thyroid disorders, thera- peutic effects of thyroid hormones in major depression, and the effects of anti-depressant treatments on the thyroid axis.

Physiology of the thyroid axis

Thyrotropin-releasing hormone (protirelin, thyroliberin, or TRH), which is secreted by the hypothalamus, stimulates the synthesis and release of thyroid-stim- ulating hormone (thyrotropin or TSH) by the pituitary gland. All processes in the thyroid gland, from the uptake of iodine to the release of T4 and T3, are stimulated by TSH. Most of T3 and all of the biologically inactive rT3 are produced by deiod- ination of T4 in peripheral tissues (DeGroot et al., 1996).

Circulating thyroid hormones are reversibly bound and transported by plasma proteins: primarily T4-binding inter-α globulin (TBG) for T4 and T3, T4-binding pre-albumin (TBPA) for some of T4, and albumin for a minimal amount of T4 and T3. Metabolic effects are produced by the unbound, free fraction of the thyroid hormones, which is 10 times higher for T3 than for T4 (0.3% vs. 0.03%) due to the stronger affinity of the main carrier, thyroid-binding globulin, TBG, for T4 than for T3. The availability of free T3 is a function of the concentration of free T4, the activity of deioidinases for the generation of T3, and the concentration of the pro- teins transporting thyroid hormones (TBG, TBPA and albumin).

Deiodinases, which are iodine-cleaving enzymes, play an important role in the action of thyroid hormones in the brain. The brain takes up T4 from transthyretin which carries T4 across the blood–brain barrier (Hendrick et al., 1998). Three types of deiodinases have been found; they differ in their substrate of preference, tissue location, and responsiveness to T3 (Larsen, 1997). In the brain 5'deiodinase type II converts T4 to T3. This enzyme is specific to the pituitary and the cerebral cortex and the brain can autoregulate T3 conversion (Hendrick et al., 1998). Type III deiodinase is found in the brain and produces rT3 (Lasser & Baldessarini, 1997). Deiodinases are responsible for generating 80% of plasma T3 and for providing intracellular T3. Additionally, deiodinases inactivate all thyroid hormones.

The effects of thyroid hormones can be mediated by nuclear and by non-nuclear mechanisms (DeGroot et al., 1989; Lazar, 1993; Davis & Davis, 1996; Motomura & Brent, 1998). Most of these non-nuclear actions occur in seconds to minutes, up to an hour, after exposure either to T4, T3, or metabolites such as rT3 and diiodothyronine (T2). Although the intensity of non-genomic effects is modest compared to that of genomic, nuclear-mediated effects, their final action may be significant through increases in the generation and activity of second messengers.

The nuclear mechanism, the genomic pathway, includes the interaction of T3 with specific nuclear receptors and the formation of hormone-receptor complexes, which by acting on the promoter region of target genes either stimulate or inhibit gene transcription (Oppenheimer, 1983; Larsen et al., 1986; DeGroot, 1991; Motomura & Brent, 1998). Thus, for example, T3 stimulates transcription of the gene encoding rat growth hormone (Brent et al., 1989) and inhibits transcription of the genes encoding for the alpha and the beta subunits of TSH (Chin et al., 1993) and TRH (Hollenberg et al., 1995), among others. Currently, four different thyroid hormone receptor subtypes have been described; three have been found in humans and rats (Sap et al., 1986; Weinberger et al., 1986; Nakai et al., 1988; Sakurai et al., 1989), and a fourth, pituitary-specific, in rats (Hodin et al., 1989). Of interest is the finding that these receptors subtypes are structurally related to other receptors of the steroid receptor superfamily, which includes receptors for glucocorticoids, estrogens, mineralocorticoids, progesterone, vitamin D3, and retinoic acid (for review see Evans, 1988).

Regulation

The HPT axis is regulated by a negative feedback mechanism. TRH and TSH play stimulatory roles on the pituitary and thyroid gland, respectively. T4 and T3 inhibit TSH secretion by determining the pituitary 'set point' for TRH stimulation and by regulating both the synthesis of TRH in the hypothalamus (Iriuchijima et al., 1984; Segerson et al., 1987; Utiger 1987; Hollenberg et al., 1995) and its degradation (Bauer, 1987; Suen & Wilk, 1987, 1989). TRH is a tripeptide, produced by post-translational cleavage of a larger molecule, pro-TRH (Lechan et al., 1986).

Neuropeptides, neurotransmitters, and other hormones modulate the activity of the HPT axis. Inhibitory effects on TSH secretion have been reported for somatostatin, cortisol, gamma-amino butyric acid and dopamine, while noradrenergic input appears to stimulate the secretion of TRH as well as TSH. The effects of other compounds like serotonin, histamine, melatonin and cholecystokinin are contradictory (Morley, 1981; Martin & Reichlin, 1987; DeGroot et al., 1996).

Thyroid hormones appear to regulate the expression of the pro-TRH gene. In hypothyroid rats the expression of the gene in the paraventricular nuclei is increased (Segerson et al., 1987). Although this effect has not been demonstrated in other parts of the brain, a regulatory role for thyroid hormones on the biosynthesis of TRH is supported by the finding that hypothyroidism increases the content of TRH and TRH-precursors in rat pancreas, adrenals, prostate and other organs not known to be involved in the regulation of the HPT axis (Wolf et al., 1984; Simard et al., 1989).

TRH and its receptors are widely distributed in the body. TRH-immunoreactive cell bodies have been found not only in the thyrotropic area of the hypothalamus, the paraventricular nuclei (Aizawa & Greer, 1981), but also in other areas of the rat nervous system, such as the olfactory bulb, pyriform cortex, entorhinal cortex, hippocampus, amygdaloid complex, striatum, nucleus accumbens, hypothalamus, substantia nigra, medula oblongata (including the raphe nuclei) and spinal cord, and in other organs including pancreas and stomach (Hokfelt et al., 1989). In humans, the highest concentration of TRH receptors is found in the rhinencephalon (hippocampus and amygdala), which is known to contain low levels of TRH; conversely, the hypothalamus, with one of the highest concentrations of TRH, has low concentrations of TRH receptors (Manaker et al., 1986). A similar dissociation between TRH and its receptors has also been found in rats (Manaker et al., 1985). After binding to its receptor, the initial steps of TRH action involves the association of the TRH-receptor complex to a G protein and consequent activation of phospholipase C and hydrolysis of phosphatidylinositol 4,5-bisphosphate (PIP2; Straub & Gershengorn, 1986; Gershengorn, 1986).

Effects of HPT-axis hormones on the brain: TRH and metabolites

Although the ultimate goal of the hypothalamic–pituitary–thyroid (HPT) axis is the provision of thyroid hormones to meet the metabolic demand, its hypothalamic component, TRH, has many other biological effects besides the stimulation of TSH synthesis and release. Many of these actions are excitatory in nature and are not restricted to the brain, and therefore TRH has been conceptualized as an 'ergotropic' substance (Metcalf & Dettmar, 1981). Actions of TRH on pain perception, blood pressure, heart rate, catecholamine turnover, dopamine metabolism, serotonin receptors, respiration, acetylcholine, thermoregulation, and glucose regulation are some of the effects described (Keller et al., 1974; Morley, 1979; Brown, 1981; Jackson, 1982; Griffiths & Bennett, 1983; Griffiths, 1985; Kabayama et al., 1985; Zadina et al., 1986; Amir, 1988; Metcalf & Jackson, 1989).

The metabolism of TRH involves biotransformation to form acid-TRH and histidyl prolineamide (His–Pro–NH_2). Following its formation, His–Pro–NH_2 is immediately cyclicized to form cyclo (His–Pro), probably by a non-enzymatic reaction (Prasad & Peterkofsky, 1976). His–Pro is likely also produced from other sources, such pre-pro-TRH or the aminoacid pool, since its distribution differs from that of TRH and since it is present even after TRH-containing tissues are destroyed (Mori et al., 1983; Lamberton et al., 1984; Lechan & Jackson 1985; Prasad et al., 1987).

The administration of TRH metabolites to both animals and humans have produced brain effects. Acid-TRH produces 'wet dog shakes' and cyclo (His–Pro) has shown many actions, some similar and others opposed to those produced by TRH (Prasad et al., 1977; Bauer et al., 1978; Peterkofsky et al., 1982; Mori et al., 1982b; Peters et al., 1985; Prasad, 1989). A receptor for cyclo (His–Pro) has not yet been characterized; however, many of its actions appear to involve a dopaminergic mechanism, probably at the presynaptic site, inhibiting (Na+–K+) ATP-ase activity (Prasad et al., 1978; Battaini & Peterkofsky 1980; Prasad et al., 1980; Brabant et al., 1981). Elevated levels of cyclo (His–Pro) have been reported in the serum of hypothyroid patients (Mori et al., 1982a), as well as in the spinal cord tissue of patients with amyotrophic lateral sclerosis (Jackson et al., 1987). Increased levels of the dipeptide have also been found in the CSF of patients with neurologic/neuropsychiatric disorders, but a relationship with a specific disorder has not been established (Iriuchijima et al., 1987). Recently, elevated cyclo (His–Pro) in the CSF of untreated schizophrenic patients has been noted (Prasad et al., 1991).

The formation of a third TRH metabolite, histidyl proline, has been observed in vitro (Browne & O'Cuinn, 1983; Coggins et al., 1987a). In rats, histidyl proline, also known as His–Pro, binds specifically to brain membranes (Coggins et al., 1987b) and produces behavioral effects (Coggins et al., 1986).

The HPT axis in the elderly

The aging process brings changes both in the structure of the gland and the physiology of the HPT axis (DeGroot et al., 1996; Solomon, 1991). The volume of the thyroid gland remains stable until the sixth decade and then gradually loses up to 20% of its maximum volume when increased nodularity and cellular infiltration occur (Ingbar, 1985; Ogiu et al., 1997). The incidence of anti-thyroid antibodies is increased in aging (Ingbar, 1985; DeGroot et al., 1996), but in healthy centenarians the prevalence of anti-thyroid antibodies is decreased (Mariotti et al., 1993; Pinchera et al., 1995). It appears that age-associated diseases may play a role since anti-thyroid antibodies occur more frequently in the sick or hospitalized elderly. Alternatively, findings in centenarians could reflect an age-associated decline in the immune system.

Thyroid function remains normal until advanced age (Solomon; 1991, Mooradian & Wong, 1994). Between the sixth and eighth decade, serum levels of free T4 remains unchanged while levels of free T3 and TSH gradually decline (Mariotti et al., 1993; Muller, 1994; Erfurth & Hagmar, 1995; Monzani et al., 1996).

Reverse T3 levels increase with aging but without reaching the levels found in non-thyroidal illnesses (Mariotti et al., 1993).

The absence of a reciprocal increment in TSH when free T3 is decreased may reflect changes in the set-point of the pituitary thyrotrophs or in the hypothalamus. This possibility is supported by decrements in the response of TSH to TRH that occurs in aging (Snyder et al., 1974; Erfurth & Hagmar, 1995) even when free T3 is decreasing. This possibility is also supported by age-associated alterations in the circadian rhythm of TSH. Monzani et al. (1996) reported a significant diurnal decrement of TSH in subjects aged 65–80 years that was absent in subjects aged 81–92 years.

Mood disorders related to the HPT axis in the elderly

A relationship between the HPT axis and mood disorders is supported by (a) the occurrence of psychiatric symptoms in the setting of thyroid dysfunction, (b) HPT axis-related hormone abnormalities in affective disorders, (c) the therapeutic effects of HPT axis-related hormones in mood disorders, and (d) the effect of treatment modalities for affective disorders on the HPT axis.

Hypothyroidism

The prevalence of primary hypothyroidism in the elderly ranges between 0.5% and 15%; females are most commonly affected. Methodologic variations, such as clinical vs. subclinical hypothyroidism, T4 vs. TSH levels, and iodine supply, may influence the reported prevalence rates (DeGroot et al., 1996, Chiovato et al., 1997, Wang & Crapo, 1997). The most common causes are autoimmune diseases and iatrogenically produced after-treatment for Graves' disease.

Symptoms and signs attributed to aging, as well as silent non-thyroidal illnesses, may mask the manifestations of hypothyroidism. The most frequent symptoms of hypothyroidism are fatigue, weakness, mental slowing, dry skin, cold intolerance, constipation, hyporeflexia, and hearing loss (Hornick & Kowal, 1997). Neurologic signs such as ataxia, carpal tunnel syndrome, and peripheral neuropathy commonly occur, as well. Mental symptoms can be significant and include depression and cognitive impairment (Samuels, 1998, Hickie et al., 1996, Ganguli et al., 1996).

Laboratory tests reveal an elevated TSH and low thyroid hormones levels in clinical hypothyroidism. In addition, hypercholesterolemia, normo- or macrocytic anemia, hyponatremia, and elevations of creatine phosphokinase, lactic dehydrogenase (LDH), and glutamic–oxalacetic transaminase (SGOT) may be seen with testing. The treatment of hypothyroidism in the elderly consists of replacement with L-thyroxine, in doses 20% to 30% lower than that for younger patients (Rosenbaum & Barzel, 1982), i.e. about 0.11mg/day (Sawin et al., 1983).

Women have a significantly higher rate of hypothyroidism, both overt and sub-clinical. Elderly men have a fairly constant prevalence of elevated TSH by age, somewhere around 2% to 5% (Samuels, 1998). In contrast, the prevalence of elevated TSH is about 4% in young women and increases to 18% in women over the age of 74 years (Samuels, 1998). The significantly higher rate of hypothyroidism in women may reflect the stimulating effect of female reproductive hormones on immunologic function, producing greater rates of autoimmune disease in women and/or the lower levels of androgens which may suppress autoimmune disease. Autoimmune thyroid disease is marked by the presence of anti-thyroid antibodies. Anti-thyroid antibodies increase with age, while fully expressed autoimmune thyroid disease does not (Mariotti et al., 1998). In general, the presence of anti-thyroid antibodies is associated with diminished thyroid function (Hendrick et al., 1998). The prevalence of anti-thyroid antibodies does not appear to be greater in depressed populations compared with controls when adjustments are made for sex and prior lithium exposure (Hendrick et al., 1998).

Hyperthyroidism

In the elderly, the prevalence of hyperthyroidism ranges between 0.5% and 2.3%, more often occurring in females than in males (DeGroot et al., 1996; Hornick & Kowal, 1997; Chiovato et al., 1997). More often hyperthyroidism is caused by toxic multinodular goiter and toxic adenomas than by Graves' disease. Clinical presentations include weight loss, proximal weakness, dyspnea, palpitations, anorexia rather than increased appetite, and change in mental status. Mental syndromes include depression, anxiety, confusion and cognitive impairment (Mokshagundam & Barzel, 1993). Cardiovascular manifestations including tachycardia, atrial fibrillation, angina and congestive heart failure may often be the presenting symptoms of thyrotoxicosis. The risk for fractures increases as osteoporosis worsens. A particular form of thyrotoxicosis, apathetic, occurs in the elderly and is characterized by fatigue, apathy, depression, and a wasted appearance (Thomas et al., 1970; Tibaldi et al., 1986).

Treatment of hyperthyroidism includes the use of thionamides (propylthiouracil and metimazole), radioactive iodine, and surgery. In the elderly, the preferred treatment is radioactive iodine; however, other considerations, e.g. a large goiter that may require surgery, are taken into account. To prevent sudden decompensation, preoperatory preparation may require the use of thionamides and beta-blockers.

Hyperthyroidism has been linked to depression, and a commonly observed abnormality in thyroid function among depressed patients is a relative increase of total or free T4 and a relative decrease of T3 levels (Hendrick et al., 1998). The increased T4 levels may result from decreased peripheral conversion of T4 to T3, or the increased T4 activity may reflect compensatory homeostatic mechanisms to maintain normal brain function (Hendrick et al., 1998). As patients achieve remission, T4 and free T4 levels have been observed to drop. Some antidepressants, such as fluoxetine and tranylcypromine, appear to induce an increase in deiodinase activity in the brain. This increased activity could result in increased central T3 levels, with increased uptake of T4 from the periphery and lower serum T4 (Hendrick et al., 1998).

Euthyroid sick syndrome (ESS)

Abnormalities in the concentration of thyroid hormones and TSH have been described during the course of non-thyroidal illnesses (Wartofsky & Burman, 1982; McIver & Gorman, 1997). The syndrome is characterized by decrements in plasma levels of T3, rT3 and T4, and TSH, the latter even in the presence of low T3 and T4. ESS has been noted in trauma (Phillips et al., 1984), infections (Hamblin et al., 1986), surgery (Holland et al., 1991, Girvent et al., 1998), malignancy (Wehmann et al., 1985), and inflammatory diseases (Herrmann et al., 1989), among other conditions. The hormonal pattern has been attributed to a homeostatic mechanism aimed at the conservation of energy and proteins during the diseases process or to a maladaptive hormonal response to the concurrent disease. Abnormalities at the thyroid gland, pituitary, and hypothalamic levels as well as in the regulation of peripheral thyroid hormone, including binding proteins and deiodinases, are suspected. An important role appears to be played by proteins involved in inflammatory process, in particular interleukin-6 (Bartalena et al., 1998, Girvent et al., 1998, Davies et al., 1996) and the tumor necrosis factor alpha (van der Poll et al., 1990; Poth et al., 1991; Mooradian et al., 1990, 1991). ESS is reversible in the majority of cases. However, in severe cases, mortality can be predicted by the degree of thyroid dysfunction. Whether ESS should be treated remains controversial (Tibaldi & Surks, 1985; McIver & Gorman, 1997).

Geriatric depression

The HPT axis affects neurotransmitters known to be involved in mood, such as the catecholamine system and the serotonin system (Lasser & Baldessarini, 1997). In the rat brain, hypothyroidism is associated with decreased functional sensitivity of β-adrenergic receptors, but the effect on α-adrenergic receptors is inconsistent (Lasser & Baldessarini, 1997). Thyroid hormone modulates turnover of serotonin and dopamine in some areas of rat brain (Lasser & Baldessarini, 1997). In general, thyroid hormones are thought to increase adrenergic function, though the CNS demonstrates more complex effects.

Research has shown that baseline levels of TSH, T4, T3, free T4, and free T3 are not different in elderly major depressives when compared to age and sex-matched normal controls (Tsuboyama et al., 1999, unpublished data). In normal controls, but not in depressives, however, free T3 increases with aging (Tsuboyama et al., 1999, unpublished data). The TSH response to TRH decreases in both controls and depressed subjects as they age, and it significantly correlates with baseline TSH levels (Baumgartner et al., 1986). Lower TSH after TRH administration has been confirmed (Molchan et al., 1991).

Thyroid axis abnormalities in major depression have been thoroughly reviewed (Whybrow & Prange, 1981; Kirkegaard & Faber, 1981; Loosen & Prange, 1982; Prange & Loosen, 1984; Baumgartner et al., 1988; Nemeroff 1989; Nemeroff & Evans, 1989). In short, serum T4 levels have been found to be normal or elevated but still within normal range. Serum reverse T3 (rT3) elevations have been noted. All levels decrease following recovery T4, free T4, and rT3 (Whybrow et al., 1972; Loosen & Prange, 1980; Kirkegaard & Faber, 1981; Baumgartner et al., 1988; Brady & Anton, 1989; Scott et al., 1990).

In depressed patients, basal TSH secretion is normal or decreased (Vogel et al., 1977). Such decreased baseline levels of TSH persist throughout a 24-hour period (Duval et al., 1990). The normal nocturnal surge of TSH is attenuated or absent in depressed patients (Weeke & Weeke, 1980; Sack et al., 1985; Bartalena et al., 1990; Duval et al., 1990).

In approximately half of the patients with major depression, the TSH response to TRH administration (TRH test) is abnormal. Blunted TSH response occurs in about a third of depressed patients (Prange et al., 1972; Loosen & Prange, 1982), and more often in those patients with subnormal morning TSH levels (Bartalena et al., 1990). Such responses suggest there is an elevation of thyroid hormone function in the CNS with alteration of central regulatory mechanisms resulting in blunted TSH response. Exaggerated TSH response to TRH, which suggests hypothyroidism, have been reported in 15% of major depressives (Targum et al., 1982).

The usefulness of a blunted TSH response to TRH as a state or a trait marker for depression has been discussed. Loosen and Prange (1982) reviewed 13 studies addressing this issue, five of which favored a role for the blunted response as a state or a trait marker. A blunted TSH response (which was supported by Brambilla et al., 1980) might represent a trait marker in some cases. Loosen and Prange (1982) reached this conclusion after a finding of blunted TSH response to TRH in two of six unaffected first-degree relatives of a depressed subject. Baumgartner et al. (1988), however, did not establish that a blunted response was a marker for a depressive state. There is controversy since, in thyroidal illnesses, a blunted TSH response to TRH may remain unchanged for several months after treatment (Sanchez-Franco et al., 1974; Emrich et al., 1976). Baumgartner and colleagues (1988) expressed doubts that the test could be used as either a state or a trait marker for depression.

An association between the TSH response to TRH and depressive subtypes, severity of illness, or specific symptoms of depression has also been sought. Although there are suggestions that some features of depression, like unipolar course (Extein et al., 1981; Gold et al., 1981), endogenous symptom profile (Calloway et al., 1984), and high symptom severity (Agren & Wide, 1982), may be associated with a blunted response, there is no consensus. Most investigators have not found an association between particular clinical features and blunted TSH response to TRH (Loosen & Prange, 1982; Sternbach et al., 1984; Rubin et al., 1987; Loosen, 1988; Calloway, 1989). It is possible that hyperfunctioning of the HPT axis represents a non-specific stress response, while hypofunctioning may be more relevant to mood disorders.

The TRH test has also been used to predict outcome. Kirkegaard and collaborators (1975, 1978) have found that patients are less likely to relapse in the next 6 months if their TSH response to TRH when clinically recovered is at least $2.0\mu U/ml$ higher than their TSH post-TRH when depressed. If, upon recovery, the TSH response to TRH is persistently low, tricyclic antidepressants diminish the likelihood of relapse (Krog-Meyer et al., 1984; Langer et al., 1986).

The behavioral effects of TRH in geriatric depressed patients have received little investigation, probably due to technical difficulties. have not been well studied. Most investigations on the effects of TRH on depression have included younger patients, with at mean age of less than or about 50 years. Findings from these studies cannot be extrapolated to geriatric depression because the nature of geriatric depression may differ from that of depression in early life, and because of aging-associated changes in the HPT axis.

TRH concentrations in human fluids have also received little investigation, probably due to technical difficulties. Although there have been doubts about the specificity of assays for TRH in plasma (Iversen, 1986), the concentration of TRH-like immunoreactivity in plasma of depressed patients is reportedly decreased (Itoh et al., 1987). Previously, Kirkegaard and collaborators (1979) reported that TRH in the CSF of untreated depressed patients was increased. Although Banki et al. (1988), using a more specific and sensitive assay, confirmed the finding, a most recent study has failed to corroborate it (Roy et al., 1994).

Antithyroid antibodies appear to be a significant occurrence in depressed subjects. The prevalence of positive antibodies varies according to the sample studied. Antithyroid antibodies are present in up to 20% of psychiatric patients with depressive symptoms (Nemeroff et al., 1985). The prevalence rate of antithyroid antibodies decreases to 9% in a selected sample of unipolar depressives (Joffe, 1987) but is much higher (up to 60%) in depressed patients who also suffer some degree of hypothyroidism (Gold et al., 1982).

To summarize, in depressive states, T4 is elevated but still within the normal range, T3 is normal, and rT3 is elevated. Recovery from depression appears to be accompanied by decrements on T4, FT4, and rT3. TSH appears to be lower throughout the 24-hour period and lacks the normally occurring nocturnal surge; its response to TRH is blunted in about one-third of patients and exaggerated in 15% of patients. The usefulness of the TRH test as a state or trait marker, as an indicator of severity, as a correlate of subtypes of depression, or as a predictor of treatment response or of relapse, is controversial. Reports by Kirkegaard and colleagues (1979) that TRH concentration is increased in the CSF of depressives have not been confirmed.

It is possible that discrepancies among the studies are a consequence of differences in depressive subtypes studied, duration of episodes, or sensitivity of the assays used. Differences may also be related to the timing of testing; a patient early in a depressive episode could have a different hormonal profile than a patient emerging from a depressive episode.

Therapeutic effects of HPT axis-related hormones in affective disorders

Mood-elevating effects have been reported for all of the thyroid axis-related hormones, except rT3.

Treatment of depressed patients with a combination of T3 and imipramine was reported to be more advantageous than T3 or imipramine alone (Prange et al., 1968). This effect has been confirmed by other investigators (Earle, 1970; Goodwin et al., 1982), but not all (Gitlin et al., 1987), investigators. As reviewed by Extein & Gold (1989), however, 14 out of 17 studies from 1969 to 1986 reported potentiation of the effect of antidepressant drugs by T3. The improvement occurred in four of six studies in which T3 was given at the initiation of treatment and in 10 of 11 studies when thyroid hormones were used only in TCA-resistant patients. This beneficial effect of T3 has also been reported to occur in combination with phenelzine (Joffe, 1988), ECT (Stern et al., 1990), and possibly with fluoxetine (Crowe et al., 1990). High dose levothyroxine has been reported to improve depression and mania scores in patients with treatment refractory rapid cycling bipolar affective disorder (Bauer & Whybrow, 1990).

The controversy on the effectiveness of T3 as augmenting agent appears to be resolving. In a randomized, double blind, placebo-controlled study, T3 and lithium were reported as equally effective in augmenting desipramine antidepressant effects in resistant cases (Joffe et al., 1993).

The positive effect of adjunctive T3 on patients treated with ECT or lithium for mood disorders has been recently reviewed (Tremont & Stern, 1997). The findings of the study indicated that the adjunctive thyroid hormone treatment may attenuate the cognitive side effects of ECT and lithium (Tremont & Stern, 1997).

Prange and collaborators (1970) also reported that TSH accelerates the antidepressant effect of imipramine; its use however was discouraged because of lack of advantages over T3 (Wilson et al., 1974). The discovery of TRH by teams led by Guillemin (Burgus et al., 1969) and by Schally (Boler et al., 1969) enabled another thyroid axis-related hormone to be tested as antidepressant. Such an effect was reported by Plotnikoff et al. (1972). It was suggested that the effect was probably central and compatible with L-dopa potentiation (Prange et al., 1974). This report was followed by others supporting such a mood-elevating effect (Kastin et al., 1972; Lipton & Goodwin, 1975; Van den Burg et al., 1976) and also not supporting such a mood-elevating effect (Mountjoy et al., 1974; Sorensen et al., 1974; Hollister et al., 1974).

Current research is looking into the effects of TRH on mood in the elderly and its relationship with TSH responses (Tsuboyama, unpublished data). Of interest is the 'subjective improvement' with TRH reported by patients suffering from amyotrophic lateral sclerosis. In a double-blind crossover trial, 25 patients received 25 mg of TRH subcutaneously every day for 3 months. Ten patients reported subjective benefits; 10 complained of deterioration when TRH was stopped; and 17 knew they were receiving TRH because of 'beneficial effects.' No objective benefits from TRH were observed, however (Mitsumoto et al., 1986). Similarly, in the study by Caroscio et al. (1986), 11 of 12 patients who received TRH reported subjective improvement in function. Again, the objective response to TRH, as assessed by motor and functional ratings, was poor. The fact that this 'subjective improvement' was reported by patients with a progressive and incurable disease and experiencing shivering, nausea, and diaphoresis, supports the notion that TRH positively affects the feeling of well being.

Relationship between treatment modalities for affective disorders and the thyroid axis

Changes in biogenic amines, their receptors and metabolites, as well as in dynamic responses (i.e. GH post-clonidine, adenylate cyclase activity) have been shown to occur with antidepressant treatment. Their mechanism of action, however, remains unclear (Snyder & Peroutka, 1984; Deakin, 1986; Heninger & Charney, 1987; Murphy et al., 1987).

Nevertheless, all antidepressant modalities have in common a variety of interactions with the HPT axis. A synergistic interaction with TCA on the noradrenergic system, like the potentiation of the hyperthermic effect of TRH in mice following the administration of imipramine or amitriptyline (Desiles et al., 1980; Przegalinski et al., 1989), has been reported. Antidepressants may also have a direct effect on the synthesis and/or release of TRH, as demonstrated by increased TRH concentration in the rat nucleus accumbens following chronic amitriptyline administration (Lighton et al., 1985).

Additionally, increments in TRH could also be secondary to decrements in thyroid hormones occurring with antidepressant treatments like TCA (Fischetti, 1962; Schlienger et al., 1980; Joffe et al., 1984) or ECT (Tauboll et al., 1987). ECT produces changes in neurotransmitters, their metabolites, and receptors (Modigh, 1976; APA, 1978; NIMH, 1985), as well as increments in TRH levels in limbic and cortical structures (Walczak et al., 1983; Kubek et al., 1985, 1989; Sattin et al., 1987; Sattin, 1987).

Sleep deprivation is another treatment modality for depression (Pflug & Tolle, 1971). Elevation of TSH levels following sleep deprivation has been described in normal subjects (Parker et al., 1976, 1987). TSH, total and free T4 and T3, rT3, and cortisol all increase during sleep deprivation in depressed patients, but the relationship between increments in TSH and clinical improvement is not clear yet (Baumgartner & Meinhold, 1986; Sack et al., 1988; Baumgartner et al., 1990a, b).

Since synthesis and release of TSH are stimulated by TRH (Utiger, 1987), it is possible that the elevation in TSH found during treatment with lithium, carbamazepine, and sleep deprivation are mediated by increments in TRH secretion.

Exposure to bright light can have antidepressant effects. Bright light inhibits the synthesis and release of melatonin (Klein & Weller, 1972; Woolf & Lee, 1977; Lewy et al., 1980). Although an inhibitory role of melatonin on TRH synthesis and/or secretion has not been clearly established, decrements in serum TSH following intraventricular administration of melatonin in rats has been observed (Relkin, 1972).

The anti-thyroid effects of lithium are well established. Initially, lithium decreases both the 131-I uptake by the thyroid gland and the secretion of thyroid hormones; later the 131-I uptake increases, secondary to an increased TSH secretion (Schou et al., 1968; Sedvall et al., 1969; Cooper et al., 1970; Lazarus & Bennie, 1972). Treatment with carbamazepine causes reduction in T4 (total and free) and T3, and an increase in TSH. Responders to treatment have larger decrements on thyroid hormones than non-responders (Roy-Byrne et al., 1984). Combined treatment with lithium exaggerates the antithyroid effects of carbamazepine (Kramlinger & Post, 1990).

Deiodinases – enzymes that cleave iodine from thyroid hormones – play a crucial role in the intraneuronal generation of T3 (Larsen, 1997). The human brain seems to contain only deiodinases II and III, and their properties are similar to those in rats (Campos-Barros et al., 1996). In rats, lithium (Baumgartner et al., 1994b), carbamazepine (Baumgartner et al., 1994a), and fluoxetine (Baumgartner et al.,

1994c) increased the activity of deiodinase II and decreased the activity of deiodinase III, causing an increment in the concentration of T3 in the brain. A similar effect of desipramine on deiodinase II has also increased T3 concentration in the rat brain (Campos-Barros et al., 1994; for review see Kirkegaard & Faber, 1998).

In summary, most treatment modalities for depression also affect the HPT axis, as do treatments which are mood stabilizing or antimanic. Direct or indirect stimulation of synthesis and release of TRH could be a critical factor in obtaining an antidepressant effect. As previously stated, the hormonal variations obtained in these studies could be influenced by the stage of the illness episode when the studies were conducted.

Cognitive effects of HPT axis in aging

The HPT axis is involved in cognition and hypothyroidism is a rare cause of dementia in the elderly. While treatment of clinical hypothyroidism improves cognitive function in the elderly, there is no evidence that hypothyroidism is a completely reversible cause of dementia (Dugbartey, 1998). Less well understood are subtle abnormalities of the HPT axis on cognition in the aged. Some studies of subclinical hypothyroidism suggest that it is associated with memory impairment that may improve with treatment, though this is not supported by all studies (Samuels, 1998).

In the community-based elderly, TSH levels were related to episodic memory performance, independent of age and education (Wahlin et al., 1998) T4 levels were unrelated to cognitive performance. In female goiter patients with subclinical hypothyroidism, decrease in memory, but no decrease in mood, was found when compared with euthyroid patients (Baldini et al., 1997). Treatment with T4 demonstrated improvement in some memory measures (Baldini et al., 1997).

Treatment-resistant depressed hypothyroid patients on replacement doses of T4 have benefited from the addition of T3 (Cooke et al., 1992). A recent study on hypothyroid patients suggests that T3 rather than T4 may have a significant role on mood and cognition regulation since cognition, depression, and anxiety scores improved when replacement T4 was partially substituted with T3 (Bunevicius et al., 1999). The study compared the therapeutic effects of T4 alone with those of T4 plus T3 in 31 women and 2 men (mean age = 46) with hypothyroidism (Bunevicius et al., 1999). Over two 5-week periods, patients were given his or her usual dose of T4 for one 5-week period and during the other, a regimen in which 50 μg of the usual dose of T4 was replaced by 12.5 μg of T3. Patients had lower serum-free and total T4 concentrations and higher serum total T3 concentrations after treatment with T4 plus T3 than after T4 alone, and they scored better after the combined treatment on cognitive tests measuring for episodic memory performance. This suggested that partial substitution of T3 for T4 may improve memory in hypothyroid patients (Bunevicius et al., 1999).

Even within normal ranges, thyroid functioning appears to influence behavior through normal neurophysiological adaptive mechanisms (Wahlin et al., 1998). A study of non-demented elderly men and women by Wahlin et al. (1998) investigated the relationship of normal ranges of T4 and TSH to cognitive performance. Test results indicated that T4 was unrelated to performance while TSH was positively related to episodic memory performance, with effects independent of the influence of age, education, and depressive mood symptoms. There was no reliable relationship between TSH and either verbal fluency, short-term memory, perceptual–motor speed or visuospatial functioning (Wahlin et al., 1998).

The field of neurocognitive functioning with hypothyroidism has been recently reviewed by Dugbartey (1998), who concluded that hypothyroidism is associated with psychomotor slowing and deficits in memory, visuoperceptual skills, and construction skills, none of which shows a consistent pattern of recovery following replacement. On the other hand, sustained auditory attention, language comprehension and motor functions such as grip strength do not seem to be impaired in hypothyroidism (Dugbartey, 1998). Hyperthyroidism is associated with confusion in 8% to 52% of elderly patients while confusion is not a presenting sign of hyperthyroidism in young adults (Samuels, 1998).

Summary and conclusions

Over the last 20 years an impressive and complex body of knowledge has been built on the interactions between the HPT axis and major depressive illness. While depressive mood more frequently occurs in hypothyroidism than in hyperthyroidism, the hormonal pattern in depressives, i.e. high normal T4 and low baseline and blunted TSH post-TRH, is more reminiscent of hyperthyroidism than of hypothyroidism. On the therapeutic front, the picture is clearer. A significant effect of T3 in augmentation strategies for depression has been confirmed. Moreover, the observation that both mood and cognition scores of T4-replaced hypothyroid patients improve when T4 is partially replaced by T3 lends significant support to the idea that T3 is an important regulator of mood and cognition in the elderly. In this regard it is important to note that the generation of intraneuronal T3 depends on the activity of deiodinases, and that some antidepressant treatments have shown to increase the activity of those enzymes.

Most studies on the interactions of the HPT axis and major depression interactions have focused on populations of a wide-age range; reports that specifically center on elderly depressives are limited. Moreover, the increased occurrence of medical illnesses in the elderly and the consequent development of eurothyroid sick syndrome may obscure findings in this population. The development of standardized measures to define a healthy elderly individual may assist in clarifying findings pertaining to the HPT axis in the elderly population. Criteria such as those currently utilized in gerontoimmunologic studies and ·the SENIEUR protocol (Ligthart et al., 1984, Stohlawetz et al., 1998) may be a helpful step in that direction.

ACKNOWLEDGMENT

Supported by the US Federal Government through the grant MH 01038 from the National Institute of Mental Health.

REFERENCES

Agren, H. & Wide, L. (1982). Patterns of depression reflected in pituitary–thyroid and pituitary–adrenal endocrine changes. *Psychoneuroendocrinology*, 7, 309.

Aizawa, T. & Greer, M. A. (1981). Delineation of the hypothalamic area controlling thyrotropin secretion in the rat. *Endocrinology*, 109, 1731.

American Psychiatric Task Force on ECT. (1978). Electroconvulsive therapy. Washington, DC: American Psychiatric Association.

Amir, S. (1988). Thyrotropin-releasing hormone (TRH): insulin-like action on glucoregulation. *Biochemical Pharmacology*, 37, 4245.

Artunkal, S. & Togrol, B. (1964). Psychological studies in hyperthyroidism. In *Brain–Thyroid Relationships*, ed. M. P. Cameron & M. O'Connor. Boston: Little, Brown & Co.

Asher, R. (1949). Myxodematous madness. *British Medical Journal*, 2, 555.

Baldini, I. M., Vita, A., Mauri, M. C., Amodei, V., Carrisi, M., Bravin, S. et al. (1997). Psychopathological and cognitive features in subclinical hypothyroidism. *Progress in Neuro-Psychopharmacology and Biological Psychiatry*, 21(6), 925–35.

Banki, C. M., Bissette, G., Arato, M. & Nemeroff, C. (1988). Elevation of immunoreactive CSF TRH in depressed patients. *American Journal of Psychiatry*, 145, 1526.

Bartalena, L., Bogazzi, F., Brogioni, S., Grasso, L. & Martino, E. (1998). Role of cytokines in the pathogenesis of the euthyroid sick syndrome. *European Journal of Endocrinology*, 138(6), 603.

Bartalena, L., Placidi, G. F., Martino, E., Falcone, M., Pellegrini, L., Dell'osso, L., Pacchiarotti, A. & Pinchera, A. (1990). Nocturnal serum thyrotropin surge and the TSH response to TSH-releasing hormone: dissociated behavior in untreated depressive. *Journal of Clinical Endocrinology and Metabolism*, 71, 650.

Battaini, F. & Peterkofsky, A. (1980). Histidyl-proline diketopiperazine. an endogenous brain peptide that inhibits Na^+/K^+ ATPase. *Biochemical and Biophysical Research Communications*, 94, 240.

Bauer, K. (1987). Adenohypophysial degradation of thyrotropin releasing hormone is regulated by thyroid hormones. *Nature*, 330, 375.

Bauer, M. S. & Whybrow, P. C. (1990). Rapid cycling bipolar affective disorder. II. Treatment of refractory rapid cycling with high-dose levothyroxine: a preliminary study. *Archives of General Psychiatry*, 47, 435.

Bauer, K., Graf, K. J., Faivre-Bauman, A., Beier, S., Tixier-Vidal, A. & Kleinhauf, H. (1978). Inhibition of prolactin secretion by histidyl-proline diketopiperazine. *Nature*, 274, 174.

Baumgartner, A. & Meinhold, H. (1986). Sleep deprivation and thyroid hormone concentrations. *Psychiatry Research*, 19, 241.

Baumgartner, A., Campos-Barros, A., Gaio, U., Hessenius, C., Flechner, A. & Meinhold, H. (1994a). Carbamazepine affects triiodothyronine production and metabolization in rat hippocampus. *Life Sciences*, 54(23), 401.

Baumgartner, A., Campos-Barros, A., Gaio, U., Hessenius, C., Frege, I. & Meinhold, H. (1994b). Effects of lithium on thyroid hormone metabolism in rat frontal cortex. *Biological Psychiatry*, 36(11), 771.

Baumgartner, A., Dubeyko, M., Campos-Barros, A., Eravci, M. & Meinhold, H. (1994c). Subchronic administration of fluoxetine to rats affects triiodothyronine production and deiodination in regions of the cortex and in the limbic forebrain. *Brain Research*, 635(1–2), 68.

Baumgartner, A., Graf, K-J., Kurten, I. & Meinhold, H. (1988). The hypothalamic–pituitary–thyroid axis in psychiatric patients and healthy subjects: parts 1–4. *Psychiatry Research*, 24, 271.

Baumgartner, A., Graf, K-J., Kurten, I., Meinhold, H. & Scholz, P. (1990a). Neuroendocrinological investigations during sleep deprivation in depression. I. Early morning levels of thyrotropin, TH, cortisol, prolactin, LH, FSH, estradiol, and testosterone. *Biological Psychiatry*, 28, 556.

Baumgartner, A., Hahnenkamp, L. & Meinhold, H. (1986). Effects of age and diagnosis on thyrotropin response to thyrotropin-releasing hormone in psychiatric patients. *Psychiatric Research*, 17, 285.

Baumgartner, A., Riemann, D. & Berger, M. (1990b). Neuroendocrinological investigations during sleep deprivation in depression. II. Longitudinal measurement of thyrotropin, TH, cortisol, prolactin, GH, and LH during sleep and sleep deprivation. *Biological Psychiatry*, 28, 569.

Boler, J., Enzmann, F., Folkers, K., Bowers, C. Y. & Schally, A. V. (1969). The identity of chemical and hormonal properties of the thyrotropin releasing hormone and pyroglutamyl-histidyl-proline amide. *Biochemical and Biophysical Research Communications*, 37, 705.

Brabant, G., Wicking, E. J. & Neischlag, E. (1981). The TRH-metabolite histidyl-proline-diketopiperazine (DKP)inhibits prolactin secretion in male rhesus monkeys. *Acta Endocrinologica*, 98, 189.

Brady, K. T. & Anton, R. F. (1989). The thyroid axis and desipramine treatment in depression. *Biological Psychiatry*, 25, 703.

Brambilla, F., Smeraldi, E., Bellodi, L. et al. (1980). Neuroendocrine correlates and monoaminergic hypothesis in primary affective disorders (PAD). In *Progress in Psychoneuroendocrinology*, ed. F. Brambilla, G. Racagni & D. de Wied, pp. 235–45. New York: Elsevier/North-Holland.

Breese, G. R., Moore, R. & Howard, J. (1972). Central actions of 6-hydroxydopamine and other phenylethylamine derivatives on body temperature in the rat. *Journal of Pharmacology and Experimental Therapy*, **180**, 591.

Brent, G. A., Larsen, P. R., Harney, J. W., Koenig, R. J. & Moore, D. D. (1989). Functional characterization of the rat growth hormone promoter elements required for induction by thyroid hormone with and without a co-transfected beta type thyroid hormone receptor. *Journal of Biological Chemistry*, **264**(1), 178.

Brown, M. R. (1981). Thyrotropin releasing factor: a putative CNS regulator of the autonomic nervous system. *Life Sciences*, **28**, 1789.

Browne, P. & O'Cuinn, G. (1983). An evaluation of the role of a pyroglutamyl peptidase, a post-proline cleaving enzyme and a post-proline dipeptidyl aminopeptidase, each purified from the soluble fraction of guinea-pig brain, in the degradation of thyroliberin in vitro. *European Journal of Biochemistry*, **137**, 75.

Bunevicius, R., Kazanavicius, G., Zalinkevicius, R. & Prange, A. J. Jr. (1999). Effects of thyroxine as compared with thyroxine plus triiodothyronine in patients with hypothyroidism. *New England Journal of Medicine*, **340**, 424.

Burgus, R., Dunn, T., Desiderio, D. & Guillemin, R. (1969). Structure moleculaire du facteur hypothalamique hypophysiotrope TRF d'origine ovine: mise en evidence par spectrometric de masse de la sequence PCA–His–Pro–NH$_2$. *Comptes Rendus de l'Academie des Sciences*, **269**, 1870.

Calloway, S. P. (1989). Thyroid function in depression. In *Modern Perspectives in the Psychiatry of Affective Disorders: Modern Perspectives in Psychiatry*, vol. 13, ed. J. G. Howells, pp. 85–105. New York: Brunner/Mazel.

Calloway, S. P., Dolan, R. J., Ronagy, P., DeSouza, V. F. & Wakeling, A. (1984). Endocrine changes and clinical profiles in depression. II. The thyrotropin-releasing hormone test. *Psychological Medicine*, **14**, 759.

Campos-Barros, A., Hoell, T., Musa, A., Sampaolo, S., Stoltenburg, G., Pinna, G., Eravci, M., Meinhold, H. & Baumgartner, A. (1996). Phenolic and tyrosyl ring iodothyronine deiodination and thyroid hormone concentrations in the human central system. *Journal of Clinical Endocrinology and Metabolism*, **81**(6), 2179.

Campos-Barros, A., Meinhold, H. Stulla, M., Muller, F., Kohler, R., Eravci, M., Putzien, O. & Baumgartner, A. (1994). The influence of desipramine on thyroid hormone metabolism in rat brain. *Journal of Pharmacology and Experimental Therapy*, **268**(3), 1143.

Caroscio, J. T., Cohen, J. A., Zawodniak, J., Takai, V., Shapiro, S., Blaustein, S., Mulvihill, M. N., Loucas, S. P., Gudesblatt, M., Rube, D. & Yahr, M. D. (1986). A double-blind, placebo-controlled trial of TRH in amyotrophic lateral sclerosis. *Neurology*, **36**, 141.

Chin, W. W., Carr, F. E., Burnside, J. & Darling, D. S. (1993). Thyroid hormone regulation of thyrotropin gene expression. *Recent Progress in Hormone Research*, **48**, 393.

Chiovato, L., Mariotti, S. & Pinchera, A. (1997). Thyroid diseases in the elderly. *Balliere's Clinical Endocrinology and Metabolism*, **11**(2), 251.

Clarfield, A. M. (1988). The reversible dementias: do they reverse? *Annals of Internal Medicine*, **109**(6), 476.

Coggins, P. J., McDermott, J. R., Snell, C. R. & Gibson, A. M. (1987a). Thyrotropin releasing hormone degradation by rat synaptosomal peptidases: production of the metabolite His–Pro. *Neuropeptides*, **10**, 147.

Coggins, P. J., McDermott, J. R. & Snell, C. R. (1987b). High affinity specific binding of the thy-rotropin releasing hormone metabolite histidylproline to rat brain membranes. *Neuropeptides,* **9**, 83.

Coggins, P. J., Sahgal, A., McDermott, J. R., Snell, C. R., Keith, A. B. & Edwarson, J. A. (1986). Histidyl-proline, a rapidly degraded metabolite of thyrotropin releasing hormone, has behav-ioural activity. *Pharmacology, Biochemistry, and Behavior,* **24**, 1229.

Cohen, K. L. & Swigar, M. E. (1979). Thyroid function screening in psychiatric patients. *Journal of the American Medical Association,* **242**, 254.

Cooke, R. G., Joffe, R. T. & Levitt, A. J. (1992). T3 augmentation of antidepressant treatment in T4-replaced thyroid patients. *Journal of Clinical Psychiatry,* **53**(1), 16.

Cooper, T. B., Wagner, B. M. & Kline, N. S. (1970). Contribution to the mode of action of lithium on iodine metabolism. *Biological Psychiatry,* **2**, 273.

Crowe, D., Collins, J. P. & Rosse, R. B. (1990). Thyroid hormone supplementation of fluoxetine treatment (letter). *Journal of Clinical Psychopharmacology,* **10**, 150.

Davies, P. H., Black, E. G., Sheppard, M. C. & Franklyn, J. A. (1996). Relation between serum interleukin-6 and thyroid hormone concentrations in 270 hospital in-patients with non-thy-roidal illness. *Clinical Endocrinology,* **44**(2), 199.

Davis, P. J. & Davis, F. B. (1996). Nongenomic actions of thyroid hormone. *Thyroid,* **6**, 497.

Deakin, J. F. W. (1986). *The Biology of Depression.* Gaskell Psychiatric Series, London.

DeGroot, L. J. (1991). Mechanism of thyroid hormone action. *Advances in Experimental Medicine and Biology,* **299**, 1.

DeGroot, L. J., Larsen, P. R. & Hennemann, G. (1996). *The Thyroid and Its Diseases.* Churchill & Livingstone.

DeGroot, L. J., Nakai, A., Sakurai, A. & Macchia, E. (1989). The molecular basis of thyroid hormone action. *Journal of Endocrinology Investigation,* **12**(11), 843.

Denicoff, K. D., Joffe, R. T., Lakshmanan, M. C., Robbins, J. & Rubinow, D. R. (1990). Neuropsychiatric manifestations of altered thyroid state. *American Journal of Psychiatry,* **147**, 94.

Desiles, M., Puech, A. J. & Rips, R. (1980). Involvement of a central α-adrenoreceptor induced by thyrotropin releasing hormone. *British Journal of Pharmacology,* **69**, 163.

Desvergne, B., Petty, K. J. & Nikodem, V. M. (1991). Functional characterization and receptor binding studies of the malic enzyme thyroid hormone response element. *Journal of Biological Chemistry,* **266**(2), 1008.

Dugbartey, A. T. (1998). Neurocognitive aspects of hypothyroidism. *Archives of Internal Medicine,* **158**(13), 1413–18.

Duval, F., Macher, J-P. & Mokrani, M-C. (1990). Difference between evening and morning thy-rotropin responses to protirelin in major depressive episode. *Archives of General Psychiatry,* **47**, 443.

Earle, B. V. (1970). Thyroid hormone and tricyclic antidepressants in resistant depressions. *American Journal of Psychiatry,* **126**, 1667.

Emrich, D., Bahre, Zur Muhlen, A., Hesch, R. D. & Kobberling, J. (1976). Insufficient TSH stim-ulation after successful treatment for hyperthyroidism. *Hormone and Metabolic Research,* **8**, 408.

Erfurth, E. M. T. & Hagmar, L. E. (1995). Decreased serum testosterone and free triiodothyronine levels in healthy middle-aged men indicate an age effect at the pituitary level. *European Journal of Endocrinology*, 132, 663.

Esposito, S., Prange Jr, A. J. & Golden, R. N. (1997). The thyroid axis and mood disorders: overview and future prospects. *Psychopharmacology Bulletin*, 33, 205–17.

Evans, R. M. (1988). The steroid and thyroid hormone receptor superfamily. *Science*, 240, 889.

Extein, I. L. & Gold, M. (1989). Thyroid hormone potentiation of tricyclic antidepressants. In *Treatment of Tricyclic-Resistant Depression*, ed. I. L. Extein [*Progress in Psychiatry*, series ed. D. Spiegel]. Washington, DC: American Psychiatric Press, Inc.

Extein, I., Pottash, A. L. & Gold, M. S. (1981). The thyrotropin-releasing hormone test in the diagnosis of unipolar depression. *Psychiatry Research*, 5, 311.

Fischetti, B. (1962). Pharmacological influences on thyroid activity. *Archivio Italiano di Scienze Farmacologiche*, 12, 33.

Friedman, T. C. & Wilk, S. (1986). Delineation of a particulate thyrotropin-releasing hormone-degrading enzyme in rat brain by the use of specific inhibitors of prolyl endopeptidase and pyroglutamyl peptide hydrolase. *Journal of Neurochemistry*, 46, 1231.

Ganguli, M., Burmeister, L. A., Seaberg, E. C., Belle, S. & DeKosky, S. T. (1996). Association between dementia and elevated TSH: a community-based study. *Biological Psychiatry*, 40(8), 714.

Gershengorn, M. C. (1986). Mechanism of thyrotropin releasing hormone stimulation of pituitary hormone secretion. *Annual Review of Physiology*, 48, 515.

Girvent, M., Maestro, S., Hernandez, R., Carajol, I., Monne, J., Sancho, J. J., Gubern, J. M. & Sitges-Serra, A. (1998). Euthyroid sick syndrome, associated endocrine abnormalities, and outcome in elderly patients undergoing emergency operation. *Surgery*, 123(5), 560.

Gitlin, M. J., Weiner, H., Fairbanks, L., Hershman, J. M. & Friedfield, N. (1987). Failure of T3 to potentiate tricyclic antidepressant response. *Journal of Affective Disorders*, 13, 267.

Gold, M. S. (1983). Hypothyroidism – or is it depression? *Psychosomatics*, 24, 646.

Gold, M. S., Pottash, A. L. C. & Extein, I. (1982). Symptomless autoimmune thyroiditis in depression. *Psychiatry Research*, 6, 261.

Gold, M. S., Pottash, A. L. & Mueller, E. A. III. (1981). Grades of thyroid failure in 100 depressed and anergic psychiatric inpatients. *American Journal of Psychiatry*, 138, 253.

Goodwin, F. K., Prange, A. J., Post, R. M., Muscettola, G. & Lipton, M. A. (1982). Potentiation of antidepressant effects by 1-triiodothyronine in tricyclic nonresponders. *American Journal of Psychiatry*, 139, 34.

Griffiths, E. C. (1985). Thyrotropin releasing hormone: endocrine and central effects. *Psychoneuroendocrinology*, 10, 225.

Griffiths, E. C. & Bennett, G. W. (1983). *Thyrotropin-releasing Hormone*. New York: Raven Press.

Griffiths, E. C. & McDermott, J. R. (1983). Enzymic inactivation of hypothalamic regulatory hormones. *Molecular and Cellular Endocrinology*, 33, 1.

Hamblin, P. S., Dyer, S. A., Mohr, V. S., Le Grand, B. A., Lim, C. F., Tuxen, D. V., Topliss, D. J. & Stockigt, J. R. (1986). Relationship between thyrotropin and thyroxine changes during recovery from severe hypothyroxinemia of critical illness. *Journal of Clinical Endocrinology and Metabolism*, 62, 717.

Harding, P. P. & Duester, G. (1992). Retinoic acid activation and thyroid hormone repression of the human alcohol dehydrogenase gene ADH3. *Journal of Biological Chemistry*, **267**, 14145.

Haupt, M. & Kurz, A. (1993). Dementia in hypothyroidism. *Fortschritte Der Neurologie-Psychiatrie*, **58**, 175.

Hauser, P., Soler, R., Brucker-Davis, F. & Weintraub, B. D. (1997). Thyroid hormones correlate with symptoms of hyperactivity but not inattention in attention deficit hyperactivity disorder. *Psychoneuroendocrinology*, **22**(2), 107–14.

Hendrick, V., Altshuler, L. & Whybrow, P. (1998). Psychoneuroendocrinology of mood disorders. The hypothalamic–pituitary–thyroid axis. *Psychiatric Clinics of North America*, **21**(2), 277–92.

Heninger, G. R. & Charney, D. S. (1987). Mechanism of action of antidepressant treatments: implication for the etiology and treatment of depressive disorders. In *Psychopharmacology: The Third Generation of Progress*, ed. H. Y. Meltzer, pp. 535–44. New York: Raven Press.

Herrmann, F., Hambsch, K., Sorger, D., Hantzschel, H., Muller, P. & Nagel, I. (1989). [Low T3 syndrome and chronic inflammatory rheumatism]. *Zeitschrift Fur Die Gesamte Innere Medizin Und Ihre Grenzgebiete*, **44**(17), 513–18.

Hickie, I., Bennett, B., Mitchell, P., Wilhelm K. & Orlay, W. (1996). Clinical and subclinical hypothyroidism in patients with chronic and treatment-resistant depression. *Australian and New Zealand Journal of Psychiatry*, **30**(2), 246.

Hodin, R. A., Lazar, M. A., Wintman, B. I., Darling, D. S., Koenig, R. J., Larsen, P. R., Moore, D. D. & Chin, W. W. (1989). Identification of a thyroid hormone receptor that is pituitary-specific. *Science*, **244**, 76.

Hokfelt, T., Tsuruo, Y., Ulfhake, B., Cullheim, S., Arvidsson, U., Foster, G. A., Schultzberg, M., Schalling, M., Arborelius, L., Freedman, J., Post, C. & Visser, T. (1989). Distribution of TRH-like immunoreactivity with special reference to coexistence with other neuroactive compounds. In *Thyrotropin-releasing Hormone: Biomedical Significance*, ed. G. Metcalf & I. M. D. Jackson, 553, 76. New York: Annals of the New York Academy of Sciences.

Holland, F. W. II, Brown, P. S. Jr., Weintraub, B. D. & Clark, R. E. (1991). Cardiopulmonary bypass and thyroid function: a 'euthyroid sick syndrome'. *Annals of Thoracic Surgery*, **52**(1), 46.

Hollenberg, A. N., Monden, T., Flynn, T. R., Boers, M. E., Cohen, O. & Wondisford, F. E. (1995). The human thyrotropin-releasing hormone gene is regulated by thyroid hormone through two distinct classes of negative thyroid hormone response elements. *Molecular Endocrinology*, **9**(5), 540.

Hollister, L. E., Berger, P., Ogle, F. L., Arnold, R. C. & Johnson, A. (1974). Protireline (TRH) in depression. *Archives of General Psychiatry*, **31**, 468.

Hornick, .T. R. & Kowal, J. (1997). Clinical epidemiology of endocrine disorders in the elderly. *Endocrinology and Metabolism Clinics of North America*, **26**(1), 145.

Ingbar, S. H. (1985). The thyroid gland. In *Textbook of Endocrinology*, ed. J. D. Wilson & D. W. Foster, pp. 682–815. Philadelphia: Saunders.

Iriuchijima, T., Prasad, C., Wilber, J. F., Jayaraman, A., Rao, J. K., Robertson, H. J. F. & Rogers, D. J. (1987). Thyrotropin-releasing hormone and cycle (His–Pro)-like immunoreactivities in the cerebrospinal fluids of 'normal' infants and adults, and patients with various neuropsychiatric and neurologic disorders. *Life Sciences*, **41**, 2419.

Iriuchijima, T., Rogers, D. & Wilber, J. F. (1984). L-triiodothyronine (L-T3) can inhibit thyrotropin-releasing hormone (TRH) secretion from rat hypothalami *in vitro*. *Clinical Research*, 32, 865A.

Itoh, N., Matsui, N., Fuwano, S., Yaginuma, H., Miyashita, O. & Sakai, M. (1987). Serial DST, TRH test, and TRH-like immunoreactivity measurements in major affective disorders. *Biological Psychiatry*, 22, 559.

Iversen, E. (1986). Thyrotropin-releasing hormone cannot be detected in plasma from normal subjects. *Journal of Clinical Endocrinology and Metabolism*, 63, 516.

Jackson, I. M. D. (1982). Thyrotropin-releasing hormone. *New England Journal of Medicine*, 306, 145.

Jackson, I. M. D., Adelman, L. S., Munsat, T. L., Forte, S. & Lechan, R. M. (1987). Amyotrophic lateral sclerosis. TRH and histidyl-proline diketopiperazine in the spinal cord and cerebrospinal fluid. *Neurology*, 36, 1218.

Joffe, R. T. (1987). Antithyroid antibodies in major depression. *Acta Psychiatrica Scandinavica*, 76, 598.

Joffe, R. T. (1988). Triiodothyronine potentiation of the antidepressant effect of phenelzine. *Journal of Clinical Psychiatry*, 49(10), 409.

Joffe, R. T., Roy-Byrne, P. P., Uhde, T. W. & Post, R. M. (1984). Thyroid function and affective illness: a reappraisal. *Biological Psychiatry*, 19, 1685.

Joffe, R. T., Singer, W., Levitt, A. J. & MacDonald, C. (1993). A placebo-controlled comparison of lithium and triiodothyronine augmentation of tricyclic antidepressants in unipolar refractory depression. *Archives of General Psychiatry*, 50(5), 387.

Josephson, A. M. & Mackenzie, T. B. (1980). Thyroid-induced mania in hypothyroid patients. *British Journal of Psychiatry*, 137, 222.

Kabayama, T., Kato, T., Tojo, K., Shinatsu, A., Ohta, H. & Imura, H. (1985). Central effects of DN1417, a novel TRH analog, a plasma glucose and catecholamines in conscious rats. *Life Sciences*, 36, 1287.

Kastin, A. J., Ehrensing, R. H., Schalch, D. S. & Anderson, M. S. (1972). Improvement in mental depression with decreased thyrotropin response after administration of thyrotropin-releasing hormone. *Lancet*, ii, 740.

Kathol, R. G. & Delahunt, J. W. (1986). The relationship of anxiety and depression of symptoms of hyperthyroidism using operational criteria. *General Hospital Psychiatry*, 8, 23.

Keller, H. H., Bartholine, G. & Pletscher, A. (1974). Enhancement of cerebral noradrenaline turnover by thyrotropin-releasing hormone. *Nature*, 24, 528.

Kirkegaard, C. & Smith, E. (1978). Continuation therapy in endogenous depression controlled by changes in the TRH stimulation test. *Psychological Medicine*, 8, 501.

Kirkegaard, C. & Faber, J. (1981). Altered serum levels of thyroxine, triiodothyronine and diiodothyronines in endogenous depression. *Acta Endocrinologica*, 96, 199.

Kirkegaard, C. & Faber, J. (1998). The role of thyroid hormones in depression. *European Journal of Endocrinology*, 138, 1.

Kirkegaard, C., Faber, J., Hummer, L. & Rogowski, P. (1979). Increased levels of TRH in cerebrospinal fluid from patients with endogenous depression. *Psychoneuroendocrinology*, 4, 227.

Kirkegaard, C., Korner, A. & Faber, J. (1990). Increased production of thyroxine and inappropriately elevated serum thyrotropin levels in endogenous depression. *Biological Psychiatry*, 27, 472.

Kirkegaard, C., Norlem, N., Lauridsen, U. B. & Bjorum, N. (1975). Prognostic value of thyrotropin releasing hormone stimulation test in endogenous depression. *Acta Psychiatrica Scandinavica*, 52, 170.

Klein, D. C. & Weller, J. L. (1972). Rapid light-induced decrease in pineal serotonin N-acetyltransferase activity. *Science*, 177, 532.

Kleinschmidt, H. J. & Waxenberg, S. E. (1956). Psychophysiology and psychiatric management of thyrotoxicosis. A two year follow-up study. *Journal of the Mount Sinai Hospital*, 23, 131.

Kramlinger, K. G. & Post, R. M. (1990). Addition of lithium carbonate to carbamazepine: hematological and thyroid effects. *American Journal of Psychiatry*, 147, 615.

Krog-Meyer, I., Kirkegaard, C., Kijne, B., Lumholtz, B., Smith, E., Lykke-Olesen, L. & Bjorum, N. (1984). Prediction of relapse with the TRH test and prophylactic amitriptyline in 39 patients with endogenous depression. *American Journal of Psychiatry*, 141(8), 945–8.

Kubek, M. J., Low, W. C., Sattin, A., Morzorati, S. L., Meyerhoff, J. L. & Larsen, S. H. (1989). Role of TRH in seizure modulation. In *Thyrotropin-releasing Hormone: Biomedical Significance*, ed. G. Metcalf & I. M. D. Jackson, 553, 286. New York: Annals of the New York Academy of Sciences.

Kubek, M. J., Meyerhoff, J. L., Hill, T. G., Norton, J. A. & Sattin, A. (1985). Effects of subconvulsive and repeated electroconvulsive shock on thyrotropin-releasing hormone in rat brain. *Life Sciences*, 36, 315.

Lamberton, R. P., Lechan, R. M. & Jackson, I. M. D. (1984). Ontogeny of TRH and histidyl-proline diketopiperazine in the rat CNS and pancreas. *Endocrinology*, 115, 2400.

Langer, G., Koining, G., Matzinger, R., Schonbeck, G., Resch, F. et al. (1986). TRH-TSH test as predictor of outcome. *Archives of General Psychiatry*, 43, 861.

Larsen, P. R. (1997). Update on the human iodothyronine selenodeiodinases, the enzymes regulating the activation and inactivation of thyroid hormone. *Biochemical Society Transaction*, 25(2), 588.

Larsen, P. R., Harney, J. W. & Moore, D. D. (1986). Sequences required for cell-specific thyroid hormone regulation of rat growth hormone promoter activity. *Journal of Biological Chemistry*, 261, 14373.

Lasser, R. A. & Baldessarini, R. J. (1997). Thyroid hormones in depressive disorders: a reappraisal of clinical utility. *Harvard Review of Psychiatry*, 4, 291–305.

Lazar, M. A. (1993). Thyroid hormone receptors. Multiple forms, multiple possibilities. *Endocrine Reviews*, 14, 184.

Lazarus, J. H. & Bennie, E. H. (1972). Effect of lithium on thyroid function in man. *Acta Endocrinologica*, 70, 266.

Lechan, R. M. & Jackson, I. M. D. (1985). TRH but not histidyl-proline diketopiperazine is depleted from rat spinal cord following 5,7-dihydroxytryptamine treatment. *Brain Research*, 326, 152.

Lechan, R. M., Wu, P. W., Jackson, I. M. D., Wolf, H., Cooperman, S., Mandel, G. & Goodman,

R. (1986). Thyrotropin-releasing hormone precursor: characterization in rat brain. *Science*, **231**, 159.

Lewy, A. J., Wehr, J. A., Goodwin, F. K., Newsom, D. A. & Markey, S. P. (1980). Light suppresses melatonin secretion in humans. *Science*, **210**, 1267.

Lighton, C., Bennett, G. W. & Marsden, C. A. (1985). Increase in levels and *ex vivo* release of thyrotropin releasing hormone (TRH) in specific regions of the rat CNS by chronic antidepressant treatment. *Neuropharmacology*, **24**, 401.

Ligthart, G. J., Corberand, J. X., Fournier, C., Galanaud, P., Hijmans, W., Kennes, B., Muller-Hermelink, H. K. & Steinmann, G. G. (1984). Admission criteria for immunogerontological studies in man: the SENIEUR protocol. *Mechanisms of Ageing & Development*, **28**, 47.

Lipton, M. A. & Goodwin, F. K. (1975). A controlled study of thyrotropin-releasing hormone in hospitalized depressed patients. *Psychopharmacology Bulletin*, **11**, 28.

Loosen, P. T. (1988). The TRH test in psychiatric disorders. In *Affective Disorders: Directions in Psychiatry, Monograph Series*, No. 2, ed. F. Flach, pp. 52–63. New York, London: W.W. Norton & Co.

Loosen, P. T. (1992). Effects of thyroid hormones on central nervous system in aging. *Psychoneuroendocrinology*, **17**(4), 355.

Loosen, P. T. & Prange, A. J. Jr. (1980). Thyrotropin releasing hormone (TRH): a useful tool for psychoneuroendocrine investigation. *Psychoneuroendocrinology*, **5**, 63.

Loosen, P. & Prange, A. J. Jr. (1982). Serum thyrotropin response to thyrotropin-releasing hormone in psychiatric patients: a review. *American Journal of Psychiatry*, **139**, 405.

McIver, B. & Gorman, C. A. (1997). Euthyroid sick syndrome: an overview. *Thyroid*, **7**(1), 125–32.

Manaker, S., Eichen, A., Winokur, A., Rhodes, C. H. & Rainbow, T. C. (1986). Autoradiographic localization of thyrotropin releasing hormone receptors in human brain. *Neurology*, **36**, 641.

Manaker, S., Winokur, A., Rhodes, C. H. & Rainbow, T. C. (1985). Autoradiographic localization of thyrotropin-releasing hormone (TRH) receptors in the rats CNS. *Journal of Neuroscience*, **5**, 167.

Mariotti, S., Barbesino, G., Caturegli, P., Bartalena, L., Sansoni, P., Fagnoni, F., Monti, D., Fagiolo, U., Franceschi, C. & Pinchera, A. (1993). Complex alteration of thyroid function in healthy centenarians. *Journal of Clinical Endocrinology and Metabolism*, **77**, 1130.

Mariotti, S., Chiovato, L., Franceschi, C. & Pinchera, A. (1998). Thyroid autoimmunity and aging. *Experimental Gerontology*, **33**(6), 535–41.

Martin, J. B. & Reichlin, S. (1987). *Clinical Neuroendocrinology*, 2nd edn, p. 130. Philadelphia: F.A. Davis Co.

Metcalf, G. & Dettmar, P. W. (1981). Is thyrotropin-releasing hormone an endogenous substance in the brain? *Lancet*, **i**, 586.

Metcalf, G. & Jackson, I. M. D. (1989). *Thyrotropin-Releasing Hormone: Biomedical Significance*, vol. 553. New York: Annals of the New York Academy of Sciences.

Mitsumoto, H., Salgado, E. D., Negroski, D., Hanson, M. R., Salanga, V. D., Wilber, J. F., Wilbourn, A. J., Breuer, A. C. & Leatherman, J. (1986). Amyotrophic-lateral sclerosis: effects of acute intravenous and chronic subcutaneous administration of thyrotropin-releasing hormone in controlled trials. *Neurology*, **36**, 152.

Modigh, K. (1976). Long term effects of electroconvulsive shock therapy on synthesis, turnover, and uptake of brain monoamines. *Psychopharmacology*, **49**, 179.

Mokshagundam, S. & Barzel, U. S. (1993). Thyroid disease in the elderly. *Journal of the American Geriatric Society*, **41**, 1361.

Molchan, S. E., Lawlor, B. A., Hill, J. L., Mellow, A. M., Davis, C. L., Martinez, R. & Sunderland, T. (1991). The TRH stimulation test in Alzheimer's disease and major depression: relationship to clinical and CSF measures. *Biological Psychiatry*, **30**(6), 567.

Monzani, F., Del Guerra, P., Caraccio, N., Del Corso, L., Casolaro, A., Mariotti, S. & Pentimone, F. (1996). Age-related modifications in the regulation of the hypothalamic–pituitary–thyroid axis. *Hormone Research*, **46**(3), 107.

Mooradian, A. D. & Wong, N. C. W. (1994). Age-related changes in thyroid hormone action. *European Journal of Endocrinology*, **131**(5), 451.

Mooradian, A. D., Reed, R. L., Osterweil, D., Schiffman, R. & Scuderi, P. (1990). Decreased serum triiodothyronine is associated with increased concentrations of tumor necrosis factor. *Journal of Clinical Endocrinology and Metabolism*, **71**(5), 1239.

Mooradian, A. D., Reed, R. L., Osterweil, D. & Scuderi, P. (1991). Detectable serum levels of tumor necrosis factor alpha may predict early mortality in elderly institutionalized patients. *Journal of the American Geriatric Society*, **39**(9), 891.

Mori, M., Mallik, T., Prasad, C. & Wilber, J. F. (1982a). Histidyl-proline diketopiperazine, cyclo (His–Pro). Measurement by radioimmunoassay in human blood in normal and in patient with hyper- and hypothyroidism. *Biochemical and Biophysical Research Communications*, **109**, 541.

Mori, M., Pegues, J., Prasad, C., Wilber, J., Peterson, J. & Githens, S. (1983). Histidyl-proline diketopiperazine cyclo (His–Pro). Identification and characterization in rat pancreatic islets. *Biochemical and Biophysical Research Communications*, **115**, 281.

Mori, M., Prasad, C. & Wilber, J. F. (1982b). Chronic alcohol consumption increases cycle (His–Pro)-like immunoreactivity in the rat brain. *Journal of Neurochemistry*, **38**, 1785.

Morley, J. E. (1979). Extrahypothalamic thyrotropin releasing hormone (TRH): its distribution and its functions. *Life Sciences*, **25**, 1539.

Morley, J. E. (1981). Neuroendocrine control of thyrotropin secretion. *Endocrine Review*, **2**, 396.

Motomura, K. & Brent, G. A. (1998). Mechanisms of action of thyroid hormone. *Endocrinology and Metabolism Clinics of North America*, **27**, 1.

Mountjoy, C. Q., Weller, M., Hall, R., Price, J. S., Hunter, P. & Dewar, J. H. (1974). A double-blind crossover sequential trial of oral thyrotropin-releasing hormone in depression. *Lancet*, i, 958.

Muller, M. J. (1994). Thyroid and ageing. *European Journal of Endocrinology*, **130**, 242.

Murphy, D. L., Aulakh, C. S., Garrick, N. A. & Sunderland, T. (1987). Monoamine oxidase inhibitors as antidepressants: implications for the mechanism of action of antidepressants and the psychobiology of the affective disorders and some related disorders. In *Psychopharmacology: The Third Generation of Progress*, ed. H. Y. Meltzer, pp. 545–52. New York: Raven Press.

Myers, L. & Hays, J. (1991). Myxedema coma. *Critical Care Clinics*, **7**(1), 43.

Nakai, A., Seino, S., Sakurai, A., Szilak, I., Bell, G. I. & DeGroot, L. J. (1988). Characterization of a thyroid hormone receptor expressed in human kidney and other tissues. *Proceedings of the National Academy of Sciences*, USA, **85**, 2781.

Nemeroff, C. B. (1989). Clinical significance of psychoneuroendocrinology in psychiatry: focus on the thyroid and adrenal. *Journal of Clinical Psychiatry*, **50**(Suppl), 13.

Nemeroff, C. B. & Evans, D. L. (1989). Thyrotropin-releasing hormone (TRH), the thyroid axis and affective disorder. In *Thyrotropin-releasing Hormone: Biomedical Significance*, ed. G. Metcalf G & I. M. D. Jackson, 553, 304. New York: Annals of the New York Academy of Sciences.

Nemeroff, C. B., Simon, J. S., Haggerty, J. J. Jr. & Evans, D. L. (1985). Antithyroid antibodies in depressed patients. *American Journal of Psychiatry*, **142**, 840.

Nicoloff, J. T. & LoPresti, J. S. (1993). Myxedema coma. A form of decompensated hypothyroidism. *Endocrinology and Metabolism Clinics of North America*, **22**(2), 279.

NIMH Consensus Development Conference on Electroconvulsive Therapy. (1985). *Journal of the American Medical Association*, **245**, 2103.

Ogiu, N., Nakamura, Y., Ijiri, I., Hiraiwa, K. & Ogiu, T. (1997). A statistical analysis of the internal organ weights of normal Japanese people. *Health Physics*, **72**(3), 368.

Oppenheimer, J. H. (1983). The nuclear receptor–triiodothyronine complex: relationship to thyroid hormone distribution, metabolism, and biological action. In *Molecular Basis of Thyroid Hormone Action*, ed. J. H. Oppenheimer & H. H. Samuels, pp. 1–34. New York: Academic Press.

Parker, D. C., Pekary, A. E. & Hershman, J. M. (1976). Effects of normal and reversed sleep–wake cycles upon nyctohemeral rhythmicity of plasma thyrotropin: evidence suggestive of an inhibitory influence in sleep. *Journal of Clinical Endocrinology and Metabolism*, **43**, 318.

Parker, D. C., Rossman, L. G., Pekary, A. E. & Hershman, J. M. (1987). Effects of 64-hour sleep deprivation on the circadian wave-form of thyrotropin (TSH). further evidence of sleep-related inhibition of TSH release. *Journal of Clinical Endocrinology and Metabolism*, **64**, 157.

Peterkofsky, A., Battaini, F., Koch, Y., Takahara, Y. & Dannies, P. (1982). Histidyl-proline diketopiperazine: its biological role as a regulatory peptide. *Molecular and Cellular Biochemistry*, **42**, 45.

Peters, J., Foord, S., Dieguez, C., Salvader, J., Hall, R. & Scanlon, M. F. (1985). Lack of effect of the TRH related dipeptide histidyl-proline diketopiperazine on TSH and prolactin secretion in normal subjects, in patients with microprolactinomas and in primary hypothyroidism. *Clinical Endocrinology*, **23**, 289.

Pflug, B. & Tolle, R. (1971). Disturbance of the 24-hour rhythm in endogenous depression and the treatment of endogenous depression by sleep deprivation. *Internal Pharmacopsychiatry*, **6**, 1877.

Phillips, R. H., Valente, W. A., Caplan, E. S., Connor, T. B. & Wiswell, J. G. (1984). Circulating thyroid hormone changes in acute trauma: prognostic implications for clinical outcome. *Journal of Trauma*, **24**(2), 116.

Pinchera, A., Mariotti, S., Barbesino, G., Bechi, R., Sansoni, P., Fagiolo, U., Cossarizza, A. & Franceschi, C. (1995). Thyroid autoimmunity and ageing. *Hormone Research*, **43**, 64.

Plotnikoff, N. P., Prange, A. J. Jr., Breese, G. R., Anderson, M. S. & Wilson, I. C. (1972). Thyrotropin releasing hormone: enhancement of Dopa activity by a hypothalamic hormone (TRH). *Science*, **178**, 417.

Poth, M., Tseng, Y. C. & Wartofsky, L. (1991). Inhibition of TSH activation of human cultured thyroid cells by tumor necrosis factor: an explanation for decreased thyroid function in systemic illness? *Thyroid*, 1, 235–40.

Prange, A. J. Jr. (1996). Novel uses of thyroid hormones in patients with affective disorders. *Thyroid*, 6(5), 537–43.

Prange, A. J. Jr. & Lipton, M. A. (1962). Enhancement of imipramine mortality in hyperthyroid mice. *Nature*, 196, 588.

Prange, A. J. Jr. & Loosen, P. T. (1984). Findings in affective disorders relevant to the thyroid axis, melanotropin, oxytocin, and vasopressin. In *Neuroendocrinology and Psychiatric Disorder*, ed. G. M. Brown, S. H. Koslow & S. Reichlin, pp. 191–200. New York: Raven Press.

Prange, A. J. Jr., Lipton, M. A. & Love, G. N. (1963). Diminution of mortality in hypothyroid mice. *Nature*, 197, 1212.

Prange, A. J. Jr., Wilson, I. C., Breese, G. R. & Lipton, M. A. (1976). Hormonal alterations of imipramine response: a review. In *Hormones, Behavior and Psychopathology*, ed. E. S. Sachar, pp. 41–67. New York: Raven Press.

Prange, A. J. Jr., Wilson, I. C., Knox, A. E., McClane, T. K. & Lipton, M. A. (1970). Enhancement of imipramine by thyroid stimulating hormone: clinical and theoretical implications. *American Journal of Psychiatry*, 127, 191.

Prange, A. J. Jr., Wilson, I. C., Lara, P. P., Alltop, L. B. & Breese, G. R. (1972). Effects of thyrotropin-releasing hormone in depression. *Lancet*, ii, 999–1002.

Prange, A. J. Jr., Wilson, I. C., Lara, P. P. & Alltop, L. B. (1974). Effects of thyrotropin-releasing hormone in depression. In *The Thyroid Axis, Drugs, and Behavior*, ed. A. J. Prange Jr., pp. 135–45. New York: Raven Press.

Prange, A. J. Jr., Wilson, I. C., Rabon, A. M. & Lipton, M. A. (1968). Enhancement of imipramine by triiodothyronine in unselected depressed patients. *Excerpta Medica International Congress*, 180, 532.

Prasad, C. (1989). Neurobiology of Cyclo (His–Pro). In *Thyrotropin-releasing Hormone Biomedical Significance*, ed. G. Metcalf & I. M. D. Jackson. *Annals of the New York Academy of Sciences*, 553, 232.

Prasad, C. & Peterkofsky, A. (1976). Demonstration of pyroglutamyl peptides and amidase activities towards TRH in hamster hypothalamic extracts. *Journal of Biological Chemistry*, 251, 3229.

Prasad, C., Hilton, C. W., Lohr, J. B., & Robertson, H. J. R. (1991). Increased cerebrospinal fluid cyclo (His–Pro) content in schizophrenia. *Neuropeptides*, 20, 187.

Prasad, C., Jayaraman, A., Robertson, H. G. F. & Rao, J. K. (1987). Is all cyclo (His–Pro) derived from thyrotropin-releasing hormone? *Neurochemistry Research*, 12, 767.

Prasad, C., Matsui, T. & Peterkofsky, A. (1977). Antagonism of ethanol narcosis by histidyl-proline diketopiperazine. *Nature*, 268, 142.

Prasad, C., Matsui, T., Williams, J. & Peterkofsky, A. (1978). Thermoregulation in rats: opposing effects of TRH and its metabolite histidyl-proline-diketopiperazine. *Biochemical and Biophysical Research Communications*, 85, 1582.

Prasad, C., Wilber, J. F., Akerstrom, V. & Banerji, A. (1980). Cyclo (His–Pro): a selective inhibitor of rat prolactin secretion *in vitro*. *Life Sciences*, 27, 1979.

Przegalinski, E., Baran, L. & Siwanowicz, J. (1989). The effect of repeated treatment with anti-depressant drugs on the thyrotropin-releasing hormone (TRH)-induced hyperthermia in mice. *Journal of Pharmacy and Pharmacology*, **41**, 639.

Relkin, R. (1972). Rat pituitary and plasma prolactin levels after pinealectomy. *Journal of Endocrinology*, **53**, 179.

Rosenbaum, R. L. & Barzel, U. S. (1982). Levothyroxine replacement dose for primary hypothyroidism decreases with age. *Annals of Internal Medicine*, **96**(1), 53.

Roy, A., Wolkiwitz, O.M., Bissette, G. & Nemeroff, C. B. (1994). Differences in CSF concentrations of thyrotropin-releasing hormone in depressed patients and normal subjects: negative findings. *American Journal of Psychiatry*, **151**(4), 600–2.

Roy-Byrne, P. P., Joffe, R. T., Ulide, T. W. & Post, R. M. (1984). Carbamazepine and thyroid function in effectively ill patients. *Archives of General Psychiatry*, **41**, 1150.

Rubin, R. T., Poland, R. E., Lesser, I. M. & Martin, D. J. (1987). Neuroendocrine aspects of primary endogenous depression-IV: pituitary–thyroid axis activity in patients and matched control subjects. *Psychoneuroendocrinology*, **12**, 333.

Sack, D. A., James, S. P., Rosenthal, N. E. & Wehr, T. A. (1985). TSH is lower at night in depression. 138th Annual Meeting of the American Psychiatric Association, Dallas, Texas (New Research Section, Abstract 86).

Sack, D. A., James, S. P., Rosenthal, N. E. & Wehr, T. A. (1988). Deficient nocturnal surge of TSH secretion during sleep and sleep deprivation in rapid cycling bipolar illness. *Psychiatry Research*, **23**, 179.

Sakurai, A., Nakai, A. & DeGroot, L. J. (1989). Expression of three forms of thyroid hormone receptor in human tissues. *Molecular Endocrinology*, **3**, 392.

Samuels, M. H. (1998). Subclinical thyroid disease in the elderly. *Thyroid*, **8**(9), 803–13.

Sanchez-Franco, F., Garcia, M. D. & Cacicedo, L. (1974). Transient lack of TSH response to thyrotropin-releasing hormone (TRH) in treated hyperthyroid patients with normal or low serum thyroxine (T4) and triiodothyronine (T3). *Journal of Clinical Endocrinology and Metabolism*, **38**, 1098.

Sap, J., Munoz, A., Damm, K., Goldberg, Y., Ghysdael, J., Leutz, A., Beug, H. & Vennstrom, B. (1986). The c-erb-A protein is a high-affinity receptor for thyroid hormone. *Nature*, **324**, 635.

Sattin, A. (1987). A possible role for thyrotropin releasing hormone (TRH) in antidepressant treatment. *Advances in Experimental Medical Biology*, **221**, 549.

Sattin, A., Hill, T. G., Norton, J. A. & Kubek, M. J. (1987). The prolonged increase in thyrotropin-releasing hormone in rat limbic forebrain regions following electroconvulsive shock. *Regulatory Peptides*, **19**, 13.

Sawin, C. T., Herman, T., Molitch, M. E., London, M. H. & Kramer, S. M. (1983). Aging and the thyroid: decreased requirement for thyroid hormone in older hypothyroid patients. *American Journal of Medicine*, **75**(2), 206.

Schlienger, J. L., Kapfer, M. T., Singer, L. & Stephan, F. (1980). The action of clomipramine on thyroid function. *Hormone and Metabolic Research*, **12**, 481.

Schou, M. A., Amdisen, S., Jensen, E. & Olsen, T. (1968). Occurrence of goitre during lithium treatment. *British Medical Journal*, **3**, 710.

Scott, A. I. F., Milner, J. B., Shering, P. A. & Beckett, G. J. (1990). Fall in free thyroxine after ECT: real effect or an artifact of assay? *Biological Psychiatry*, 27, 784.

Sedvall, G., Jonsson, B. & Pettersson, U. (1969). Evidence of an altered thyroid function in man during treatment with lithium carbonate. *Acta Psychiatrica Scandinavica*, 207(Suppl.), 59.

Segerson, T. P., Kauer, J. K., Wolfe, H. C., Mobtaker, H., Wu, P., Jackson, I. M. D. & Lechan, R. M. (1987). Thyroid hormone regulates TRH biosynthesis in the paraventricular nucleus of the rat hypothalamus. *Science*, 238, 78.

Simard, M., Pekary, A. E., Smith, V. P. & Hershman, J. M. (1989). Thyroid hormones modulate thyrotropin–releasing hormone biosynthesis in tissues outside the hypothalamic-pituitary axis of male rats. *Endocrinology*, 125, 524.

Snyder, S. H. & Peroutka, S. J. (1984). Antidepressants and neurotransmitter receptors. In *Frontiers of Clinical Neuroscience Series*, vol. 1, ed. R. M. Post & J. C. Ballenger, series ed. J. H. Wood & B. R. Brooks, pp. 686–97. Baltimore and London: Williams & Wilkins.

Snyder, P. J., Jacobs, L. S., Rabello, M. M., Sterling, F. H., Shore, R. N., Utiger, R. D. & Daughaday, W. H. (1974). Diagnostic value of thyrotrophin-releasing hormone in pituitary and hypothalamic diseases: assessment of thyrotrophin and prolactin secretion in 100 patients. *Annals of Internal Medicine*, 81, 751.

Solomon, D. H. (1991). Effect of aging on thyroid hormone metabolism. In *Thyroid Hormone Metabolism*, ed. S. Y. Wu, pp. 267–92. Oxford: Blackwell Scientific.

Sorensen, R., Svendsen, K. & Schou, M. (1974). TRH in depression (letter). *Lancet*, ii, 865.

Stern, R. A., Nevels, C. T., Shelhourse, M. E., Prohaska, M. L. & Prange, A. J. Jr. (1990). Combined thyroid hormone and ECT treatment. American Psychiatric Association 143rd Annual Meeting, New York (New Research Section, Abstract NR 443).

Sternbach, H. A., Gwirtsman, H. E. & Gerner, R. H. (1984). Biological tests in the diagnosis and treatment of affective disorders. In *Psychoneuroendocrine dysfunction*, ed. N. S. Shah & A. G. Donald, pp. 383–98. New York and London: Plenum Medical Book Co.

Stohlawetz, P., Hahn, P., Koller, M., Hauer, J., Resch, H., Smolen, J. & Pietschmann, P. (1998). Immunophenotypic characteristics of monocytes in elderly subjects. *Scandinavian Journal of Immunology*, 48(3), 324.

Straub, R. E. & Gershengorn, M. C. (1986). Thyrotropin-releasing hormone and GTP activate inositol trisphosphate formation in membranes isolated from rat pituitary cells. *Journal of Biological Chemistry*, 261, 2712.

Suen, C-S. & Wilk, S. (1987). Regulation of a thyrotropin-releasing hormone-degrading enzyme in GH3 cells: induction of pyroglutamyl peptidase I by 3,5,3'-triiodothyronine. *Endocrinology*, 121, 770–5.

Suen, C-S. & Wilk, S. (1989). Regulation of thyrotropin releasing hormone degrading enzymes in rat brain and pituitary by L-3,5,3'-triiodothyronine. *Journal of Neurochemistry*, 52, 884.

Targum, S. D., Sullivan, A. C. & Byrnes, S. M. (1982). Neuroendocrine interrelationships in major depressive disorder. *American Journal of Psychiatry*, 139, 282.

Tauboll, E., Gjerstad, L., Stokke, K. T., Lundervold, A. & Telle, B. (1987). Effects of electroconvulsive therapy (ECT) on thyroid function parameters. *Psychoneuroendocrinology*, 12, 349–54.

Thomas, F. B., Mazzaferri, E. L. & Skillman, T. G. (1970). Apathetic thyrotoxicosis. A distinctive clinical and laboratory entity. *Annals of Internal Medicine*, 72(5), 679.

Tibaldi, J. M. & Surks, M. I. (1985). Effects of nonthyroidal illness on thyroid function. *Medical Clinics of North America*, **69**(5), 899.

Tibaldi, J. M., Barzel, U. S., Albin, J. & Surks, M. (1986). Thyrotoxicosis in the very old. *American Journal of Medicine*, **81**(4), 619.

Tremont, G. & Stern, R. A. (1997). Use of thyroid hormone to diminish the cognitive side effects of psychiatric treatment. *Psychopharmacology Bulletin*, **33**(2), 273–80.

Utiger, R. D. (1987). Thyrotropin-releasing hormone and thyrotropin secretion. *Journal of Laboratory and Clinical Medicine*, **109**, 327.

van den Burg, W., van Praag, H. M., Bos, E. R. H., Piers, D. A., van Zanten, A. K. & Doorenbos, H. (1976). TRH by slow, continuous infusion. an antidepressant? *Psychological Medicine*, **6**, 393.

van der Poll, T., Romijn, J. A., Wiersinga, W. M. & Sauerwein, H. P. (1990). Tumor necrosis factor: a putative mediator of the sick euthyroid syndrome in man. *Journal of Clinical Endocrinology and Metabolism*, **71**(6), 1567.

Vardarli, I., Schmidt, R., Wdowinski, J. M., Teuber, J., Schwedes, U. & Usadel, K. H. (1987). [The hypothalamo-hypophyseal thyroid axis, plasma protein concentrations and the hypophyseo-gonadal axis in low T3 syndrome following acute myocardial infarct]. *Klinische Wochenschrift*, **65**(3), 129.

Vogel, H. P., Benkert, O., Illig, R., Muller-Oerlinghausen, B. & Poppenberg, A. (1977). Psychoendocrinological and therapeutic effects of TRH in depression. *Acta Psychiatrica Scandinavica*, **56**(3), 223.

Wahlin, A., Wahlin, T. B., Small, B. J. & Backman, L. (1998). Influences of thyroid stimulating hormone on cognition functioning in very old age. *Journal of Gerontology: Psychological Sciences*, **53B**(4), 234–9.

Walczak, D., Meyerhoff, J., Bates, V. E., Lynch, T. & Kubek, M. J. (1983). Effect of partial and fully generalized kindled seizures on thyrotropin releasing hormone levels in specific cortical and subcortical regions of rat brain. *Society of Neuroscience*, **9**(Abstr), 485.

Wang, C. & Crapo, L. M. (1997). The epidemiology of thyroid disease and implications for screening. *Endocrinology and Metabolism Clinics of North America*, **26**(1), 189.

Wartofsky, L. & Burman, K. D. (1982). Alterations in thyroid function in patients with systemic illness: the 'euthyroid sick syndrome.' *Endocrine Review*, **3**(2), 164.

Weeke, A. & Weeke, J. (1980). The 24-hour pattern of serum TSH in patients with endogenous depression. *Acta Psychiatrica Scandinavica*, **62**, 69.

Wehmann, R. E., Gregerman, R. I., Burns, W. H., Saral, R. & Santos, G. W. (1985). Suppression of thyrotropin in the low-thyroxine state of severe nonthyroidal illness. *New England Journal of Medicine*, **312**(9), 546.

Weinberger, C., Thompson, C. C., Ong, E. S., Lebo, R., Gruol, D. J. & Evans, R. (1986). The c-erb-A gene encodes a thyroid hormone receptor. *Nature*, **234**, 641.

Whybrow, P. & Ferrell, R. (1974). Thyroid state and human behavior. contributions from a clinical perspective. In *The Thyroid Axis, Drugs, and Behavior*, ed. A. J. Prange, pp. 5–28. New York: Raven Press.

Whybrow, P. C. & Prange, A. J. Jr. (1981). A hypothesis of thyroid–catecholamine–receptor interaction: its relevance to affective illness. *Archives of General Psychiatry*, **38**, 106.

Whybrow, P. C., Coppen, A., Prange, A. J., Noguera, R. & Baily, J. E. (1972). Thyroid function and the response to liothyronine in depression. *Archives of General Psychiatry*, 26, 242.

Whybrow, P. C., Prange, A. J. Jr. & Treadway, C. R. (1969). Mental changes accompanying thyroid gland dysfunction. *Archives of General Psychiatry*, 20, 48.

Wilson, I. C., Prange, A. J. Jr., & Lara, P. (1974). L-Triiodothyronine alone and with imipramine in the treatment of depressed women. In *The Thyroid Axis, Drugs and Behavior*, ed. A. J. Prange, pp. 49–62. New York: Raven Press.

Wolf, B., Aratan-Spire, S. & Czernichow, P. (1984). Hypothyroidism increases pancreatic thyrotropin-releasing hormone concentrations in adult rats. *Endocrinology*, 114, 1334.

Woolf, P. D. & Lee, L. (1977). Effect of the serotonin precursor, tryptophan, on pituitary hormone secretion. *Journal of Clinical Endocrinology and Metabolism*, 45, 123.

Zadina, J. E., Banks, W. A. & Kastin, A. J. (1986). Central nervous system effects of peptides, 1980–1985: a cross-listing of peptides and their central actions from the first six years of the journal *Peptides. Peptides*, 7, 497.

5

Estrogen and depression in aging women

Mary F. Morrison and Kathryn Tweedy

Introduction

Although the prevalence of major depression decreases in aging women, there is an increased prevalence of non-major depressive disorders in women after the age of 65. These minor depressive syndromes are two to three times as common in older women as in men of the same age. The reasons for this sex difference in the prevalence of depressive symptoms are not known. Aging women experience significant changes in social role and relationships, health status, family composition and economic status, all of which may present intense psychological challenges that could contribute to depression.

Aging women also undergo distinct biological changes, the impact of which on mood remains to be clarified. These biological changes, which are the focus of this book, include decreasing levels of hormones such as estradiol, testosterone, dehydroepiandrosterone, progesterone, insulin-like growth factor, and growth hormone. Estrogen deficiency, in particular, has been suggested as one cause of the non-major depressive disorders in elderly women. Moreover, estrogen replacement, including use of the specific estrogen receptor modulators tamoxifen and raloxifene, is increasingly recommended for disease prevention after menopause. The psychological consequences of such treatments are not well understood. If we are to consider the use of estrogen and other sex hormones to prevent or treat depressive symptoms in aging women, it will be important to understand the psychological, pharmacological, and biochemical effects of these agents.

Epidemiology of depressive disorders in aging

Gender differences in the epidemiology and phenomenology of depression may be informative about the neurobiology of depressive disorders. One of the most striking and consistent findings in psychiatric epidemiology is that women have a two to three times higher rates of depression than men (Weissman et al., 1991, 1996; Seeman, 1997). Some psychiatric epidemiologists believe that the sex difference in major depression ends at age 50 to 54 years, consistent with the theories that implicate the menstrual cycle in the increased risk of depression in women (Burvill, 1995). The prevalence of major depression is significantly lower in the geriatric population than in the young adults, but there is still a female predominance (1.4% vs. 0.4%; Weissman et al., 1991). The peak risk of developing major depression occurs at age 30 for women and 40 for men, and both women and men have a smaller peak in incidence at age 55 (Eaton et al., 1997). Although there is a decrease in major depression in the elderly, the prevalence of 'minor' depression is increased (Romanoski et al., 1992). There is also a female predominance in other minor depressions among the elderly (Blazer et al., 1987; Stallones et al., 1990; Judd et al., 1994). The term 'minor depression' or 'subsyndromal depression' is used to designate a condition that does not fulfill the DSM-IV criteria for major depression. This does not mean that minor depression is clinically insignificant. Subsyndromal depressions are associated with significant increases in social dysfunction and disability (Broadhead et al., 1990; Judd et al., 1994; Beekman et al., 1997; Rapaport & Judd, 1998). Milder depressive symptoms are appropriate targets for therapeutic interventions. The presence of minor depression or milder depressive symptoms appears to be a risk factor for the development of major depression (Parmelee et al., 1992). Treatment of these disorders can represent an important approach to preventing more severe psychiatric illness and may improve psychosocial functioning (Rapaport & Judd, 1998). There is a need to understand the mechanisms by which gender influences mood, so that optimal therapeutic approaches can be developed.

The estrogen deficiency hypothesis of depression

Because affective symptoms have been noted in women undergoing changes in reproductive endocrinology, differences in sex steroids have been investigated as factors that may contribute to the differential susceptibility to depression between women and men. The increased prevalence of depressive symptoms in premenopausal women raises the possibility that estrogen might be a causative agent in depression, but this supposition does not stand up to scrutiny. For example, it does not explain why postmenopausal women have a higher prevalence of depression than do men their age (Weissman et al., 1991). Much of the data on natural and surgical menopause, as well as clinical observations in women receiving antiestrogen therapy for breast cancer, suggest that estrogen deficiency may actually contribute to depressive symptoms and lack of response to antidepressant medication observed in aging women (Sherwin & Gelfand, 1985; Halbreich, 1990; Shariff et al., 1995; Lopez-Jaramillo et al., 1996; Schneider et al., 1998). In an unblinded, placebo-controlled study, premenopausal women without psychiatric history, who were rendered temporarily hypogonadal by gonadotropin releasing hormone (GnRH) agonist therapy, had an increase in depressive symptoms 11 days after GnRH injection (Toren et al., 1996). However, the depressive symptoms persisted even when estradiol levels were then markedly increased. Mood observations in women with estrogen deficiency states induced by various means suggest that estrogen deficiency may increase depressive symptoms. Thus, estrogen deficiency may cause minor depression in aging women. Whether exogenous estrogen use and high estrogen levels can protect against depressive symptoms will be discussed in the next sections.

Epidemiologic evidence that estrogen use is protective against depression

It is not yet clear that menopause is associated with an increased incidence of depression (for review see Kaufert et al., 1992). A community survey in Seattle found that a history of premenstrual syndrome, postpartum depression and vasomotor symptoms correlated with reports of consistently depressed mood at midlife (age 35 to 55; Woods & Mitchell, 1996), suggesting that those with previous vulnerability to changes in reproductive hormones and those with vasomotor symptoms which can be associated with insomnia are at increased risk of depressions at midlife. The prevalence of depressive symptoms in premenopausal women in Finland is much lower than that observed in the United States (Lehtinen & Joukamaa, 1994). In addition, there is an increased prevalence of depressive disorders in women in their mid-40s and a higher prevalence in women aged 60 to 64. Finland has a more homogenous population compared with the United States and these data may suggest age-related biological changes in mood (at least in Caucasian women) that are obscured in US studies with heterogenous populations. Follow-up data from the Baltimore site of the Epidemiologic Catchment Area study cited above, suggest that there may be an increased incidence of depression in women in their mid-40s and another vulnerable period around ages 55 to 60 (Eaton et al., 1997). In an older population in California (women age 50 to 90), estrogen use was associated with a decreased likelihood of depressive symptoms (Palinkas & Barrett-Connor, 1992). In this cross-sectional study of 1190 white women, 25% were currently using estrogen. The prevalence of scores of 13 or more on the Beck Depression Inventory was 9%. Mean scores increased steadily with age in the untreated women, while no significant increase in scores was seen in the estrogen treated group. This finding is consistent with the hypothesis that ongoing estrogen deficiency increases the likelihood of developing depressive symptoms and that estrogen therapy is protective. However, in the youngest group (age 50 to 59), treated women had significantly higher scores than untreated women of the same age. The reason for this is not known but either reflects a referral bias in this age group (e.g. depressed women at this age are more likely to get ERT than older women) or that estrogen given to women who are in the early postmenopausal period may lower mood. Epidemiologic data suggest that an increased incidence and prevalence of depressive symptoms occurs for women in the mid-40s and again at an age between 55 to 64. One possibility for these age-related increases in depressive symptoms are gonadal steroid changes, with the mid-40s increase being the perimenopausal period with fluctuating estrogen levels and age 55 to 64 representing the 'younger' postmenopausal period with low and stable estrogen levels. There are increasing data to suggest that, in aging women with low estrogen levels, estrogens may play an important role in maintaining brain function which will be discussed further in the next section.

Neuroprotective role of estrogen in aging women

Estrogen has been shown to enhance neuron growth (Brinton et al., 1997) and to exert a neuroprotective effect on certain neurons in the CNS (Green et al., 1997; Azcoitia et al., 1998). Like antidepressants, estrogen increased the expression of nerve growth factors and their receptors in cellular models (Sohrabji et al., 1994; Joffe & Cohen, 1998). Ovariectomy in rats reduced brain derived nerve growth factor (BDNF) in parts of the hippocampus and the frontal and temporal cortex, while estrogen replacement reversed this in some but not all regions (Simpkins et al., 1997; Joffe & Cohen, 1998). Estrogen's protective effect on memory and cognitive functioning may be due to its ability to preserve hippocampal neuron circuits and prevent neuron death. This effect is supported by in vitro studies using SK-N-SH human neuroblastoma cells (cells that carry the protein message for nerve growth factor; Green et al., 1997) and in vivo rodent studies using a neuronal excitotoxin, kainic acid (Azcoitia et al., 1998). This subject is further reviewed in Chapters 8 and 9.

Although the involvement of estrogen and nerve growth factors require further study, these studies and others suggest that estrogen may exert an antidepressant effect through its effects on nerve growth factors (further discussed in Joffe & Cohen, 1998) and prevent neuronal degeneration in older women (Brinton et al., 1997). The clinical evidence that estrogen may improve mood in aging women will be reviewed in the next section.

Estrogen therapy for mood disorders

Interest in estrogen therapy for mood disorders in women of all ages has been long-standing and a thorough review has recently been published summarizing the relevant literature in women in their premenopausal and midlife years (Joffe & Cohen, 1998). This section will concentrate on the literature addressing populations of aging women and medical populations relevant to estrogen deficiency. The studies of estrogen in the 1970s discussed below were mainly investigations of estrogen's utility as an antidepressant augmentation strategy. More recent studies have focused on populations with and without significant mood disturbance in the perimenopause; surgically menopausal; and non-surgically postmenopausal group. Clinical studies of estrogen therapy for mood disorders in aging women have been characterized by methodological problems. These have included inconsistencies in the choice of subjects, failure to monitor estrogen levels, failure to control for the possible dysphoric effects of progestin administered to women with intact uteri, variability in the composition of the therapeutic estrogen preparations, and the application of possibly inappropriate outcomes measures. The result of all these methodological problems is that variability in outcome may have obscured a therapeutic effect.

Inappropriate selection of subjects has been the most problematic methodological flaw. Many studies have included both perimenopausal and postmenopausal women in the same study. Whereas perimenopausal women have fluctuating levels of estrogen, postmenopausal women demonstrate stable, low levels of estrogen. Severity of hot flushes in these two groups has not been assessed routinely and could potentially confound results. There are few studies of estrogen's mood effects in women older than 65. The older group of postmenopausal women may not experience beneficial effects on mood, even if younger postmenopausal women do. If these older women are not analyzed separately, their lack of responsiveness might dilute the apparent therapeutic effect of estrogen replacement. Inclusion of surgically menopausal women with those who have undergone natural menopause may also have led to invalid conclusions. Women who recently have experienced surgical menopause tend to be younger and have had an abrupt decline in both estradiol and testosterone levels. Women with natural menopause have had a gradual decline in estradiol levels and minimal reductions in testosterone levels. It is possible that the responsiveness of the mood disorder to estrogen therapy in these two circumstances is different, again leading to a dilution of the apparent therapeutic effect.

Few studies have included determinations of serum estrogen levels. This would complicate comparison of mood effects of different estrogenic preparations, which might result in different serum estrogen levels. Failure to include serum estrogen levels also might tend to obscure therapeutic effects by failing to distinguish between women whose mood disorder was associated with the lowest baseline serum estrogen levels and those in whom baseline estrogen levels were higher. The etiology of depression and its responsiveness to estrogen might be different in these two groups.

A prominent hypothesis concerning the role of sex hormones in female depression holds that progesterone has a dysphoric effect (Halbreich, 1997). Studies that employ such combination therapies may miss a therapeutic effect of estrogen if it is counteracted by a dysphoric effect of progesterone. If that were the case, inclusion of studies using such combination replacement therapies together with studies using only estrogen in a meta-analysis might obscure a therapeutic effect.

Another potential confounder of clinical studies is that estrogen effects on mood are likely to be mild, whereas the assessment instruments used in the studies were developed and validated on subjects with more severe depressive disorders. Whether these instruments, such as the Hamilton Depression scale, are sensitive enough to assess minor changes in mood states remains to be determined.

Early attempts to determine if estrogen affects mood

In the early 1970s, estrogen was increasingly prescribed to women for menopausal symptoms and beneficial effects on mood were noted anecdotally (Michael et al., 1970). At the same time, there was increasing recognition that oral contraceptives were associated with depressive symptoms in younger women. These apparently contradictory observations suggested the need for more formal investigations to whether estrogen really does affect mood. A preliminary study in depressed pre-menopausal women compared the antidepressant effects of imipramine (IMI) plus ethinyl estrogen with those of IMI plus placebo (Prange et al., 1972). Two doses of estrogen were used, 0.025 mg and 0.050 mg/day. The IMI dose in all groups was 150 mg/day. At 2 and 3 weeks, women receiving IMI plus high dose estrogen showed less antidepressant effect than women taking either IMI plus low dose estrogen or IMI alone did. All three groups had similar depression scores at 6 weeks. In this study, premenopausal women on imipramine plus high dose estrogen did not have as robust an antidepressant effect as the other imipramine groups and there was no apparent benefit from estrogen treatment. On the other hand, in a clinical sample of young *post*menopausal women, a four week open trial of ERT suggested that estrogen may have a non-therapeutic mood elevating effect (Schneider et al., 1977). Non-depressed women had increased feelings of well-being and slightly lower depression scores on estrogen than before treatment, but depression scores did not improve in previously depressed women. An opposite conclusion was drawn from a prospective placebo-controlled clinical trial of supraphysiologic doses of estrogen in treatment-resistant depressed women (Klaiber et al., 1979). Both pre- and postmenopausal women were included. The estrogen-treated group improved from severely depressed to moderately depressed, while the placebo group was unchanged. Thus, early clinical trials of ERT failed to arrive at a consensus about the effects of estrogen on depression.

Recent clinical trials of estrogen replacement to improve mood

Current data suggest that, in both perimenopausal women and surgically meno-pausal women, ERT results in improved mood. However, in unselected groups of postmenopausal depressed women, studies have shown a high placebo response and no clear estrogen-placebo difference.

A prospective, placebo-controlled trial in perimenopausal women with depression and no hot flushes suggested that estrogen produces significant improvement in symptoms of tearfulness, emotional numbness, mood instability, and Center for Epidemiologic studies and Beck Depression Inventory Scores (Schmidt et al., 1994). In another study, perimenopausal women were randomly given one of three treatments for depressive symptoms: estradiol 50 mg, estradiol 50 mg plus testosterone 100 mg, or placebo (Appleby et al., 1981). Both hormonal treatments were significantly better than placebo at 2 months. However, at 4 months, depression scores increased somewhat in both hormonal groups. The response in the perimenopausal women can be contrasted with the postmenopausal women in the same study discussed below.

Surgical menopause has been studied as a clinical model for the effects of estrogen on mood in women who develop menopause through normal, age-related ovarian failure. Oophorectomized premenopausal women received supraphysiologic doses of either estrogen, androgen or a combination and attained lower depression scores coincident with their higher plasma estrogen and testosterone levels (Sherwin & Gelfand, 1985). When hormones were withdrawn, depression scores of all oophorectomized women were higher than those of the hysterectomy/no oophorectomy control group, although no scores were in the range of major depression. Thus, estrogens and androgens both appear to improve depressive symptoms in these women. The relevance of this study to the mood and cognitive changes seen in women with non-surgical menopause is debated.

In non-surgically postmenopausal women, studies have been conducted on estrogen and depression. In addition, estrogen's effect on quality of life and insomnia is relevant to estrogen's effect on mood. Estrogen improves affect and quality of life in euthymic young postmenopausal women. In a randomized placebo-controlled trial, transdermal estradiol improved quality of life in young (45 to 65 years) postmenopausal women (Wiklund et al., 1993). The frequency of health-related quality of life complaints, involving sex life, family life, employment, housework and hobbies, was significantly reduced after 3 months of unopposed ERT (without progesterone). In young (45 to 60) Hispanic postmenopausal women without depression and hot flushes, two different doses of unopposed oral conjugated estrogens (0.625 mg and 1.25 mg) demonstrated a significant improvement in Beck Depression scores. Apparently, beneficial effects could be achieved in non-depressed women by replacement doses of estrogen.

Insomnia is more common in women than men and increases with age (Polo-Kantola et al., 1998). Insomnia related to vasomotor symptoms and the aging process, may increase the vulnerability of postmenopausal women to depressive disorders (Joffe & Cohen, 1998). In a randomized, placebo-controlled, crossover study in young postmenopausal women (ages 47 to 65 years) with insomnia and no hot flushes, estrogen produced significant, mild-moderate improvement in insomnia ($P = 0.019$) and morning tiredness ($P = 0.040$; Polo-Kantola et al., 1998). In the women with vasomotor symptoms (hot flushes and sweating), there was a modest correlation (r range 0.29 to 0.37, p range 0.003 to 0.023) between severity of vasomotor symptoms and anxiety and depressive symptoms. Thus estrogen appears to be beneficial in the treatment of insomnia in postmenopausal women with and without vasomotor symptoms. However, because women who are experiencing significant hot flushes are likely to have symptoms of depression and anxiety, the effect on insomnia could not be separated from an effect on depression.

The most inconsistent findings have been those in studies of the therapeutic antidepressant effects of estrogen in postmenopausal women. In an open study of the effectiveness of 0.06 mg/day of ethinyl estradiol in postmenopausal and premenopausal women with endogenous depression, seven of ten postmenopausal patients achieved a decrease of at least 12 points in Hamilton Depression scores (Holsboer et al., 1983; Young & Korszun, 1998). These findings must be interpreted with caution, however, not only because the study was small and not blinded, but because many of the studies of the effect of estrogen treatment on postmenopausal mood changes have been characterized by unusually high placebo responses. In one study referred to above, 31 postmenopausal women were randomly given one of three treatments for menopausal symptoms (not all subjects had depressive symptoms): estradiol 50 mg, estradiol 50 mg plus testosterone 100 mg, or placebo (Appleby et al., 1981). Both active and placebo groups responded to the treatment interventions in the postmenopausal women. Mean scores on psychological symptoms at 4 months (assessed by Symptom Rating Test) demonstrated a decrease of approximately 49% in the placebo group, 25% in the estradiol group, and 51% in the estradiol plus testosterone group. The perimenopausal subjects in the same study responded significantly better to hormonal treatment than to placebo. Either estrogen had a specific effect to block the unusually high placebo effect in postmenopausal women or estrogen had an independent dysphoric effect that is equal in magnitude to the placebo effect in this population. However, in a more recent study, no difference was found between the efficacy of transdermal estradiol therapy and placebo in treating menopausal depression. Postmenopausal women (age 45 to 60) who met criteria for major depression were recruited from a menopause clinic and were assigned to a 3-month treatment with unopposed estradiol or placebo (Saletu et al., 1995). There was no difference between placebo and estrogen in scores on the Hamilton Depression Rating Scale and the Kupperman Index (a rating scale of menopausal symptomatology). Sixty-five percent of the placebo group and 63% of the estradiol group were responders on the Hamilton Depression scale. In this study, only estrogen-treated patients demonstrated changes on EEG mapping, the significance of which is unknown. A randomized, double blind, placebo-controlled, pilot study of ERT for involutive depression was conducted in 20 postmenopausal women without previous affective disorder history, who were selected from a population of 138 postmenopausal women because they initially demonstrated an improvement in mood on open label trial of ERT (Lopez-Jaramillo et al., 1996). Beck depression scores decreased from 30 ± 4 to 16 ± 2 after one month of 1.25 mg/day conjugated equine estrogens. Beck scores in the placebo group changed little, from 29 ± 3 to 26 ± 4. This study demonstrates that there is a subgroup of postmenopausal women who experience mood improvement from estrogen in a blinded study. This study will be discussed further below as nitric oxide subunits were measured in these women. Our group has been conducting a randomized, placebo-controlled trial of transdermal estradiol for mild to moderate depressions (HAM-D scores of 8 to 20) in postmenopausal women from ages 50 to 90. Preliminary analysis of the first 30 subjects suggests a high placebo response, despite excluding early placebo responders, and no estrogen-placebo difference. Thus it is not clear from the literature whether estrogen is an antidepressant, a depressant or a blocker of the unusually high placebo effect in the majority postmenopausal women. Either the studies themselves were flawed, or there are as yet undetermined causes for heterogeneity in antidepressant response to estrogen, particularly in the postmenopausal population.

Mania been described in association with ERT, but it is an uncommon side effect. For example, an 85-year-old woman without previous psychiatric history developed mania after ERT was started for osteoporosis (Young et al., 1997). Withdrawal of estrogen was followed by the disappearance of the mania. A 70-year-old woman with treatment resistant depression was given a supraphysiologic dose of estrogen titrated over 1 month. The estrogen induced new onset rapid cycling mood disorder (Oppenheim, 1984). A causative role in mania in postmenopausal women might argue in favor of a role for estrogen as an antidepressant.

Selective estrogen receptor modulators

Different actions of estrogens are mediated by different receptors. If we are to refine our ability to use estrogenic drugs as psychotherapeutic agents, it will be necessary to be able to activate individual estrogen receptor types. Some progress toward that goal has been made recently. Selective estrogen receptor modulators (SERMs) are pharmaceuticals developed to produce beneficial estrogen-like effects on bone and lipid metabolism, while acting as estrogen antagonists in the breast and uterus, where estrogen can be carcinogenic. Since estrogen appears to have beneficial effects on the CNS of aging women, the identification of SERMs with beneficial CNS effects is an important next step. SERMs evolved out of the search for an antiestrogen that would be an effective treatment for breast cancer. Clinical trials of antiestrogens have revealed that they do not work simply. Based on their selective capacity to inhibit or stimulate estrogen receptor sites, a distinction emerged between partial antiestrogens and pure antiestrogens.

Administration of pure antiestrogens, such as MER 25 and ICI 164,384, blocks all estrogenic activity while partial antiestrogens (including tamoxifen and raloxifene) act as both agonists and antagonists (Bryant & Dere, 1998), depending on the target tissue. Because traditional hormone replacement therapy has been limited by unwanted side effects, the potential of SERMs for disease prevention is a promising area of development.

Tamoxifen

Tamoxifen has been used to treat breast cancer for over 30 years. However, its use as a preventive measure for breast cancer has only recently been discovered. The National Surgical Adjuvant Breast and Bowel Project study (NSABBP; $N > 13\,000$ women) proved that in women with a high risk of breast cancer, tamoxifen treatment significantly reduced their chances of developing the disease (Fisher et al., 1998). Given these data and the high incidence of breast cancer in the United States, prophylactic tamoxifen treatment will be increasingly used for breast cancer prevention.

Tamoxifen's effects on CNS have not been well characterized. Anecdotal clinical experiences of oncologists suggest that tamoxifen increases depressive symptoms in some women with breast cancer. Published studies that address depression as a side effect have not used well recognized, validated scales for depression (Powles et al., 1990; Love et al., 1991; Cathcart et al., 1993). In an unblinded assessment of depressive symptoms in node negative women with breast cancer, 15% of the tamoxifen group had depressive symptoms compared with 3% of the no tamoxifen group (Cathcart et al., 1993). Postmenopausal women with early stage breast cancer ($N = 42$, mean age $= 65$) and no psychiatric history were given tamoxifen. Seventeen percent of the women developed clinically significant increases in their scores on the IPAT depression scale (Shariff et al., 1995). In a retrospective analysis from four clinical trials of women with metastatic breast cancer treated with tamoxifen, mood changes (6% vs. 2%, $P = 0.03$) and anorexia (22% vs. 14%, $P = 0.04$) were more common in older (>65) cohorts than in younger ones. Preliminary data from the NSABBP study suggests that tamoxifen use does not cause a significant increase in depressive symptoms in either premenopausal or postmenopausal women (Personal communication, P. Ganz, PhD, 12/98). An intriguing finding from a retrospective analysis of data from a nursing home in New York (only women older than 65 were analyzed) was that women who received tamoxifen were more successful at basic activities of daily living (ADLs such as eating, transferring, and toileting), and the risk of Alzheimer's disease was 32.6% lower compared with women not on tamoxifen (Breuer et al., 1998). Tamoxifen appears to cause a deterioration in mood in a small percentage of women. The preliminary data on tamoxifen and risk of Alzheimer's disease suggest that tamoxifen has estrogen agonist effects in the CNS that were previously unrecognized.

Raloxifene

Initial trials with raloxifene, the first antiestrogen to be labeled as a SERM, demonstrated that it also prevents bone loss and lowers serum cholesterol levels. Unlike other estrogenic compounds, raloxifene exerts its beneficial effects without the increased risk of uterine cancer seen with tamoxifen (Mitlak & Cohen, 1997). Raloxifene has also been shown to prevent mammary tumors (Bryant & Dere, 1998). There are very few data regarding central nervous system functioning and raloxifene. Preliminary basic evidence suggests that raloxifene has less CNS protective effect when compared with estrogen (Diaz-Brinton, 1998). However, Bryant, in unpublished data, has observed estrogen agonist effects from raloxifene on trkA (a nerve growth factor; Nickelsen et al., 1998). In a randomized, double blind, placebo-controlled study, raloxifene was not associated with any changes in mood or cognition in postmenopausal women after 1 year. Raloxifene does not cause adverse CNS effects in women and whether beneficial CNS effects compare to those of estrogen will require further study.

Neurotransmitters that mediate estrogen's effects on mood

Serotonin

A fundamental tenet of modern psychopharmacology is that the neurotransmitter serotonin (5–HT) plays a central role in regulating mood. Therefore, it would be expected that, if estrogen has affects on mood, these might be mediated through interactions with serotonergic mechanisms. There is now considerable evidence for such interactions. The overall activity of 5–HT in the brain appears to decrease with aging (for review see Meltzer et al., 1998). Post-mortem human studies have suggested an aging-dependent reduction with in the number of 5–HT1A, 5–HT 1B/D and 5–HT2A receptors in the frontal lobe, occipital lobe and the hippocampus. The 5–HT1A and 5–HT2B receptors and the 5–HT transporter are the most frequently targeted loci for antidepressant drugs. The 5–HT transporter is a protein found on the membrane of 5–HT nerve terminals and is responsible for reuptake of released 5–HT into the terminals. Levels of 5–HT transporter have not been shown to decrease with aging in humans though the data are inconsistent (Meltzer et al., 1998).

Estrogen acts on the serotonin neurotransmitter mechanisms in the brain, affecting 5–HT synthesis, uptake and receptor modulation (Maswood et al., 1995; Osterlund & Hurd, 1998; Pecins-Thompson et al., 1998). Some investigators have hypothesized that estrogen is important in modulating serotonergic effects on mood (Sherwin & Suranyi-Cadotte, 1990; Halbreich et al., 1995). There is conflicting evidence from animal studies and limited clinical trials as to the direction, magnitude, and significance of these findings.

Basic scientific evidence

Estrogen administration to ovariectomized, estrogen-deficient monkeys increased the synthesis of tryptophan hydroxylase, which is the rate-limiting enzyme in the synthesis of serotonin, and significantly increased the expression of tryptophan hydroxylase mRNA in the dorsal raphe (approximately ten-fold higher than spayed animals; Pecins-Thompson et al., 1996). Thus, estrogen may increase intraneuronal levels of tryptophan hydroxylase, which could result in increased levels of brain serotonin. Chronic estradiol treatment of ovariectomized rats significantly increased ^{3}H-imipramine binding and ^{3}H-serotonin binding in their hypothalamus and frontal cortex, suggesting that estrogens also up-regulate the expression of serotonin receptors (Rehavi et al., 1987). Estrogen increased the binding of a highly selective 5–HT ligand, RP62203, in several areas of the female rat brain that are thought to regulate mood and cognition; anterior frontal, anterior cingulate and primary olfactory cortex, and nucleus accumbens (Fink & Summer, 1996). Thus, estrogen increases serotonergic binding in critical brain areas for affective function.

Estrogen and 5–HT1A receptors

Agonists that bind to 5–HT1A receptors have been shown to have anxiolytic (Hen, 1998) and possibly antidepressant properties (Osterlund & Hurd, 1998). Acute estradiol treatment down-regulated 5–HT1A receptor mRNA in the limbic system of female rats (but not in the hippocampus or cingulate; Osterlund & Hurd, 1998; Sumner & Fink, 1995), which resulted in reduced 5–HT synthesis, turnover, and release into target areas (Osterlund & Hurd, 1998). This suggests that acute administration of estradiol might decrease the anxiolytic effects of 5–HT1A expression.

Estrogen and 5–HT2 receptors

5–HT2A receptors have been implicated in depression (Fink et al., 1998) and suicide (Mann et al., 1998). However, although aging has been associated consistently with reduced levels of 5–HT2A receptors, no consistent association has been found between depression and 5–HT2A receptor levels (Meltzer et al., 1998). Long-term administration of imipramine caused a decrease in 5–HT2 (but not beta adrenergic) receptor binding in rat cerebral cortex (Kendall et al., 1981). This effect was not seen in ovariectomized animals. The imipramine-induced reduction of 5–HT2 receptor binding was restored by administration of estradiol and/or progesterone. This study was seen as evidence that the presence of estrogen is important in brain serotonergic function. However, ovariectomy did not affect the interaction of other drugs with the serotonin system, such as trazodone, pargyline and mianserin (a blocker of postsynaptic 5–HT2 receptors; Kendall et al., 1982). Thus the presence of estrogen (or progesterone) was required for the action of imipramine in reducing the density of 5–HT2 receptors, but estrogen did not have a general effect on the actions of other drugs that affect serotonin function. Also, the effect is not specific to estrogen. The mechanism by which imipramine affects 5–HT2 levels is not clear, since this drug has complex pharmacological actions. Nor did these experiments determine whether estrogen has a direct effect on 5–HT2 receptors. More recently, acute administration of estradiol benzoate to ovariectomized rats significantly increased the density of 5–HT2A receptors, as measured by ^{3}H-ketanserin binding (in the presence of prazosin), in brain areas that are thought to be involved in mood and cognition: the anterior frontal, anterior cingulate and pyriform cortex, the olfactory tubercle, the nucleus accumbens, and the lateral dorsal raphe nucleus (Fink & Sumner, 1996). These findings are consistent with the view that estrogen may affect mood by increasing the concentration of 5–HT2 receptors in key areas of the brain.

Estrogen and the serotonin transporter

There are conflicting data in rodents about the effects of estrogen on the 5–HT transporter. Tritiated paroxetine is a highly selective PET radioligand for the 5–HT transporter (Meltzer et al., 1998). There is scant literature on the effects of aging on the 5–HT transporter, but there appeared to be no age effect in two reports using ^{3}H-paroxetine binding (Meltzer et al., 1998). Thus, it appears that the 5–HT axonal plexus is unaffected by normal aging, despite the previously discussed age-related decline in the density of postsynaptic serotonin receptors. In gonadectomized male and female rats, chronic administration of estradiol benzoate decreased ^{3}H-paroxetine binding in several regions of hippocampus, but not neocortex (Mendelson et al., 1993). For some of the regions, the effect was greater in the female rats than in the males. Since blockade at 5–HT uptake has an antidepressant effect, the fact that chronic estradiol administration was associated with reduced serotonin transporter density is consistent with the theory that estrogen has an antidepressant effect. On the other hand, a more recent study showed that the injection of estradiol benzoate into acutely ovariectomized female rats significantly increased 5–HT transporter levels in several regions of the brain, including lateral septum, basolateral amygdala, ventral nucleus of thalamus and ventromedial hypothalamic nucleus. Estrogen produced a slight reduction in paroxetine binding in periaqueductal central grey (McQueen et al., 1997). In the same study, 5–HT transporter mRNA expression was increased in the dorsal raphe. The discrepancy between the findings of the Mendelson and McQueen studies might be due to the difference between acute and chronic gonadectomy or to the regions of the brain that were studied. Basic evidence supports the possibility that estrogen modulates the serotonergic system at the 5–HT1A and 5–HT2A receptors and the 5–HT transporter. The interaction of estrogen and 5–HT2A receptors provides the strongest evidence for an antidepressant effect of estrogen being mediated by serotonin.

Clinical evidence

Clinical research suggests that estrogen increases serotonergic functioning as measured by peripheral and central markers. Preliminary data on central markers will be discussed below. Non-depressed women who had undergone bilateral oophorectomy were given supraphysiologic doses of estrogen in order to study the relationship between depressive symptoms, estrogen levels and platelet ^{3}H-imipramine binding (Sherwin & Suranyi-Cadotte, 1990). Non-depressed premenopausal women treated with a gonadotropin releasing hormone agonist for 12 days had decreased estradiol levels and an increase in depressive symptoms (Eyal et al., 1996). ^{3}H-imipramine binding to platelets decreased in association with the decrease in estradiol levels and increase in depressive symptoms. Although all mood scores were in the normal range for both studies above, higher estrogen levels were associated with a more positive mood and increased ^{3}H-imipramine binding. In postmenopausal women, oral and transdermal estradiol produced increases in urinary 5-hydroxyindole acetic acid levels (5–HIAA, a serotonin metabolite; Lippert et al., 1996). Estrogen replacement augments the cortisol response to the serotonergic agonist *m*-CPP (metachlorophenylpiperzine) in postmenopausal women, which suggests estrogen increases serotonin responsivity (Halbreich et al., 1995).

Estrogen and serotonergic antidepressant response

Whether estrogen increases serotonergic antidepressant efficacy in postmenopausal women is not yet clear, although a retrospective analysis of sertraline response in depressed postmenopausal women suggested that estrogen may improve serotonin-specific reuptake inhibitor (SSRI) response in this population. Two large studies of fluoxetine for late life major depressive disorder did not achieve good remission rates on intent to treat analysis (35% and 21%; Roose & Suthers, 1998) Sertraline achieved better response rates in other studies (51% and 45% in a chronic major depression study; Roose & Suthers, 1998). Geriatric psychiatrists have been debating about whether the antidepressant response to SSRIs is less in aged populations and whether estrogen status makes a difference in the antidepressant response of postmenopausal women. The available data is retrospective and has limitations. In a retrospective analysis of a large multicenter study of geriatric women with major depression treated with the selective serotonin reuptake inhibitor fluoxetine for 6 weeks, women on estrogen replacement therapy (ERT) experienced greater fluoxetine–placebo difference than women not on estrogen (Schneider et al., 1997). These data are difficult to interpret. The fluoxetine women did not respond well to fluoxetine, whether they were on ERT (41.9% clinical response) or they were not (35.7%). The fluoxetine–placebo difference in the women on ERT was driven by a low placebo response in the women on estrogen (17.1%). In another retrospective analysis of the antidepressant response in postmenopausal (aged 60 or older) depressed women who participated in one of two multicenter studies of sertraline, women on estrogen alone ($N = 34$, women taking medroxyprogesterone were excluded) were compared with women who were not on estrogen ($N = 93$). In this analysis, estrogen appeared to increase response to sertraline as assessed by CGI (Clinical Global Impression Improvement Scale) and Hamilton Depression (HAM-D) scores ≤ 7 (Schneider et al., 1998). Seventy nine percent of women on estrogen were responders to sertraline by CGI at endpoint compared with 58% women on sertraline without estrogen ($P = 0.04$). Forty-nine percent of women on estrogen were sertraline responders by HAM-D compared with 32% women without estrogen (P value borderline at 0.092). Thus, the presence of estrogen may be important to serotonergic antidepressant response in postmenopausal women, but prospective studies of estrogen vs. placebo combined with a serotonergic antidepressant are needed.

Imaging data

Functional imaging data suggests that women may have lower rates of serotonin synthesis than men and that ERT may increase 5–HT2 receptor binding in postmenopausal women. Functional imaging techniques, including PET and SPECT (single photon emission tomography), permit in vivo characterization of regional blood flow, cerebral metabolism (PET only), neuroreceptor and transporter concentration, and neurotransmitter synthesis in normal aging and in depressive states (Meltzer et al., 1998). For PET, there are now specific radioligands: [^{18}F]altanserin for selective 5–HT2A receptor ligand, [^{11}C]WAY-100635 5–HT1A receptor marker, and [^{11}C]McN-5652X, a highly potent blocker of the 5HT reuptake site (Meltzer et al., 1998). [^{11}C]methyl-L-tryptophan has been used as a PET tracer to measure serotonin synthesis in human brain (Nishikawa et al., 1997). The mean rate of serotonin synthesis is 52% higher in the brains of young adult men compared with young women (Nishizawa et al., 1997). Female subjects not only had a lower baseline serotonin synthesis rate compared to men, but demonstrated a significantly reduced rate of serotonin synthesis after tryptophan depletion. Thus the differential regulation of serotonin synthesis may contribute to the increased vulnerability of women to depressive disorders. There is limited experience with direct imaging of 5–HT receptors in patients with depression. With SPECT, there is increased 5–HT2A receptor binding (measured by [^{123}I]ketanserin) in the parietal cortex of depressed subjects compared to controls (D'Haenen et al., 1992). With PET, there is a preliminary study of eight patients (women and men, mean age = 48 years) with major depression who were compared with 22 controls using [^{18}F]altanserin to assess 5–HT2A receptor binding (Biver et al., 1997). The subjects with major depression were found to have decreased [^{18}F]altanserin uptake in the right orbito-insular cortex compared to controls. Preliminary unpublished data from the University of Pittsburgh demonstrated a possible estrogen effect on serotonin in one postmenopausal euthymic woman on no medications in her early 50s (G. Smith, B. Pollack & E. Moses, personal communication, 10/98). Three [^{18}F]altanserin scans were performed: prior to ERT, after 8 weeks of estradiol 1 mg, and after 2 weeks of combined estradiol/progestin (medroxyprogesterone 10 mg/day) treatment. The study is ongoing but in this one subject the following brain regions showed an increase greater than 20% in [^{18}F]altanserin binding after 10 weeks of hormone treatment: lateral temporal association, lateral orbitofrontal, orbitofrontal, parietal and sensimotor cortices. These findings, if confirmed, suggest that ERT may upregulate central 5–HT2 receptors in postmenopausal women.

Clinical data suggests that estrogen increases serotonergic function at least in women with low estrogen. Low serotonin may contribute to the increased vulnerability of women to affective disorders. The beneficial effects of estrogen on mood, if present, appear to be mild.

Estrogen and norepinephrine

Estrogen's effects on mood through changes in noradrenergic function have received less attention. Circulating estrogen concentrations influences the release of norepinephrine within specific hypothalamic nuclei (Simonian & Herbison, 1997). ERT in postmenopausal women significantly decreases plasma norepinephrine (Blum et al., 1996). The effect of estrogen alone and estrogen plus progesterone on the expression of the norepinephrine transporter (NET) was examined in the locus coeruleus (LC) of ovariectomized monkeys (Schutzer & Bethea, 1997). Expression of mRNA for NET was unchanged in the LC due to either steroid treatment. In addition, the noradrenergic neurons of the primate LC lack nuclear receptors for ovarian steroids. Estrogen affects norepinephrine release in the hypothalamus and the periphery. Estrogen does not affect expression of norepinephrine transporter in the LC of a primate.

ERT is known to affect levels of monoamine oxidase (MAO), the enzyme that degrades catecholamines and serotonin. Most literature has suggested that estrogen is a MAO inhibitor (Klaiber et al., 1979; Holsboer et al., 1983). In a study of non-depressed postmenopausal women (mean age = 53.3), 60% of women had increases in platelet MAO activity and 40% had decreases during HRT compared with placebo (Klaiber et al., 1996). Women with short menopause duration and high pretreatment serum testosterone levels were more likely to have increased MAO activity. Platelet MAO activity was inversely correlated with scores on the Hamilton Depression scale after two cycles of HRT ($r = -0.36$, $P < 0.05$). Estrogen's salutory effects on mood may result from inhibition of MAO.

Nitric oxide

Preliminary data suggest that increased nitric oxide release may be involved in the beneficial mood effects of estrogen in some depressed postmenopausal women. ERT demonstrated mood improvement in a randomized, double blind, placebo-controlled, study for depression in postmenopausal women described above. (Lopez-Jaramillo et al., 1996). Nitric oxide (NO) metabolites (NO_2 and NO_3) were measured before and after treatment. There was a significant increase in the sum of the levels of the two subunits in the estrogen group (from 138.3 μmole/l $\pm$ 11.8 to 161.8 $\pm$ 15.2, $P < 0.05$) and no significant change or baseline differences in the placebo group. The significance of these findings for the possible antidepressant effect of estrogen is not clear but NO has many neuromodulatory functions in the central and peripheral nervous systems. It is thought to play a role in memory by mediating long-term potentiation at certain glutamatergic synapses in the hippocampus (Moncada & Higgs, 1993). In the rat hypothalamus, neurons expressing nitric oxide synthase mRNA are located in close proximity to neurons expressing GnRH mRNA (Grossman et al., 1994). Estrogen's beneficial effects on coronary vasculature are thought to be partly mediated through an increase in NO and will be discussed more below (Best et al., 1998). The preliminary report of Lopez-Jaramillo suggests that, in the subset of postmenopausal depressed women who experience mood improvement with ERT, increased nitric oxide levels may be involved.

Interactions between estrogen and other hormones in regulating mood

Progestin

Mood effects of progestins have clinical importance to a discussion of the mood effects of estrogens. Progestins are prescribed to postmenopausal women on ERT to prevent endometrial cancer that has been associated with unopposed estrogen.

Certain metabolites of progesterone are known to bind to the GABA–A receptor and produce sedative effects. Progestins have been noted to produce dysphoric effects in some women (Sherwin, 1991). However, there has been little study of the mood effects of progestins.

Medroxyprogesterone alone did not appear to decrease mood in a small study of young postmenopausal women (median age = 54; Prior, 1994). In a preliminary study, varying doses (25 to 100 mg) of IM progesterone were given to premenopausal and postmenopausal women (deWit, 1998). Postmenopausal women reported sedative effects from progesterone while premenopausal women noted little effect. Both groups had comparable plasma progesterone concentrations. This suggests that postmenopausal women may be more sensitive to the sedative effects of progesterone. A meta-analysis of the effect of hormone replacement therapy on depressed mood suggested that while estrogen alone demonstrated a moderate effect in reducing depressed mood (effect size (ES) = 0.69), progesterone alone (ES = 0.39) and in combination with estrogen (ES = 0.45) was associated with smaller reductions in depressed mood (Zweifel & O'Brien, 1997). The mean age for subjects in this meta-analysis was very young, 49.5 years, and thus may not be generalizable to older women. Progestins alone may not cause mood deterioration in aging women. Prior estrogen exposure may be required for adverse mood effects. The impact of progestins in the oldest postmenopausal women and the degree to which progestins cause a decline in mood requires further study.

The role of the HPA and HPG axes in mood

Hypothalamic–pituitary–adrenal (HPA) axis function and hypothalamic–pituitary–gonadal (HPG) function are closely intertwined, with the HPA axis inhibiting the HPG axis and products of the HPG axis increasing corticotropin releasing hormone (CRH) production. Products of the HPA axis directly inhibit the HPG axis, through inhibition of gonadotropins and GnRH release (Handa et al., 1994). Estradiol increases CRH production (Vamvakopoulos & Chrousos, 1994). CRH inhibits the GnRH neuron of the hypothalamic arcuate nucleus via beta-endorphin (Ferin et al., 1984). Thus estradiol is likely to inhibit GnRH through this mechanism. HPA axis and HPG axis interaction will be discussed further in Chapter 13, 'Estrogens, stress, and psychoneuroimmunology in women over the lifespan' and Chapter 14, 'Gender differences in immune function at the cellular level.' There seems to be a connection among affective illness, female sex and abnormalities in the cortisol, thyroid and gonadal axes (Whybrow, 1993). Whybrow suggested that the connection may lie in a gene c-erb, located on chromosome 17. C-erb is part of a 'super-family' of genes that encode steroid receptors, including those for estradiol, cortisol and thyroid hormones. The thyroid responsive element that is necessary for the modulation of transcription of target genes has a nearly identical sequence to that of the estrogen responsive element (Whybrow, 1993). Thus, there is a potential for 'cross-talk' among the receptors and their genes.

Systemic effects of estrogen replacement therapy

Physiology and biochemistry of estrogen

Genomic and non-genomic actions of estrogen

The hormonal effects of estrogen and its metabolites are complex and involve both genomic and non-genomic actions of estrogen and estrogen metabolites. The genomic actions are slow, while the non-genomic actions appear to be immediate. Estrogen acts on target cells or tissues by binding to intracellular estrogen receptor (ER) proteins. Aided by estrogen response elements, the hormone–receptor complex then binds to DNA sites within the cell nucleus, altering messenger RNA (mRNA) transcription, mediating protein synthesis, and thereby regulating physiological response (Nelson, 1995; Lindsay et al., 1997). The discovery that anti-estrogens can selectively stimulate or inhibit different gene encoding activities suggests the presence of multiple transcriptional pathways and novel estrogen response elements that modulate hormone-receptor binding to DNA, as well as the possibility of estrogen receptor subtypes (Bryant & Dere, 1998). Estrogen-mediated delayed genomic responses take minutes to hours to become apparent (Lindsay et al., 1997). However, the ability of estrogen to exert immediate (milliseconds to minutes) effects on target organs has led to the exploration of non-genomic pathways of action. These non-transcriptional pathways include binding to membrane receptors and activation of second messenger systems (Moss et al., 1997).

Estrogen metabolism

A knowledge of estrogen metabolic pathways is important, not only to understand the mechanisms by which this hormone is inactivated, but because some of the metabolites of estrogen also have biological activity, although their importance is not yet fully understood. A potent C-18 steroid hormone, estrogen is produced by the aromatization (enzymatic cleaving of carbon atoms) of testosterone and androstenedione. Aromatization of androgens to estrogens occurs most extensively in the ovaries but aromatase activity is also present in the brain, liver, adipose tissue, fibroblasts and mammary glandular cells (Zhu & Conney, 1998). Ultimate control of gonadal hormone production lies in the hypothalamically induced release of tropic hormones, such as LH and FSH, from the anterior pituitary. Estrogenic hormones are metabolized in the liver through oxidative and conjugative metabolism.

The major enzymes catalyzing β-nicotinamide adenine dinucleotide phosphate (NADPH)-dependent hydroxylation of estrogens are the cytochrome P450 enzymes (Zhu & Conney, 1998). Some P450 isoforms are also available in extrahepatic tissue, including the mammary gland, uterus and brain, for metabolism of endogenous estrogens (estradiol and estrone; Zhu & Conney, 1998). Research suggests that estrogen metabolites in, or near, these target tissues may intensify and/or facilitate the actions of estrogens by mechanisms that are not understood. C-2 estradiol metabolites have demonstrated relatively little activity, while the C-4 and C-16 metabolites had similar potency to estradiol (Martucci & Fishman, 1993). Different estrogen metabolites have different biological activities, some even producing carcinogenic effects on certain tissues (Zhu & Conney, 1998; Martucci & Fishman, 1993).

Symptoms of menopause

The average life expectancy for women in the United States is 80 years. Thus, a woman may spend one-third of her life or more in the hypoestrogenic postmenopausal state. By the year 2000, one-third of all women in the United States will be postmenopausal (Diaz-Brinton, 1998). In the next 20 years, 40 million women will be postmenopausal (Diaz-Brinton, 1998). The CNS and peripheral effects of low estrogen levels, therefore, have significant public health importance. The physical symptoms of menopause – hot flushes or flashes, vaginal dryness, and urinary incontinence – are a direct result of declining levels of estrogen. The hot flush is a hypothalamic response resulting from a change in estrogen status. There are hormonal correlates of flush activity, such as an increase in serum LH and plasma pro-opiomelanocortin (POMC) peptides (such as adrenocorticotropin hormone), but these occurrences are thought to be epiphenomena and not related to its origin (Lobo, 1997). Mental symptoms associated with menopause – sleep disturbances, mood swings, depression, anxiety, and memory problems – are also attributed to estrogen deficiency. Estrogen replacement therapy (ERT) is also used for treatment of menopause and has become a standard treatment for women undergoing oophorectomy to ease the abrupt hormonal transition of surgical menopause.

Effects of estrogen on peripheral target tissues

Estrogen's role in the prevention of heart disease (CAD) and osteoporosis has established the importance of estrogen replacement in the maintenance of health in postmenopausal women. The effects of various estrogens on different tissues are summarized in Table 5.1. Estrogen protects women against coronary heart disease by favorable alteration of lipids (Guetta et al., 1997) and vasodilatation of the coronary arteries through an increase in nitric oxide (Guetta et al., 1997; Best et al., 1998). However, estrogen does not appear to prevent myocardial infarction in

Table 5.1. Tissue-specific actions of estrogens

Estrogen type	Brand names	Cardio-vascular effects	Skeletal effects	CNS effects	Mammary tissue	Uterine tissue
Estradiol		Agonist	Agonist	Agonist	Agonist	Agonist
Oral	Estrace					
Injectable	DepGynogen					
Topical	Estraderm					
Vaginal	Estrace					
Conjugated estrogens		Agonist	Agonist	Agonist	Agonist	Agonist
Oral	Premarin					
Injectable						
Vaginal						
Estrone		Agonist	Agonist	Agonist	Agonist	Agonist
Injectable	Gynogen					
Vaginal	Oestrilin					
Ethinyl estradiol		Agonist	Agonist	Agonist	Agonist	Agonist
Oral	Estinyl					
Antiestrogens SERMs	ICI-164, 384	Antagonist	Antagonist	Unknown	Antagonist	Antagonist
Oral	Tamoxifen	Agonist	Agonist	?Agonist	Antagonist	Partial agonist
	Raloxifene	Agonist	Agonist	?Weak agonist or weak antagonist	Antagonist	Antagonist

women with established coronary artery disease (Hulley et al., 1998). Estrogen prevents bone loss associated with osteoporosis by decreasing bone resorption (Lindsay et al., 1997). Data increasingly suggest that ERT reduces the risk of colon cancer (Calle et al., 1995; Griffing, 1998). Finally, estrogen also increases collagen (the elasticizing agent of skin), thereby reversing vaginal hypertrophy, and possibly preventing urinary incontinence (Griffing, 1998).

Estrogen replacement therapy regimens

There is a wide variety of ERT regimens with equivalent effectiveness. These include oral tablets, transdermal patches, subcutaneous injections and implants, and percutaneous gels or creams, all of which deliver varying concentrations of estradiol or estrone. Oral estrogens are the most commonly prescribed and consist of conjugated (for example, Premarin) or esterified (for example, Estratab) estrogens. Therapeutic doses range from 0.3 to 1.25 mg/day. Because oral estrogens are first metabolized in the liver, transdermal and subcutaneous preparations more closely resemble endogenous hormone activity. Transdermal patches are more expensive than oral forms. Alternatively, local estrogen preparations such as creams, pessaries, and vaginal inserts can help relieve local dryness and atrophy but they have negligible systemic effects. Finally, subcutaneous injections and implants are quite effective, elevating hormone levels well beyond premenopausal ranges.

Risks and benefits of hormone replacement therapy

The major concerns of women taking estrogen replacement therapy (ERT) are the long-term risk of breast cancer and the inconvenience of vaginal bleeding in those women who have not had a hysterectomy. Most side effects associated with estrogen therapy, such as breast tenderness or enlargement, bloating, nausea, and headache, resolve within approximately 2 months (McKinney & Thompson, 1998). The irritation or rash experienced by 10% of transdermal patch users is easily managed. However, the more serious side effects, such as exacerbation of gallbladder disease and development of blood clots, require careful monitoring. Supraphysiologic levels of estrogen (as in the case of postmenopausal women on ERT) can precipitate endometrial hyperplasia and/or uterine cancer. Therefore, non-hysterectomized women must supplement ERT with progestin to stimulate endometrial shedding and reverse the propagative effects of estrogen. Progestin may be added to the ERT regimen either cyclically or continuously. Cyclic hormone replacement therapy regimens consist of 2 to 10 weeks of estrogen alone followed by 10 to 14 days of progestin and estrogen combined. The progestin produces withdrawal bleeding monthly or quarterly, depending on the length of the cycle. Withdrawal bleeding can complicate ERT compliance. Therefore, continuous combined estrogen–progestogen therapies have been developed to prevent cyclic bleeding. ERT may cause bleeding in 40% to 60% of patients in the first 6 months of treatment (Archer et al., 1994), but amenorrhea is usually achieved in 70% of patients after 1 year (Lindsay et al., 1997). Although the addition of progesterone to ERT regimens actually reduces a woman's chances of developing uterine cancer, patients should have annual pelvic exams. Similarly, women on ERT need annual mammograms to monitor the potential development of breast cancer.

Compliance with ERT

Approximately 40% of women who are eligible to take ERT actually do so, with the average duration of use being only 9 months (Lindsay et al., 1997). Compliance among these women is poor for several reasons. The most compelling deterrent to ERT use is fear of breast cancer (Mitlak & Cohen, 1997). Controversy remains as to whether postmenopausal ERT increases the risk of breast cancer. A review of the literature proposes that large doses and prolonged administration (20+ years) are required to induce breast cancer (Zumoff, 1998; McKinney & Thompson, 1998); some experts, however, find the risk greater (Colditz, 1998). Another obstacle to compliance is the reluctance to endure the withdrawal bleeding that is associated with cyclic estrogen/progestogen regimens (Mitlak & Cohen, 1997). Women who have had a hysterectomy are significantly (79%) more likely to comply with ERT than women with an intact uterus (43%; Salamone & Cauley, 1997). Taking ERT to prevent coronary artery disease and osteoporosis is likely to be a lifelong commitment. The patient must be educated regarding the risks and benefits of hormone therapy as it applies specifically to her, and assisted in the choice of ERT that best suits her preferences.

Conclusions

Depressive symptoms and minor depressions can cause disability in aging populations. Several lines of evidence suggest that estrogen may improve depressive symptoms, particularly in perimenopausal women who have demonstrated previous vulnerability to changes in estrogen levels. Whether estrogen is an effective treatment for a majority of non-major depressive disorders in postmenopausal women remains to be determined. Moreover, the role of estrogen in the regulation of mood in very old women may be different from its role in early postmenopausal women because of physiological changes brought about by a prolonged hypoestrogenic state. Discrepancies regarding the role of sex steroids in depression relate in part to the complexity of interactions among the various sex steroids and between them and other hormonal and neurotransmitter systems. A more detailed understanding of these interactions and more rigorous prospective clinical trials will be needed in order to determine whether manipulations of estrogens and other sex steroids can be effectively used in the treatment of depression and other mental illnesses in aging populations.

ACKNOWLEDGMENT

Supported in part by NIMH Grant KO7 MH01038 (Morrison, PI) and NIH Grant 5M01 RR00040 (W Kelley, PI).

REFERENCES

Appleby, L., Montgomery, J. & Studd, J. (1981). Oestrogens and affective disorders. *Progress in Obstetrics and Gynaecology*, ed. J. Studd, pp. 289–302. Edinburgh: Churchill-Livingstone.

Archer, D., Pickar, J. & Bottiglioni, F. (1994). Bleeding patterns in postmenopausal women taking continuous combined or sequential regimens of conjugated estrogens with medroxyprogesterone acetate: the Menopause Study Group. *Obstetrics and Gynecology*, **83**(5), 686–92.

Azcoitia, I., Wright, N., Chowen, J. & Garcia-Segura, L. (1998). Estradiol prevents hippocampal neuronal death induced by kainate. *European Journal of Neuroscience*, **10**(10), 202.

Beekman, A. T., Deeg, D. J., Braam, A. W., Smit, J. H. & Tilburg, W. V. (1997). Consequences of major and minor depression in later life: a study of disability, well-being and service utilization. *Psychological Medicine*, **27**, 1397–409.

Best, P., Berger, P. B., Miller, V. & Lerman, A. (1998). The effect of estrogen replacement therapy on plasma nitric oxide and endothelin-1 levels in postmenopausal women. *Annals of Internal Medicine*, **128**, 285–8.

Biver, F., Wikler, D., Lotstra, F., Damhaut, P., Goldman, S. , Mendlewicz, J. (1997). Serotonin 5–HT2 receptor imaging in major depression: focal changes in orbito-insular cortex. *British Journal of Psychiatry*, **171**, 444–8.

Blazer, D., Hughes, D. & George, L. (1987). The epidemiology of depression in an elderly community population. *The Gerontologist*, **27**(3), 281–7.

Blum, I., Vered, Y., Lifshitz, A., Harel, D., Blum, M., Nordenberg, Y. et al. (1996). The effect of estrogen replacement therapy on plasma serotonin and catecholamines of postmenopausal women. *Israel Journal of Medical Sciences*, **32**, 1158–62.

Breuer, B., Wallenstein, S. & Anderson, R. (1998). *The Effects of Tamoxifen on Independence in ADLs and the Risk of Developing Alzheimers Disease in Nursing Home Residents*. Philadelphia: Gerontological Society of America.

Brinton, R., Proffitt, P., Tran, J. & Luu, R. (1997). Equilin, a principal component of the estrogen replacement therapy premarin, increases the growth of cortical neurons via an NMDA receptor-dependent mechanism. *Experimental Neurology*, **147**, 211–20.

Broadhead, W., Blazer, D., George, L. & Tse, C. (1990). Depression, disability days, and days lost from work in a prospective epidemiologic survey. *Journal of the American Medical Association*, **264**(19), 2524–8.

Bryant, H.U. & Dere, W. H. (1998). Selective estrogen receptor modulators: an alternative to hormone replacement therapy. *Society for Experimental Biology and Medicine*, **217**, 45–52.

Burvill, P. W. (1995). Recent progress in the epidemiology of major depression. *Epidemiologic Reviews*, **17**(1), 21–31.

Calle, E. E., Miracle-McMahill, H. L., Thun, M. J. & Heath, C. W. (1995). Estrogen replacement therapy and risk of fatal colon cancer in a prospective cohort of postmenopausal women. *Journal of the National Cancer Institute*, **87**(7), 517–23.

Cathcart, C., Jones, S., Pumroy, C., Peters, G., Knox, S. & Cheek, J. (1993). Clinical recognition and management of depression in node negative breast cancer patients treated with tamoxifen. *Breast Cancer Research and Treatment*, **27**(3), 277–81.

Colditz, G. A. (1998). Relationship between estrogen levels, use of hormone replacement therapy, and breast cancer. *Journal of the National Cancer Institute*, **90**, 814–23.

deWit, H. (1998). *Mood effects of acute progesterone administration in women with normal menstrual cycles and in post-menopausal women*. American College of Neuropsychopharmacology, Las Croabas, Puerto Rico.

D'Haenen, H., Bossuyt, A., Mertens, J., Bossuyt-Piron, C., Gijsemans, M. & Kaufman, L. (1992). SPECT imaging of serotonin-2 receptors in depression. *Psychiatry Research*, 45(4), 227–37.

Diaz-Brinton, R. (1998). *Neurotropic action of estrogen replacement therapy: mechanisms for the maintenance and restoration of memory function in postmenopausal women*. American College of Neuropsychopharmacology, Las Croabas, Puerto Rico.

Eaton, W. W., Anthony, J. C., Gallo, J. C., Cai, G., Tien, A., Romanski, A., Lyketsos, C. & Chen, L. S. (1997). Natural history of diagnostic interview schedule/DSM-IV major depression: the Baltimore epidemiologic catchment area follow-up. *Archives of General Psychiatry*, 54, 993–9.

Eyal, S., Weizman, A., Toren, P., Dor, Y., Mester, R. & Rehavi, M. (1996). Chronic GnRH agonist administration down-regulates platelet serotonin transporter in women undergoing assisted reproductive treatment. *Psychopharmacology*, 125(2), 141–5.

Ferin, M., Van Vugt, D. & Wardlaw, S. (1984). The hypothalamic control of the menstrual cycle and the role of endogenous opioid peptides. *Recent Progress in Hormone Research*, 40, 441–85.

Fink, G. & Sumner, B. E. H. (1996). Oestrogen and mental state. *Nature*, 383(Sept. 26), 306.

Fink, G., Sumner, B., McQueen, J., Wilson, H. & Rosie, R. (1998). Central serotonin mechanisms affected by sex steroids: relevance for mood, mental state and memory. *Journal of Physiology*, 509.P, 17S–18S.

Fink, G., Sumner, B. E., Rosie, R., Grace, O. & Quinn, J. P. (1996). Estrogen control of central neurotransmission: effect on mood, mental state, and memory. *Cellular and Molecular Neurobiology*, 16(3), 325–44.

Fisher, B., Costantino, J., Wickerham, D., Redmond, C., Kavanah, M., Cronin, W., Vogel, V., Robidoux. A., Dimitrov, N., Atkins, J., Daly, M., Wieland S., Tan-Dhiu, Ford, L. & Wolkomooten (1998). Tamoxifen for prevention of breast cancer: Report of the National Surgical Adjuvant Breast and Bowel P-1 Study. *Journal of the National Cancer Institute*, 90, 1371–88.

Green, P., Bishop, J. & Simpkins, J. (1997). 17 alpha-estradiol exerts neuroprotective effects on SK-N-SH cells. *The Journal of Neuroscience*, 17(2), 511–15.

Griffing, G. T. (1998). Postmenopausal HRT: do benefits continue to outweigh the risk? *Clinical Geriatrics*, 6(5), 50–8.

Grossman, A. B., Rossmanith, W. G., Kabigting, E. B., Cadd, G., Clifton, D. & Steiner, R. A. (1994). The distribution of hypothalamic nitric oxide synthase mRNA in relation to gonadotrophin-releasing hormone neurons. *Journal of Endocrinology*, 140(2), R5–8.

Guetta, V., Quyyumi, A. A., Prasad, A., Panza, J., Myron, W. & Cannon, R. O. (1997). The role of nitric oxide in coronary vascular effects of estrogen in postmenopausal women. *Circulation*, 96(9), 2795–801.

Halbreich, U. (1990). Gonadal hormones and antihormones, serotonin and mood. *Psychopharmcology Bulletin*, 26(3), 291–5.

Halbreich, U. (1997). Role of estrogen in postmenopausal depression. *Neurology*, 48, S16–19.

Halbreich, U., Rojansky, N., Palter, S., Tworek, H., Hissin, P. & Wang, K. (1995). Estrogen augments serotonergic activity in postmenopausal women. *Biological Psychiatry*, 37, 434–41.

Handa, R. J., Burgess, L. H., Kerr, J. E. & O'Keefe, J. A. (1994). Gonadal steroid hormone receptors and sex differences in the hypothalamo-pituitary-adrenal axis. *Hormones and Behavior*, 28(4), 464–76.

Hen, R. (1998). *Increased anxiety in mice lacking the 5–HT$_{1A}$ receptor*. American College of Neuropsychopharmacology, Las Croabas, Puerto Rico.

Holsboer, F., Benkert, O. & Demisch, L. (1983). Changes in MAO activity during estrogen treatment of females with endogenous depression. *Modern Problems in Pharmacopsychiatry*, 19, 321–26.

Hulley, S., Grady, D., Bush, T., Furberg, C., Herrington, D., Riggs, B., Vittinghoff, E. et al. (1998). Randomized trial of estrogen plus progestin for secondary prevention of coronary heart disease in postmenopausal women. Heart and Estrogen/progestin Replacement Study (HERS) Research Group [see comments]. *Journal of the American Medical Association*, 280(7), 605–13.

Joffe, H. & Cohen, L. S. (1998). Estrogen, serotonin, and mood disturbance: What is the therapeutic bridge? *Biological Psychiatry*, 44(9), 798–811.

Judd, L., Rapaport, M., Paulus, M. & Brown, J. (1994). Subsyndromal symptomatic depression: a new mood disorder? *Journal of Clinical Psychiatry*, 55(4), 18–28.

Kaufert, P. A., Gilbert, P. & Tate, R. (1992). The Manitoba Project: a re-examination of the link between menopause and depression [see comments]. *Maturitas*, 14(2), 143–55.

Kendall, D., Stancel, G. & Enna, S. (1981). Imipramine: Effect of ovarian steroids on modifications in serotonin receptor binding. *Science*, 211, 1183–5.

Kendall, D., Stancel, G. & Enna, S. (1982). The influence of sex hormones on anti-depressant induced alterations in neurotransmitter receptor binding. *Journal of Neuroscience*, 2(3), 354–60.

Klaiber, E., Broverman, D., Vogel, W. & Koyabashi, Y. (1979). Estrogen therapy for severe persistent depressions in women. *Archives of General Psychiatry*, 36, 550–4.

Klaiber, E. L., Broverman, D. M., Vogel, W., Peterson, L. G. & Snyder, M. B. (1996). Individual differences in changes in mood and platelet monamine oxidase (MAO) activity during hormonal replacement therapy in menopausal women. *Psychoneuroendocrinology*, 21(7), 575–92.

Lehtinen, V. & Joukamaa, M. (1994). Epidemiology of depression: prevalence, risk factors and treatment situation. *Acta Psychiatrica Scandinavica, Supplementum*, 377, 7–10.

Lindsay, R., Dempster, D. & Jordan, V. (ed.) (1997). *Estrogens and Antiestrogens: Basic and Clinical Aspects*. Philadelphia: Lippincott-Raven.

Lippert, T. H., Filshie, M., Muck, A. O., Seeger, H. & Zwirner, M. (1996). Serotonin metabolite excretion after postmenopausal estradiol therapy. *Maturitas*, 24(1–2), 37–41.

Lobo, R. A. (1997). The postmenopausal state and estrogen deficiency. *Estrogens and Antiestrogens*, ed. R. Lindsay, D. W. Dempster & W. C. Jordan, pp. 63–72. Philadelphia: Lippincott-Raven.

Lopez-Jaramillo, P., Teran, E., Molina, G., Rivera, J. & Lozano, A. (1996). Oestrogens and depression [letter]. *Lancet*, 348(9020), 135–6.

Love, R. R., Cameron, L., Connell, B. L. & Leventhal, H. (1991). Symptoms associated with tamoxifen treatment in post-menopausal women. *Archives of Internal Medicine*, 151, 1842–7.

Mann, J., Huang, Y., Oppenhein, S., Dwork, A., Kartachov, A., Underwood, M. et al. (1998). *Serotonin Candidate Gene Expression in Suicide and Major Depression*. American College of Neuropsychopharmacology, Las Croabas, Puerto Rico.

Martucci, C. & Fishman, J. (1993). P450 enzymes of estrogen metabolism. *Pharmacology and Therapeutics*, 57(2–3), 237–57.

Maswood, S., Stewart, G. & Uphouse, L. (1995). Gender and estrous cycle effects of the 5-HT$_{1A}$ Agonist, 8-OH-DPAT, on hypothalamic sertononin. *Pharmacology, Biochemistry and Behavior*, 51(4), 807-13.

McKinney, K. & Thompson, W. (1998). A practical guide to prescribing hormone replacement therapy. *Drugs*, 56(1), 49-57.

McQueen, J. K., Wilson, H. & Fink, G. (1997). Estradiol-17 beta increases serotonin transporter (SERT) mRNA levels and the density of SERT-binding sites in female rat brain. *Brain Research. Molecular Brain Research*. 45(1), 13-23.

Meltzer, C., Smith, G., DeKosky, S., Pollock, B., Mathis, C., Moore, R., Kupfer, D. J. & Reynolds, C. F. 3rd. (1998). Serotonin in aging, late-life depression, and Alzheimer's disease: the emerging role of functional imaging. *Neuropsychopharmacology*, 18(6), 407-30.

Mendelson, S. D., McKittrick, C. R. & McEwen, B. S. (1993). Autoradiographic analyses of the effects of estradiol benzoate on [^{3}H]paroxetine binding in the cerebral cortex and dorsal hippocampus of gonadectomized male and female rats. *Brain Research*, 601, 299-302.

Michael, C. M., Kantor, H. L. & Shore, H. (1970). Further psychometric evaluation of older women. The effect of estrogen administration. *Journal of Gerontology*, 25, 337-41.

Mitlak, B. & Cohen, F. (1997). In search of optimal long-term female hormone replacement: the potential of selective estrogen receptor modulators. *Hormone Research*, 48, 155-63.

Moncada, S. & Higgs, A. (1993). The L-arginine-nitric oxide pathway. *New England Journal of Medicine*, 329(27), 2002-12.

Moss, R., Gu, Q. & Wong, M. (1997). Estrogen: nontranscriptional signaling pathway. *Recent Progress in Hormone Research*, 52, 33-69.

Nelson, R. (1995). *An Introduction to Behavior Endocrinology*. Sunderland, Massachusetts: Sinauer Associates.

Nickelsen, T., Lufkin, E. G., Riggs, B. L., Cox, D. A. & Crook, T. H. (1998). Raloxifene hydrochloride, a selective estrogen receptor modulator: safety assessment of effects on cognitive function and mood in postmenopausal women. *Psychneuroendocrinology*, 24, 115-28.

Nishizawa, S., Benkelfat, C., Young, S. N., Leyton, M., Mzengeza, S., DeMontigny, C., Blier, P. & Diksic, M. (1997). Differences between males and females in rates of serotonin synthesis in human brain. *Proceedings of the National Academy of Sciences*, USA, 94, 5308-13.

Oppenheim, G. (1984). A case of rapid mood cycling with estrogen: implications for therapy. *Journal of Clinical Psychiatry*, 45(1), 34-5.

Osterlund, M. K. & Hurd, Y. L. (1998). Acute 17 beta-estradiol treatment down-regulates serotonin 5HT1A receptor mRNA expression in the limbic system of female rats. *Molecular Brain Research*, 55(1), 169-72.

Palinkas, L. & Barrett-Connor, E. (1992). Estrogen use and depressive symptoms in postmenopausal women. *Obstetrics and Gynecology*, 80, 30-6.

Parmelee, P., Katz, I. & Lawton, M. (1992). Incidence of depression in long term care settings. *Journal of Gerontology*, 47, M189-96.

Pecins-Thompson, M., Brown, N. & Bethea, C. (1998). Regulation of serotonin re-uptake transporter mRNA expression by ovarian steroids in rhesus macaques. *Molecular Brain Research*, 53, 120-9.

Pecins-Thompson, M., Brown, N. A., Kohama, S. G. & Bethea, C. L. (1996). Ovarian steroid regulation of trytophan hydroxylase mRNA expression in rhesus macaques. *Neuroscience,* 16(21), 7021–9.

Polo-Kantola, P., Erkkola, R., Helenius, H., Irjala, K. & Polo, O. (1998). When does estrogen replacement therapy improve sleep quality? *American Journal of Obstetrics and Gynecology,* 178, 1002–9.

Powles, T., Tillyer, C. R., Jones, A. L., Ashley, S. E., Treleaven, J., Davey, J. B., & McKinna, J. A. (1990). Prevention of breast cancer with tamoxifen – an update on the Royal Marsden Hospital Pilot Programme. *European Journal of Cancer,* 26, 680–4.

Prange, A., Wilson, I. C. & Alltop, L. B. (1972). Estrogen may well affect response to antidepressant. *Journal of the American Medical Association,* 219, 143–4.

Prior, J. C. (1994). No adverse effects of medroxyprogesterone treatment without estrogen in postmenopausal women: double-blind, placebo controlled, crossover trial. *Obstetrics and Gynecology,* 83, 24–8.

Rapaport, M. H. & Judd, L. L. (1998). Minor depressive disorder and subsyndromal depressive symptoms: functional impairment and response to treatment. *Journal of Affective Disorders,* 48, 227–32.

Rehavi, M., Sepcuti, H. & Weizman, A. (1987). Upregulation of imipramine binding and serotonin uptake by estradiol in female rat brain. *Brain Research,* 410, 135–9.

Romanoski, A. J., Folstein, M. F., Nestadt, G., Chahal, R., Merchant, A., Brown, C. H., Gruenberg, E. M. & McHugh, P. R. (1992). Ascertained depression and DSM-III depressive disorders. Results from the Eastern Baltimore Mental Health Survey Clinical Reappraisal. *Psychological Medicine,* 22, 629–55.

Roose, S. P. & Suthers, K. M. (1998). Antidepressant response in late-life depression. *Journal of Clinical Psychiatry,* 59(10), 4–8.

Salamone, L. M. & Cauley, J. A. (1997). Attitudinal barriers to estrogen replacement therapy in older women. *Clinical Geriatrics,* 5(9), 72–89.

Saletu, B., Brandstatter, N., Metka, M., Stamenkovic, M., Anderer, P., Semlitsch, H., Heytmanek, G., Huber, J., Grunberger, J., Linzmayer, L. (1995). Double-blind, placebo-controlled, hormonal, syndromal and EEG mapping studies with transdermal oestradiol therapy in menopausal depression. *Psychopharmacology,* 122(4), 321–9.

Schmidt, P., Ollo, C. & Rubinow, D. (1994). Neuropsychiatric effects of perimenopausal estrogen replacement. *Biological Psychology,* 35, 662.

Schneider, L. S., Small, G. & Clary, C. (1998). *Estrogen Replacement Therapy and Antidepressant Response to Sertraline.* Toronto, Canada: American Psychiatric Association.

Schneider, L. S., Small, G. W., Hamilton, S. H., Bystritsky, A., Nemeroff, C. B. & Meyers, B. S. (1997). Estrogen replacement and response to fluoxetine in a multicenter geriatric depression trial. Fluoxetine Collaborative Study Group. *American Journal of Geriatric Psychiatry,* 5(2), 97–106.

Schneider, M. A., Brotherton, P. L. & Hailes, J. (1977). The effects of exogenous estrogens on depression in menopausal women. *Medical Journal of Australia,* 2, 162–3.

Schutzer, W. E. & Bethea, C. L. (1997). Lack of ovarian steroid hormone regulation of norepinephrine transporter mRNA expression in the non-human primate locus coeruleus. *Psychoneuroendocrinology,* 22, 325–36.

Seeman, M. V. (1997). Psychopathology in women and men: focus on female hormones. *American Journal of Psychiatry*, 154, 1641–7.

Shariff, S., Cumming, C. E., Lees, A., Handman, M. & Cumming, D. C. (1995). Mood disorder in women with early breast cancer taking tamoxifen, an estradiol receptor antagonist. An expected or unexpected effect? *Annals of the New York Academy of Sciences*, 761, 365–8.

Sherwin, B. B. (1991). The impact of different doses of estrogen and progestin on mood and sexual behavior in postmenopausal women. *Clinics in Endocrinology and Metabolism*, 72, 336–43.

Sherwin, B. & Gelfand, M. (1985). Sex steroids and affect in the surgical menopause: a double-blind, cross-over study. *Psychoneuroendocrinology*, 10(3), 325–35.

Sherwin, B. & Suranyi-Cadotte, B. (1990). Up-regulatory effect of estrogen on platelet (3)H-imipramine binding sites in surgically menopausal women. *Biological Psychiatry*, 28, 339–48.

Simonian, S. X. & Herbison, A. E. (1997). Differential expression of estrogen receptor and neuro-peptide Y by brainstem A1 and A2 noradrenaline neurons. *Neuroscience*, 76, 517–29.

Simpkins, J. W., Green, P. S., Gridley, K. E., Singh, M., de Fiebre, N. C. & Rajakumar, G. (1997). Role of estrogen replacement therapy in memory enhancement and the prevention of neuro-nal loss associated with Alzheimer's disease. *American Journal of Medicine*, 103(3A), 19S–25S.

Sohrabji, F., Greene, L. A., Miranda, R. C. & Toran-Allerand, C. D. (1994). Reciprocal regulation of estrogen and NGF receptors by their ligands in PC12 cells. *Journal of Neurobiology*, 25(8), 974–88.

Stallones, L., Marx, M. & Garrity, T. (1990). Prevalence and correlates of depressive symptoms among older U.S. adults. *American Journal of Preventive Medicine*, 6(5), 295–303.

Sumner, B. & Fink, G. (1995). Estrogen increases the density of 5-hydroxytryptamine$_{2A}$ receptors in cerebral cortex and nucleus accumbens in the female rat. *Journal of Steroid Biochemistry and Molecular Biology*, 54, 15–20.

Toren, P., Dor, J., Rehavi, M. & Weizman, A. (1996). Hypothalamic–pituitary–ovarian axis and mood. *Biological Psychiatry*, 40(10), 1051–5.

Vamvakopoulos, N. C. & Chrousos, G. P. (1994). Hormonal regulation of human corticotropin-releasing hormone gene expression: implications for the stress response and immune/inflammatory reaction. *Endocrine Reviews*, 15(4), 409–20.

Weissman, M. M., Bland, R. C., Canino, G. J., Faravelli, C., Greenwald, S., Hwu, H., Joyce, P. R., Karam, E. G., Lee, C., Lellouch, J., Lepine, J. et al. (1996). Cross-national epidemiology of major depression and bipolar disorder. *Journal of the American Medical Association*, 276(4), 293–9.

Weissman, M. M., Bruce, M., Leaf, P., Florio, L. & Holzer, C. (1991). Affective Disorders. In *Psychiatric Disorders in America. The Epidemiologic Catchment Area Study*, ed. L. Robins & D. Regier, pp. 53–80. New York: The Free Press.

Whybrow, P. (1993). *Sex Differences in Thyroid Axis Function: Treatment Implications for Affective Disorders. Toward a New Psychobiology of Depression in Women, Treatment and Gender.* Washington, DC: NIMH.

Wiklund, I., Karlber, J. & Mattsson, L. A. (1993). Quality of life of postmenopausal women on a regimen of transdermal estradiol therapy: a double-blind placebo controlled study. *American Journal of Obstetrics and Gynecology*, 168, 824–30.

Woods, N. F. & Mitchell, E. S. (1996). Patterns of depressed mood in midlife women: observations from the Seattle Midlife Women's Health Study. *Research in Nursing and Health*, 19(2), 111–23.

Young, E. & Korszun, A. (1998). Psychoneuroendocrinology of depression. Hypothalamic–pituitary–gonadal axis. *Psychoneuroendocrinology*, 21(2), 309–23.

Young, R. C., Moline, M. & Kleyman, F. (1997). Hormone replacement therapy and late-life mania [see comments]. *American Journal of Geriatric Psychiatry*, 5(2), 179–81.

Zhu, B. & Conney, A. (1998). Functional role of estrogen metabolism in target cells: review and perspectives. *Carcinogenesis*, 19(1), 1–27.

Zumoff, B. (1998). Does postmenopausal estrogen administration increase the risk of breast cancer? Contributions of animal, biochemical, and clinical investigative studies to a resolution of the controversy. *Society for Experimental Biology and Medicine*, 1998(217), 30–5.

Zweifel, J. E. & O'Brien, W. H. (1997). A meta-analysis of the effect of hormone replacement therapy upon depressed mood. *Psychoneuroendocrinology*, 22(3), 189–212.

6

The role of testosterone in male depression

Stuart N. Seidman and Steven P. Roose

Introduction

Gonadal function declines with age in both men and women. The sequelae of female gonadal hypofunction are well characterized and substantial: a growing body of evidence implicates female hypogonadism (i.e. reduction in circulating estrogen) in the pathophysiology of mood disorders, Alzheimer's disease, osteoporosis, and heart disease in aging women (Paganini-Hill & Henderson, 1994; Tang et al., 1996; Grady et al., 1992; Robinson et al., 1994). Such knowledge, and the relative ease of estrogen replacement, has led to productive therapeutics research with important public health implications.

But there is no parallel characterization of the male hypothalamic–pituitary–gonadal (HPG) axis. Although it is now known that testosterone (T) secretion declines substantially with age (Araujo et al., 1998; Villareal & Morley, 1994; Dai et al., 1981; Field et al., 1994), the medical and psychiatric sequelae of normative gonadal hypofunction and the potential therapeutic implications are mostly unexplored. Moreover, since hypogonadism commonly presents as a neuropsychiatric symptom complex, delineation of the role of the HPG axis in the psychiatric problems of aging may be of particular relevance. For example, the suicide rate in elderly white males triples from the sixth decade to the ninth decade; in elderly women, it remains unchanged after age 40 (Meehan et al., 1991). It is possible that this difference is related to untreated hypogonadism among men. In this chapter, we will review studies of the psychiatric sequelae of testosterone hyposecretion; the relationship between testosterone secretion and late life depressive illness – particularly new onset depression or dysthymia, suicide, and/or subsyndromal affective symptoms; and the neurovegetative, cognitive, affective, and sexual effects of exogenous testosterone administration.

Overview

Testosterone secretion in adult men has multiple determinants, and this androgen has neurobehavioral and metabolic actions (Bagatell & Bremner, 1996). Central nervous system (CNS) effects include organizing and activating actions on male sexual arousal and behavior, and some influence on energy and mood (Rubinow & Schmidt, 1996). In animal models, testosterone plays a role in regulating male social behaviors, particularly those related to male–male competition, dominance, and submission.

Reduction in circulating testosterone, or hypogonadism, is a common clinical syndrome with multiple etiologies, including hypothalamic, pituitary, or testicular pathology. Its prevalence in young adult men is about 5%; in older men it is about five times more common (Field et al., 1994). Postpubertal onset of hypogonadism is characterized primarily by loss of libido and lack of vigor, reduced musculoskeletal mass, and impaired fertility (Plymate, 1994). Such sequelae are reversed with testosterone replacement. Administration of moderately supraphysiologic doses of exogenous testosterone to men with normal testosterone level (i.e. eugonadal men) has mood elevating and libido enhancing effects in some men (Pope Jr et al., in press). Because of such well-accepted psychiatric effects of low testosterone and excess testosterone, and because of a presumed relationship between major depressive disorder (MDD) and low testosterone, the use of exogenous androgens to treat MDD and/or the depressive symptoms that evolve with age (i.e. male 'climacteric') has long been an area of intense speculation and anecdote (Sternbach, 1998; Rubinow & Schmidt, 1996). As yet, very few studies have systematically addressed these psychoendocrine issues using rigorous neuropsychiatric methodology.

Clinically, these issues are complex. Hypogonadal men commonly complain of diminished libido, dysphoria, fatigue, irritability, and appetite loss, and these symptoms are alleviated by testosterone replacement (Villareal & Morley, 1994; Burris et al., 1992; Luisi & Franchi, 1980; Morley et al., 1993; Weinbauer et al., 1997; Laycock & Wise, 1996). Endocrinologists who treat hypogonadal men uniformly but anecdotally agree that such a psychiatric symptom-complex exists, and remits substantially with testosterone replacement. The existence of a psychiatric syndrome of hypogonadism, however, has not been established by systematic investigation in population-based samples of men or by double blind replacement studies. Furthermore, although the symptoms of major depression overlap with those of hypogonadism, it is not known what proportion of depressed men have blunted testosterone secretion, and in those who do, whether the hypogonadism or the depression is primary.

Methodologic problems

Research in male HPG psychoendocrinology has suffered from methodological deficiencies. First, andrologists have long recognized that the most prominent symptoms of male hypogonadism are low libido, fatigue, dysphoria, irritability, and disturbed memory and concentration, and that such symptoms appear to resolve after testosterone is replaced (Burris et al., 1992; Luisi & Franchi, 1980; Morley et al., 1993). Yet, no published endocrinological study has systematically assessed the neuropsychiatric implications of hypogonadism or testosterone replacement using rigorous methodology (i.e. structured psychiatric interviews, standardized instruments, and a sensitive neuropsychological battery). Second, few clinical trials have assessed the efficacy of exogenous androgens for male MDD. In the few androgen treatment trials that rigorously diagnosed and followed MDD, most used mesterolone (an oral androgen without DHT or estrogenic activity), and were further limited by small numbers and diagnostic heterogeneity. There have been no published clinical trials reporting the double blind administration of testosterone alone for MDD, or for MDD with hypogonadism.

Male HPG physiology

Testosterone secretion

The testes and adrenals secrete several male sex hormones, called androgens. All are steroid hormones, that is hormones derived from cholesterol and containing a basic skeleton of four fused carbon rings. Testosterone is the most potent and abundant androgen. It binds to the intranuclear androgen receptor, which is distributed widely throughout the body and the central nervous system (CNS), including limbic and cortical tissue (Weinbauer et al., 1997; Laycock & Wise, 1996). Neural activity in the medial basal hypothalamus–controlled by adrenergic, dopaminergic, serotonergic, and endorphinergic inputs, and the surrounding hormonal milieu – stimulates the pulsatile release of gonadotropin-releasing hormone (GnRH), a decapeptide, into the hypothalamic–hypophysial portal system. GnRH promotes anterior pituitary release of luteinizing hormone (LH) and follicle stimulating hormone (FSH). LH stimulates the interstitial cells of Leydig in the testes to synthesize and secrete testosterone. Secretion occurs in pulsatile bursts, about six per day, with a morning peak and an early evening trough; in total, approximately 7 mg of testosterone is secreted daily. Secretion is regulated through a negative feedback on the hypothalamus and pituitary (Weinbauer et al., 1997; Laycock et al., 1996).

In the bloodstream, testosterone is converted to other molecules or broken down; its half-life is about 20 minutes. Approximately 98% of testosterone molecules are protein bound. Of this, just over half are weakly bound to albumin, and the remainder are tightly bound to sex hormone-binding globulin (SHBG; Weinbauer et al., 1997; Laycock and Wise, 1996). SHBG, a β-globulin produced in the testes and the liver, consists of different protein subunits and one androgen binding site. Circulating free testosterone, the fraction which dissociates readily from albumin, and the fraction which dissociates less readily from SHBG (i.e., through molecular configuration changes in the capillaries), all diffuse into the target cell and bind to the androgen receptor (Weinbauer et al., 1997; Laycock and Wise, 1996). This receptor is a typical steroid receptor, containing an N-terminal domain, a DNA-binding domain and a hormone-binding domain (Weinbauer et al., 1997; Laycock and Wise, 1996). The steroid-receptor complex binds to specific sequences of genomic DNA, and thereby influences the production of messenger RNA that modulates synthesis of a wide array of enzymatic, structural, and receptor proteins (Weinbauer et al., 1997; Laycock and Wise, 1996). In addition, testosterone influences cellular activity in a nongenomic manner through activation of membrane receptors, second messengers, and/or the membrane itself (Weinbauer et al., 1997; Laycock and Wise, 1996). Such non-genomic actions may be especially important in the CNS (Schmidt & Rubinow, 1997; Rubinow & Schmidt, 1996).

In target cells, testosterone is converted to two active metabolites: dihydrotestosterone (DHT) and estradiol (E_2). There is tissue variability in the concentration of the cytoplasmic enzymes required for this conversion, 5α-reductase and aromatase, respectively, and differential tissue sensitivity to each of these metabolites. Both testosterone and DHT bind to the androgen receptor; some androgen-responsive genes respond preferentially to intracellular DHT, making it the more potent androgen. For example, DHT is required for testosterone's effects on external genitalia and accessory sex glands; 5α-reductase enzymes are, therefore, abundant in reproductive tissues and skin. Estradiol binds to the estrogen receptor, and may be required for some of testosterone's CNS and metabolic effects. Aromatase is most abundant in CNS, liver, and adipose tissue (Weinbauer et al., 1997; Laycock and Wise, 1996; Bagatell et al., 1996).

Psychological, social, seasonal, and biological factors affect testosterone secretion transiently. Testosterone levels are elevated at times of decisive victory in competition, when social status is enhanced, during REM sleep, during cigarette smoking, after sexual activity or exercise, and during the autumn. They are decreased at times of defeat or submission, during physical or emotional stress, during heavy alcohol use, and in the spring (Kreuz et al., 1972; Dai et al., 1981; Kemper, 1990). Stress and chronic illness may be particularly important negative influences on testosterone level in the elderly (Paganini-Hill & Henderson, 1994). Testosterone level typically reverts to baseline soon after transient stimuli, though there is some evidence from non-human primates that losing a fight precipitates a lowering of testosterone level that persists for weeks (Rose et al., 1975). Among young men placed in a shock incarceration ('boot camp') prison program, testosterone levels remained low for two months (Dabbs et al., 1996). It is unknown whether a chronic or prolonged stimulus (such as a major depressive episode, malnutrition, alcohol abuse, or chronic illness) can lead to a new testosterone set point.

Testosterone levels through life

Testosterone secretion varies through life. Prenatally, the genital ridge, and then testes, are stimulated by chorionic gonadotropin from the placenta to produce testosterone. Such secretion begins about the seventh week of embryonic life, peaks from weeks 9 and 14, and continues until the first few weeks after birth (Weinbauer et al., 1997; Laycock and Wise, 1996). Thereafter, there is very little testosterone secretion until age ten, when nocturnal, pulsatile LH secretion begins. Between ages 11 to 14, testosterone secretion increases until adult male levels are achieved. It peaks at age 20, and slowly declines thereafter, though not significantly until about age 50 (Vermeulen et al., 1998; Dai et al., 1981; Field et al., 1994). Among men in their eighth decade, mean free testosterone level is approximately 50% of the testosterone level of young adult men (Vermeulen et al., 1998). However, there is great interindividual variability in testosterone levels among men; not all older men become hypogonadal.

In a comprehensive meta-analysis, Gray and colleagues (1991) used 44 studies which met stringent criteria for reporting the relationship between mean testosterone level and age. Overall, mean total testosterone level for adult men was 479 ($\pm$ 115) ng/dl. They demonstrated that the age-related decline in testosterone level is particularly pronounced among healthier men compared to men who have any illness: healthier men's testosterone level starts higher and falls faster. In a multiple regression model, the best predictors of both testosterone level and the slope of the age-related decline were good general health status and morning serum sampling, both of which predicted higher levels and steeper slopes. This was probably due largely to the blunting of the circadian early morning peak that occurs with age and illness. The decline in free testosterone, about 1% every year after age 40, is more than twice that of total testosterone. Finally, consistent positive predictors of baseline testosterone level include father's testosterone level, smoking, and SHBG level; obesity is the most consistent negative predictor (Dabbs et al., 1996).

The age-related decline in testosterone level – about 100 ng/dl per decade – is due primarily to a reduction in Leydig cell functioning, although there also appears to be some failure of the hypothalamic–pituitary system. Testicular responsiveness to LH is reduced, testosterone synthesis is impaired, the circadian early morning peak is blunted, and LH generally increases (Weinbauer et al., 1997; Laycock and Wise, 1996). Finally, end organ responsiveness may change with age: aging is associated with a down-regulation of androgen receptors in the rat prostate and liver

(Chatterjee & Roy, 1990; Shain & Boesel, 1977; Sternbach, 1998), which leads to androgen resistance.

Testosterone actions

Metabolic effects

The effects of testosterone are varied. During the embryonal stage, testosterone is responsible for the growth of the penis and scrotum, development of the prostate and seminal vesicles, descent of the testes, and suppression of the development of female genitalia (Weinbauer et al., 1997; Laycock and Wise, 1996; Bagatell et al., 1996). The testosterone surge of puberty causes the genitalia to enlarge about eight-fold, promotes the development and maintenance of secondary sexual characteristics, and supports anabolic activity. Testosterone affects hair distribution (including baldness), stimulates prostatic secretion and growth, masculinizes the larynx and the skin, promotes protein anabolism (leading to muscular development, bone growth, calcium retention, and an increase in basal metabolic rate), and increases red blood cell production and hemoglobin synthesis (Weinbauer et al., 1997; Laycock and Wise, 1996; Bagatell et al., 1996).

Neuropsychiatric effects

The CNS mechanisms of gonadal steroid action are not well elucidated, but likely include neurotransmitter and second messenger modulation in hypothalamic, limbic, and cortical regions. For example, in cats, testosterone stimulates an increase in the number of substance P neurons in the medial amygdala – a structure that mediates defensive and predatory rage behavior (Siegel & Demetrikopoulos, 1998). And defensive aggression in rats is readily elicited by electrical or chemical stimulation of the medial hypothalamus, where sex hormone concentrating cells are found in high density, and testosterone implantation modifies the propensity for the occurrence of an attack response (Siegel et al., 1998). Androgen sensitive neurons in the medial preoptic area of the hypothalamus regulate male sexual behavior in virtually all mammals studied (McEwen, 1998). Finally, multiple rodent studies have demonstrated that testosterone modulates serotonergic transmission. For example, in rats, the effects of serotonin agonists on sexual function and dominance, and the induction of the serotonin behavioral syndrome, are testosterone-dependent (Bonson & Winter, 1992; Popova & Amstislavskaya, 1989; Gonzalez et al., 1994).

Prenatal organizing effects

The neuropsychiatric effects of testosterone include perinatal 'organizing' effects, and postpubertal 'activating' effects. Regarding the former, it has been established in many mammalian species, that testosterone, acting during a brief developmental critical period, permanently alters brain structure and function (McEwen, 1998; Kemper, 1990; Weinbauer et al., 1997; Laycock and Wise, 1996). Such 'organizing' effects lead to behavioral predispositions in the setting of later re-exposure to testosterone. That is, T-sensitive neural networks are 'wired.' This has been demonstrated most clearly in rodents. For example, perinatal exposure of a female rat to testosterone leads to masculinized sexual, aggressive, and exploratory behavior postpubertally (particularly when activated by testosterone), and loss of the female pattern of gonadotropin secretion (Archer, 1991; McEwen, 1998; Weinbauer et al., 1997; Laycock and Wise, 1996). Perinatal castration of a male rat leads to impaired inter-male aggression when treated postpubertally with testosterone. This impairment can be prevented by perinatal testosterone replacement (McEwen, 1998; Kemper, 1990). Some evidence suggests that in rats, perinatal testosterone organizes later serotonergic transmission in limbic and striatal areas of the brain (Gonzalez et al., 1994). In humans, prenatal exposure of female fetuses to excessive androgens (as a consequence of congenital adrenal hyperplasia) is associated with the development of male-like play behavior during childhood, male-like sexual imagery and preferences in adulthood, and more aggressive behavior compared to female relatives (Berenbaum & Resnick, 1997; Money et al., 1984).

Postpubertal behavioral effects

Since both androgen and estrogen binding sites are distributed widely throughout the CNS, and in some sites (the amygdala in particular) testosterone is extensively aromatized to E_2, testosterone may influence CNS function through androgen and/or estrogen receptors. The neuropsychiatric effects of E_2 binding are therefore of importance to the study of androgen action. E_2 appears to modulate monoaminergic – particularly serotonergic – transmission and neuropeptide transmission (Schmidt & Rubinow, 1997). Low E_2 states (e.g. premenstrual, postnatal, and postmenopausal) are associated with dysphoric/irritable mood syndromes. Although studies linking post-menopausal status to major depression are equivocal, results from treatment trials suggest that estrogen replacement therapy (ERT) may have therapeutic promise. Estrogen has long been used clinically for medication-resistant MDD, with positive anecdotal reports (Klaiber et al., 1979). Moreover, elderly women who were receiving ERT had significantly better response rates to the interventions (tacrine for Alzheimer's disease; Schneider et al., 1996), and fluoxetine for MDD (Schneider et al., 1997) in secondary analyses of two recent multicenter, placebo-controlled randomized clinical trials. These findings should be considered preliminary, and clearly require prospective clinical trials. Yet, they suggest that exogenous gonadal steroid administration may have a modulatory – perhaps a permissive – effect on other psychopharmacologic treatments. In men, a clear parallel would be the use of testosterone as facilitator of response.

In adulthood, there is strong evidence that testosterone activates the sexual, aggressive, and social behaviors of rodents and of ungulates, such as cows and goats (Bouissou, 1983; Archer, 1991; Kemper, 1990; Rubinow & Schmidt, 1996). The relationship between testosterone secretion and these behaviors among primates (including humans) is less direct and complicated by social factors and learning (Archer, 1991; Rose et al., 1975; Kemper, 1990; Rubinow & Schmidt, 1996). Among human males, testosterone level has been variably associated with sexual activity and libido; antisocial behavior, dominance, and sensation seeking; educational and occupational achievement; marital discord and divorce; and the experiences of success and failure (Archer, 1991; Rose et al., 1975; Kemper, 1990; Rubinow & Schmidt, 1996). Such associations may be mediated through androgenic (or estrogenic, through CNS conversion of testosterone to estradiol) effects on sexual arousal, emotionality, cognition, and/or aggression. For example, in multiple large cohorts of young men (particularly in college, in jail, and in the military), Dabbs and colleagues have demonstrated that low testosterone level is associated with intellectually oriented, friendly, docile behavior, while high testosterone level is associated with what they have termed 'rambunctious' behavior – that is, behavior that is impulsive, aggressive, gregarious, and generally unfriendly. 'High testosterone men' reportedly rarely smile socially (Dabbs et al., 1996).

Dominance and submission

Testosterone level decreases in response to stress and failure, and increases after victory or a rise in social status (Kemper, 1990). These relationships have been demonstrated in studies of the change in testosterone levels among male tennis players in competition, in men in Officer Candidate School, and in men during medical internship (Kemper, 1990). Some studies suggest that increased testosterone level in young males is associated with low frustration tolerance, irritability, and impatience (Olweus et al., 1988) – factors that may be markers of affective 'tone.' Again, causal inferences cannot be drawn from these studies: testosterone secretion is both a cause and an effect of social interactions and should be appreciated as part of a system rather than as an isolated dependent or independent variable (Rubinow & Schmidt, 1996). For example, the change in testosterone level following competition has been demonstrated to be affected by prior success in competition, dominance relationships, and the perception of victory (Kemper, 1990; Rubinow & Schmidt, 1996). Testosterone-regulated affective and cognitive states may play some role in modulating such social interactions.

Intermale social interactions are important factors in the relationship between testosterone and behavior in non-human primates, and may play some role in human males. In rhesus monkeys, although sexual function requires circulating androgens, the extent to which suppression of testicular function eliminates sexual behavior depends on the social context. In a multimale group, testosterone suppression leads to an immediate and sustained reduction in sexual behavior; in a single-male, multiple-female group, sexual behavior declines after one month; and in a male–female pair, the reduction in sexual behavior does not occur until at least 2 months after testosterone suppression (Wallen et al., 1991).

Sexual behavior

The best established testosterone–behavior relationship in human males is with sexual function: testosterone replacement of hypogonadal men leads to a dramatic increase in sexual desire, sexual activity, and fantasy-associated and nocturnal erections (Bancroft & Wu, 1983; Davidson et al., 1979; Anderson et al., 1992). Suppression of testosterone secretion in eugonadal men leads to reduced sexual desire and activity, and a decrease in spontaneous erections (Bagatell et al., 1994b). There appears to be a threshold, which varies from person to person, below which sexual function is impaired. Even so, some data suggest that administration of exogenous testosterone to men who have clearly normal testosterone levels leads to an increase in arousability and sexual interest (Pope Jr et al., in press; O'Carroll & Bancroft, 1984; Schiavi et al., 1997), enhancement of nocturnal penile tumescence (NPT) in rigidity but not circumference (Carani et al., 1990), but has no effect on daytime, erotic erectile function (Pope Jr et al., in press; O'Carroll & Bancroft, 1984; Schiavi et al., 1997).

NPT is impaired in hypogonadal men, and improves with testosterone replacement (Cunningham et al., 1990; O'Carroll et al., 1985; Kwan et al., 1983; Carani et al., 1995; Bancroft & Wu, 1983; Pope Jr et al., in press). Schiavi and colleagues (Schiavi et al., 1992) found that low bioavailable testosterone was associated with reduced REM latency, fewer REM episodes, and worsened sleep efficiency in healthy men aged 45 to 75. These effects of testosterone on REM sleep were independent of age. However, age alone appears to explain the tandem decline in NPT and testosterone level in most men.

Aggression

Numerous correlational studies have examined the relationship between plasma testosterone level and measures of aggression in human males (Dabbs et al., 1990; Olweus et al., 1988; Archer, 1991; Kemper, 1990). Interpretation of these studies is limited by the known increase in testosterone that occurs as a result of aggressive encounters, and again by the social context (Bouissou, 1983; Dabbs et al., 1990; Olweus et al., 1988; Archer, 1991; Kemper, 1990). Furthermore, studies have differed in measures of aggression used (actual behavior vs. aggressive traits) and subject characteristics, and cannot be easily summarized. Some investigators have reported positive correlations between testosterone level and some aspects of aggression, especially among subjects selected on the basis of violent behavior, such as among male prisoners (Archer, 1991). Others have not found any correlation between testosterone level and multiple aspects of aggression (Olweus et al., 1988; Kemper, 1990). In a comprehensive review of the topic, Archer (Archer, 1991) concluded that consistent evidence suggests that violent male offenders have significantly higher testosterone levels than less violent individuals; and there is a small but statistically significant correlation between testosterone level and hostility in a variety of male populations. The correlation is stronger when aggressiveness is rated by others in the person's social environment compared to self-assessment.

Cognition

Spatial cognition – which includes visual perception, spatial attention, object identification, or visual memory processes – is a sexually dimorphic cognitive function. Women excel at tasks requiring fine motor dexterity or verbal fluency, and men excel on block rotation tasks and on embedded figures tests (Janowsky et al., 1994). Multiple naturalistic and treatment studies suggest that, in women, such spatial cognition is directly related to E_2 level. For example, during low E_2 menstrual phases, spatial cognition is enhanced (Hampson, 1990). Furthermore, in postmenopausal women with Alzheimer's disease, there is some evidence that E_2 replacement is associated with modest improvement in memory (Yaffe et al., 1998; Robinson et al., 1994). Finally, E_2 activates regional cerebral blood flow (rCBF) in the prefrontal cortices during cognitive activation (Schmidt & Rubinow, 1997).

In studies assessing the relationship between testosterone level and cognitive performance among young adult men with normal testosterone levels, four well-designed studies have demonstrated a positive correlation between spatial ability and testosterone level (Christiansen & Knussmann, 1987; Hannan Jr et al., 1991; Gouchie & Kimura, 1991; Gordon & Lee, 1986). And, one of these studies has demonstrated a negative correlation between testosterone level and verbal ability (Christiansen & Knussmann, 1987). Other studies have examined the relationship between exogenous testosterone administration and cognitive performance (Cappa et al., 1988; Kertzman et al., 1990; Vogel et al., 1971; Janowsky et al., 1994). Such studies are not easily summarized because of the variability in populations studied (e.g. handedness and age) and testing factors like tests used or time of day (Hampson & Moffat, 1994; Moffat & Hampson, 1996; Sternbach, 1998). It appears that there is an optimal testosterone level for spatial cognitive function since performance is poorer with low and high levels (Moffat & Hampson, 1996). In addition, there has been some speculation that prenatal organizational effects of gonadal steroids may affect cognitive aspects of testosterone activation (Moffat & Hampson, 1996).

In the most rigorous study of the role of exogenous testosterone in the cognitive function of older men, Janowsky and colleagues (1994) randomized 56 men (mean age 67 years) to receive testosterone or placebo patches for 3 months. Compared to men who received placebo, men who received testosterone had enhanced spatial cognition (especially visual perception and spatial constructional processes), as measured by the Block Design subtest of the WAIS-R. Of note, the decrease in E_2 level among men receiving testosterone appeared to be a better predictor of Block Design performance than the increase in testosterone level. Other tested cognitive domains were not affected. The relatively low testosterone dose employed, and the limited sensitivity of the cognitive tests limited this trial. Yet, the findings support a role for gonadal steroids in cognitive processing, and the area clearly warrants further investigation.

In summary, the testosterone–behavior relationship is complex, and modulated by experience. Response to testosterone is influenced by prenatal androgen exposure, and perhaps by idiosyncratic characteristics of androgen (or estrogen) receptor activation. In humans, testosterone may act by setting affective 'tone' rather than by directing specific behaviors. Testosterone secretion and action are part of a neurochemical context that determines the emotional, cognitive, and behavioral effects of a wide range of neuromodulators (Rubinow & Schmidt, 1996). Such a context may have implications for the study and alteration of affective states or syndromes.

Testosterone in aging men

The age-related decline in testosterone level can be considered either physiological or pathological. Currently, since age-adjusted norms are not used, it is treated as pathological. Yet, even if physiologic, such a decline may be clinically significant, as with female hypogonadism. The general effects of testosterone deficiency are similar to those of the aging process itself: decreased musculoskeletal mass, increased adipose deposition, decreased hematopoiesis, decreased facial hair growth, as well as decreased libido, and presumed decline in energy, mood, and memory (Swerdloff & Wang, 1993; Morley et al., 1997; Tenover, 1992, 1997; Lamberts et al., 1997; Vermeulen et al., 1998; Villareal & Morley, 1994). Testosterone replacement consistently reverses these sequelae in younger hypogonadal men (ages 20 to 60): body weight increases; fat-free muscle mass, muscle size and strength increase; continued bone loss is prevented; sexual function and secondary sex characteristics like facial hair are restored and maintained; and hematocrit increases (Villareal & Morley, 1994; Burris et al., 1992). The application of a testosterone replacement strategy for older men with low or low-normal testosterone levels is thought by some investigators to be especially promising for reversing the aging effects on bones and muscle mass, as well as for enhancing mood, energy, cognition, and libido (Sih et al., 1997; Morley et al., 1993, 1997; Tenover, 1992; Villareal & Morley, 1994; Luisi & Franchi, 1980). Some anecdotal reports of testosterone replacement in hypogonadal older men suggest that such treatment leads to improved mood, energy, libido, and sense of well-being; better sleep and appetite; and decreased frailty, with gains in muscle strength and lean body mass (Tenover, 1992; Villareal & Morley, 1994; Morley et al., 1993). Yet, there are only limited controlled data on the metabolic effects of testosterone replacement in men older than 60, and none which addresses psychiatric symptoms in this age group. Specific studies in aging men are particularly important, since age-related testosterone deficiency is generally more modest than the profound hypogonadism seen in testosterone replacement trials with younger men.

Despite the completion of numerous controlled testosterone replacement trials over the past three decades, none have described the prevalence of prereplacement psychiatric illness followed by systematic monitoring of psychiatric symptoms during testosterone replacement. It is unlikely that all hypogonadal men develop major depression, because there is no apparent increase in major depression among epidemiologic cohorts of aging men that parallels the decrease in testosterone levels. It is possible that a low-grade affective syndrome develops – perhaps not unlike the dysphoric/irritable/fatigue syndrome of female hypogonadism (i.e. menopause). Such subsyndromal depressive symptoms affect more than 10% of elderly men and are associated with significant functional impairment (Horwath et al., 1992). Moreover, the likelihood that testosterone replacement has positive effects on specific components of the major depressive syndrome, such as mood, appetite, and cognitive impairment, may be of relevance to the study and treatment of major depression in aging men. Specifically, it is conceivable that comorbid depression in the setting of the 'normative' hypogonadism of aging may remit or improve after testosterone replacement therapy; or that MDD with comorbid hypogonadism may respond less well to conventional antidepressant treatment if testosterone is not replaced. Finally, the use of exogenous testosterone as a psychotropic agent separate from baseline HPG functioning may hold therapeutic promise. Such possibilities are necessarily speculative, since there are no specific studies addressing testosterone administration/replacement and psychiatric symptoms in older depressed or non-depressed men.

Testosterone and male depressive illness

The role played by testosterone in the pathogenesis of MDD in men is likely to be either small or limited to specific subpopulations: a robust and pervasive effect would probably have been recognized earlier. Perhaps parallel to the subpopulation of women who develop estrogen-responsive mood disorders, evidence suggests that there may be some men who are particularly prone to developing testosterone-mediated mood problems or in whom testosterone has antidepressant-facilitating effects. A primary research challenge is to identify such men.

The therapeutic potential of exogenous testosterone may be much broader. Specifically, given testosterone's mood- and energy-enhancing properties and known neurotransmitter effects, exogenous testosterone could have numerous applications in the treatment of depressive illness by affecting specific features of male MDD. Whether or not testosterone also has broader clinical effects, such as decreasing symptom intensity, enhancing treatment response, or delaying relapse would be of enormous therapeutic importance.

Depression in hypogonadal men

Hypogonadal men commonly complain of loss of libido, dysphoria, fatigue, irritability, and appetite loss (Plymate, 1994; Anderson et al., 1992; Kemper, 1990; Rubinow & Schmidt, 1996). These symptoms generally respond to testosterone replacement (Burris et al., 1992; Luisi & Franchi, 1980; Morley et al., 1993). Although such apparent psychiatric sequelae of hypogonadism overlap with signs and symptoms of major depression, it is not known what proportion of hypogonadal men meet criteria for major depression, and when they do, which dysfunction is primary. Furthermore, it is unclear whether a specific HPG measure (e.g. total testosterone, free testosterone, LH, FSH, DHT) might be associated with psychiatric symptoms, and if so, at which absolute or relative level. For example, symptomatic hypogonadism apparently develops only when the total testosterone level drops below a certain threshold, typically 'set' between 200 and 300 ng/dl. Yet this threshold has generally been used to assess for HPG dysfunction in relatively young men. For example, young men with testosterone levels below 250 ng/dl often have symptoms of sexual dysfunction, such as impaired nocturnal erections and low libido (Burris et al., 1992). In contrast, standards for determining the relevance of decreasing testosterone levels among healthy aging men, – i.e. 'normative' gonadal hypofunction – may need to account for other age-related phenomena, such as changes in end organ responsiveness and changes in HPG secretory patterns (Villareal & Morley, 1994). Thus, it is not known at what testosterone level clinically significant symptoms begin, particularly regarding the psychiatric sequelae of gonadal hypofunction. Determination of an absolute lower threshold (or threshold relative to baseline) with respect to psychiatric impairment is therefore, an unanswered question.

Two epidemiologic studies have assessed both testosterone level and depressive symptoms: the Massachusetts Male Aging Study (MMAS) and the Veterans'

Experience Study (VES) (Dabbs et al., 1990; Mazur, 1995). The MMAS is a population-based survey of 1709 men aged 40 to 70 which included a morning testosterone level and a self-report depression instrument, the Center for Epidemiologic Studies Depression Scale (CES-D; Lewinsohn et al., 1997; Roberts & Vernon, 1983). There was no correlation between CES-D-determined 'depression' (using a cutoff of 16) and testosterone level (Odds Ratio 0.9, 95% CI = 0.75–1.1) (Araujo et al., 1998). Yet, since less than half of those identified by this CES-D cutoff likely had major depression (Roberts & Vernon, 1983), it is not clear whether a different cutoff or a more accurate diagnosis would have demonstrated a relationship between testosterone level and major depression. Moreover, the cohort of men with low testosterone level were not analyzed specifically to determine whether they were more likely to have higher scores on items assessing depressive symptoms.

The VES included a representative sample of 5236 Vietnam-era veterans (median age 37 years, 95% age range 33 to 42), and included multiple morning testosterone samples; a structured interview for depression, the Diagnostic Interview Schedule (DIS); and a self-report personality inventory, the MMPI (Dabbs et al., 1990; Mazur, 1995). Testosterone level was correlated modestly with antisocial personality, substance abuse, and gambling ($r = 0.13$–0.18, $P < .001$); and very weakly with depression, mania, obsessionality, and anxiety ($r = 0.03$–0.05, $P < 0.01$) (Mazur, 1995). The relationship with markers of deviance was strongest among men of low socioeconomic status. Thus, there is some suggestion that HPG functioning is related to psychopathology in young men. Again, analysis of the cohort of men with a testosterone level below a certain threshold might have been informative regarding the possibility of a 'below-threshold' androgen deficiency psychiatric syndrome.

Focusing specifically on men who present clinically with low testosterone level, Woodman and Williams (1996) reviewed the records of 173 hypogonadal men being treated in an endocrinology clinic. They found that 39% were being treated with medication for a psychiatric illness, although they did not report the specific medications or illnesses. This is far in excess of what would be expected from the general, or even medically ill, male population, and suggests that psychiatric sequelae of hypogonadism may be substantial. There is a need for a further descriptive psychiatric epidemiology of male hypogonadism.

The HPG axis in depressed men

Neuroendocrine studies of the HPG axis among men with well-diagnosed MDD have been few and contradictory. Most psychiatric investigators have focused on basal testosterone level alone. Yet, basal testosterone level is a limited indicator of HPG functioning. LH level and pattern of secretion, testosterone pulse amplitude and frequency, conversion to active metabolites, and end-organ responsivity may all play some role in affective symptoms. None of these other areas has been extensively studied by psychiatric researchers, although there is little evidence for impaired gonadotropin secretion among depressed men (Rubin, 1981; Amsterdam et al., 1981; Ettigi et al., 1979). For example, using GnRH stimulation tests, Amsterdam and colleagues (1981) demonstrated that pre- and poststimulation LH and FSH concentrations in 23 depressed men (mean age 33 years) were not significantly different from 18 age-matched controls; Brambilla and colleagues (1990) reported that, although nine depressed men had lower mean LH level at baseline compared to age-matched controls ($P<.05$), there was no difference in the area under the curve following GnRH stimulation.

Using testosterone levels, two types of observational studies have generally been done: studies comparing the mean testosterone level of groups of depressed men to non-depressed controls; and studies comparing the mean testosterone level of depressed men during acute illness to the mean testosterone level after remission. Findings from such studies have been inconsistent. In comparing cohorts of depressed men to non-depressed, age-matched controls, some investigators report that depressed men have lower mean testosterone levels (Levitt & Joffe, 1988; Rupprecht et al., 1988), but most report that there is no difference (Yesavage et al., 1985; Unden et al., 1988; Davies et al., 1992; Rubin et al., 1989). Multiple studies have reported a negative correlation between testosterone level and age among depressed men but not among age-matched controls, suggesting that there is blunted testosterone secretion among older depressed men (Rubin et al., 1989; Levitt & Joffe, 1988). Isolated studies have demonstrated a negative correlation between testosterone level and severity of depressive symptoms (Wexler et al., 1989; Yesavage et al., 1985; Davies et al., 1992), melancholia (Rubin et al., 1989), anxiety (Davies et al., 1992), and sexual activity (Rubin et al., 1989); these relationships were not found in other studies (Unden et al., 1988; Levitt & Joffe, 1988; Rupprecht et al., 1988; Vogel et al., 1978; Amsterdam et al., 1981). Finally, studies which determined testosterone level during acute illness compared to after remission have also been inconsistent: of five studies (n's = 6 to 15), acute mean testosterone levels were lower in three, higher in one, and not different in one (Mason et al., 1988; Steiger et al., 1993; Sachar et al., 1973; Unden et al., 1988; Rupprecht et al., 1988). The discrepancies between the various studies that have assessed testosterone levels in depressed men may be caused by the diurnal, seasonal, situational, and age-related variability in testosterone secretion; generally small sample sizes; and/or heterogeneity in depressed samples.

Since it is known that testosterone level declines with age, it is unusual that in many but not all studies this relationship was demonstrable only among depressed men and not among age-matched controls. Such evidence suggests that blunted testosterone secretion may be an aspect of male geriatric depression. For example,

Levitt and Joffe (1988) measured afternoon testosterone levels in 12 males with RDC-diagnosed major depression (mean age 32 years) and 12 age-matched controls (mean age 31 years). They found that there was no difference in testosterone level between these groups, but there was a significant correlation between testosterone level and age ($r = -0.7$, $P < 0.01$), which was not found in the control group (or not reported). The authors suggest that depressed men may be more sensitive (i.e. symptomatic) to the age-related decline in testosterone level (Levitt & Joffe, 1988). In more elaborate neuroendocrine studies, investigators have attempted to control for diurnal variability in hormone levels by using indwelling catheters to obtain multiple serum samples over many hours. Such labor-intensive methods have, however, had limited numbers of subjects. In one of the largest and most rigorous studies, Rubin, Poland, and Lesser (Rubin et al., 1989) enrolled 16 RDC-diagnosed depressed men (mean age 39 years) and 16 paired, age-matched controls. They assessed multiple measures of HPG functioning (i.e. LH, FSH, estradiol, and testosterone levels, and response to TRH, LHRH, and dexamethasone) over 26 hours, with serum sampling every 30 minutes, and found that testosterone level was significantly more negatively correlated with age among depressed men ($r = -0.70$) than among controls ($r = -0.10$); and was positively correlated with DSM-III-diagnosed melancholia ($r = 0.58$). There were no significant correlations between testosterone level and depressive symptoms.

Similar methods were used in two additional studies that support the tentative conclusion that blunted testosterone secretion is a state marker of depression in some men. Heuser (1998) compared 18 consecutively admitted male inpatients with major depression (mean 21-item HAM-D $= 29$, mean age 47 years) to 22 age- and BMI-matched controls (mean age 53 years). They collected blood every 30 minutes, and pooled samples for analysis of 24 hour, daytime (8 am to 7:30 pm), and nighttime (8 pm to 7:30 am) testosterone and cortisol levels, as well as evening (6 pm to 12 am) pulsatile LH and FSH secretion. Compared to the control group and after controlling for age, the depressed group had significantly lower testosterone level ($P < 0.01$), particularly during night-time hours, and a trend toward lower LH pulse frequency ($P < 0.07$). In a regression analysis comparing patients to controls, 24 hour mean testosterone level was not significantly correlated with age ($r = 0.11$ for patients, $r = -0.39$ for controls) or 24-hour mean cortisol ($r = 0.17$ for patients, $r = -0.33$ for controls). Similarly, Steiger and colleagues (Steiger et al., 1993) studied 12 men hospitalized with DSM III-R major depression (mean age 46 years) with hourly serum sampling while sleeping. They demonstrated that nocturnal testosterone secretion, particularly between 11 pm and 3 am, was significantly lower during the acute phase than after remission (1993). Rupprecht and colleagues (1988) found lower testosterone levels among six men during an acute episode of melancholic depression compared to 20 controls ($P < 0.07$), and compared to when they were recovered. Finally, limited data suggest that testosterone blunting during depression may parallel hypothalamic–pituitary–adrenal (HPA) axis activation: Unden and colleagues (1988) demonstrated lower basal testosterone level only among the 8 of 14 depressed men who had a non-suppressing dexamethasone suppression test.

Some evidence from neuropsychiatric studies of cerebral laterality supports the possibility that HPG function may vary by a still poorly defined depressive subtype. In a study of 18 men hospitalized with affective illness (mostly unipolar MDD, but including bipolar and schizoaffective disorders), Wexler and colleagues (1989) divided them into two equal subgroups based on subjects' responses to language-related dichotic listening tests of cerebral laterality. A combined laterality variable (CLV) was constructed to measure the extent to which subjects exhibited right ear advantage (REA) on word compared to nonsense dichotic tests, which had been validated as a reliable marker of information processing. The group with high CLV had significantly lower testosterone levels than the group with low CLV, with little overlap. Furthermore, among the high CLV group, testosterone level was negatively correlated with BPRS symptom severity, particularly measures of activation, anxiety, and suspiciousness. Among men in the low CLV group, testosterone level was positively correlated with these measures of symptom severity. In the combined group, there was no correlation between testosterone level and symptom severity. These intriguing findings have not been replicated, and should therefore be considered tentative. Yet, if supported, such diagnostic heterogeneity might explain why the demonstration of a correlation between testosterone level and symptom severity has been so inconsistent.

In summary, data suggest, but do not demonstrate, that among some men with major depression, testosterone secretion is blunted. The studies are mostly small and cross-sectional and have been unable to adequately control for the multideter-mined variability in testosterone levels found in normals. It is possible that a subgroup of depressed men in these studies are symptomatic due to hypogonad-ism alone, i.e. that their depressive symptoms are sequelae of low testosterone levels. Finally, in some cases, blunting of testosterone secretion may be a response to a depressive symptom, such as caloric restriction (a known inhibitor of GnRH), sleep disturbance, stress, or the experience of 'defeat.' Thus, it remains unclear whether lower testosterone levels among depressed men represent state-dependent HPG dysfunction or artifact.

Exogenous testosterone administration

In 1889, Brown-Sequard reported that self injections of the extracts of crushed animal testicles were rejuvenating, and improved 'all the functions depending on the power of action of the nervous centers' (Brown-Sequard, 1889; Rubinow &

Schmidt, 1996). Thereafter, thousands of men received exogenous testosterone to reverse senescence. Although many of these treatments could not have been endocrinologically active (Hamilton, 1986), men who received them routinely reported improved energy, mood, and memory. This highlights the importance of placebo response to presumed male sex hormone administration, and supports the limited interpretability of uncontrolled testosterone administration.

Androgen administration to non-depressed eugonadal men

Administration of exogenous androgens has direct behavioral effects. In animal models, it stimulates sexual activity, aggressive behavior, and dominance (Anderson et al., 1992; Archer, 1991; Rose et al., 1975; Kemper, 1990; Rubinow & Schmidt, 1996). In humans, studies of testosterone administration to eugonadal young men have demonstrated changes in sexual arousal, cognition, and mood (Yates et al., 1999; Pope Jr et al., in press; O'Carroll & Bancroft, 1984; Bagatell et al., 1994a, b; Anderson et al., 1992; Rubinow & Schmidt, 1996; Bagatell & Bremner, 1996) though not consistently in mood (Pope Jr et al., in press; O'Carroll & Bancroft, 1984; Anderson et al., 1992). In the majority of men, such effects are not easily demonstrated, even using supra-physiologic doses, and appear to have very profound effects on susceptible subpopulations. Most large studies in which moderately supraphysiologic doses of testosterone were administered to eugonadal men have demonstrated that it is relatively safe (Matsumoto, 1990), and has few obvious psychiatric effects detectable in parallel groups (Su et al., 1993; Tricker et al., 1996; World Health Organization Task Force on Methods for the Regulation of Male Fertility, 1990; Matsumoto, 1990). Yet, use of very large doses of synthetic androgens by bodybuilders has consistently been reported to induce mood changes, such as anger, hostility, irritability, and euphoria in some men (Uzych, 1992; Pope Jr & Katz, 1994).

In the few studies that systematically followed psychiatric symptoms, the effects of testosterone were difficult to detect. Tricker and colleagues (Tricker et al., 1996) randomized 43 eugonadal men ages 19 to 40 to double blind treatment with either testosterone 600 mg or placebo injections weekly for 10 weeks. They found no change in self-reported or observer-reported scales of hostility, anger, and mood during testosterone treatment. Similarly, Matsumoto administered testosterone 100 mg and testosterone 300 mg weekly for 6 months to 20 eugonadal men ($n = 10$ in each group; Matsumoto, 1990). He demonstrated that compared to a 4 to 6 month pretreatment placebo phase, supraphysiologic testosterone was associated with an increased hematocrit, weight gain, mild truncal acne, and reduced LH, FSH, and sperm count. Again, no significant psychiatric effects were detected in such parallel groups. These studies were limited by the minimal use of psychiatric interviews and furthermore did not have the power to detect minor psychiatric effects. Moreover, idiosyncratic effects, or effects in a subpopulation of men, were unlikely to be statistically significant in these designs.

Three additional clinical trials suggest that supraphysiologic doses of testosterone may produce mania in a subgroup of individuals. Su and colleagues (1993) administered a high dose of testosterone (methyltestosterone 240 mg per day) for a short time (3 days at the maximum dose) to 20 eugonadal men. One man became manic and one hypomanic, for a 10% 'response rate.' Yates and colleagues (Yates et al., 1999) administered testosterone 500 mg per week for 14 weeks to 18 men; one (6%) became manic. Finally, in the most systematic psychiatric investigation of the effects of moderately supraphysiologic testosterone in eugonadal men, Pope and colleagues (Pope Jr et al., in press) randomized 66 men aged 20 to 50 years to receive testosterone in doses rising to 600 mg per week vs. placebo for six weeks, followed by a 6-week no treatment period and then cross-over to the alternate treatment. They found that testosterone administration significantly increased the mean manic score on the Young Manic Rating Scale (YMRS) ($P=0.003$) and on daily diaries ($P=0.004$), the 'like the way I feel' score on daily diaries ($P=0.01$), and aggressive responses on the Point Subtraction Aggression Paradigm (PSAP) ($P=0.04$). The authors highlight how variable the response to testosterone was: 84% of subjects who received testosterone had minimal psychiatric effects (maximum YMRS <10), 12% became mildly hypomanic (YMRS 10 to 19), and 4% became markedly hypomanic (YMRS >20). There was no reliable predictor of such idiosyncratic effects.

There are a few well-controlled studies of testosterone administration to eugonadal men with erectile dysfunction (Benkert et al., 1979; Schiavi et al., 1997). In general, they have demonstrated that administration of physiologic doses of testosterone is no more effective than placebo for erectile dysfunction; leads to a modest increase in sexual interest; and does not lead to a change on self-report measures of mood. For example, Schiavi and colleagues (1997) enrolled 18 eugonadal men (age range 46 to 67 years) who presented with the chief complaint of erectile dysfunction in a double blind, placebo-controlled, cross-over study of testosterone 200 mg or placebo every 2 weeks for 6 weeks. They found that during the testosterone compared to placebo phase, ejaculatory frequency doubled while other measures of sexual arousal increased, but not with any statistical significance; erectile function and sexual satisfaction were unaffected; and mood, assessed by self-report instruments, was unaffected (Schiavi et al., 1997). Most subjects could not correctly identify the phase in which they received testosterone, and felt it was not helpful. The authors were unable to demonstrate that this schedule of testosterone administration led to an increase in circulating levels 2 weeks after each intramuscular injection, suggesting that this dose may have been too low to override the compensatory feedback mechanisms operating in eugonadal men.

Androgen administration to non-depressed hypogonadal men

Numerous testosterone replacement studies provide consistent support for its safety and efficacy in hypogonadism (Wang et al., 1996; Burris et al., 1992; Luisi & Franchi, 1980; Morley et al., 1993). Yet, in the endocrinologic literature, attention has only rarely been paid to psychiatric symptoms. In most testosterone replacement studies, the effects on sexual function (i.e. consistently improved libido and arousal, restoration of sleep-related erections and ejaculatory capacity) are described most consistently; other psychiatric symptoms are noted anecdotally or not at all (Wang et al., 1996; Burris et al., 1992; Luisi & Franchi, 1980; Morley et al., 1993). No testosterone replacement trial has included a systematic determination of pretreatment psychiatric diagnosis with adequate longitudinal monitoring of psychiatric symptoms. Yet, despite such methodologic flaws with regard to the psychiatric effects of hormonal replacement, investigators consistently note that such patients report enhanced relaxation, cheerfulness, well-being, and energy; and reduced irritability, anger, and tension (Wang et al., 1996; Burris et al., 1992; Luisi & Franchi, 1980; Morley et al., 1993).

In the only systematic study of the mood effects of testosterone replacement, Wang and colleagues (1996) followed 51 hypogonadal men aged 22 to 60 years during 2 to 6 months of testosterone replacement. Testosterone level at baseline was below 250 ng/dl, and many of the subjects had been withdrawn from testosterone replacement for 6 weeks to enter the study. Self-reported mood ratings were compared from pre-replacement baseline to weeks 3, 6, and 8 of testosterone replacement. On positive mood scales, there was a significant increase in self-reported friendliness, energy level, and well-being, usually evident by the first visit (treatment week 3), and persisting through 6 months of replacement. On negative mood scales, there was a significant decrease in self-reported nervousness, irritability, sadness, and anger (Wang et al., 1996).

Androgen administration to depressed men

The psychiatric effects of androgen administration in men (hypogonadal or eugonadal) who have rigorously diagnosed major depressive illness has not been systematically investigated. What evidence exists includes mostly anecdotal reports from the 1940s and 1950s (without syndromal diagnoses), and more recent clinical trials of oral androgen treatment of depressed men (Itil et al., 1978, 1984; Vogel et al., 1985) and testosterone treatment of mild to moderately depressed HIV-positive men (Rabkin et al., 1995).

Many reports from the older psychiatric literature described the 'antidepressant' effects of testosterone. These reports were generally conducted between 1935 and 1960 without standardized, syndromal psychiatric diagnoses, baseline testosterone levels, or standardized testosterone preparations. Many, but not all (Pardoll &

Belinson, 1941; Kerman, 1943), suggested that a substantial proportion of 'depressed' men responded immediately and dramatically, and relapsed when treatment was discontinued (Altschule & Tillotson, 1948; Danziger et al., 1944; Rinieris et al., 1979). For example, Reiter (1965) reported his experiences from London in the 1950s with 240 middle-aged men in whom he implanted intramuscular testosterone crystals (800 to 2400 mg) along with small doses of estradiol (20 mg), which he claimed gave a steady dose of 4 to 12 mg per day over 6 months. He rated men with an 8-point depression scale, with 8 defined as 'complete loss of confidence in carrying on the activities of living, a tendency to abandon any occupation, and even the danger of self-destruction,' at baseline, and at 2 and 4 months post treatment. He found that men who received lower testosterone doses (800 to 1800 mg) had moderate decreases in depression scores while those who received higher doses (2000 to 2400 ng/dl) generally had substantial and sustained reductions in their depression scores, from the 5 to 8 range to the 1 to 3 range. Lack of any control group limits interpretation of these data.

In the past two decades, we know of only seven androgen treatment trials for male depression in which investigators used DSM diagnoses of major depression and systematically followed depressive symptoms with a reliable interview-based instrument such as the Hamilton Depression Rating Scale (HAM-D). Most used the oral androgen mesterolone, which is a derivative of DHT and therefore lacks testosterone's non-DHT actions (i.e. testosterone-specific and estrogenic activity) (Weinbauer et al., 1997).

Itil and colleagues performed three mesterolone trials (Itil et al., 1978, 1984). First, they administered variable doses of mesterolone to 17 depressed men openly for 3 weeks, and found that 8 (47%) improved, particularly in mood and anxiety level (Itil et al., 1978). Then, in a randomized, double blind 4-week trial, low dose mesterolone (i.e. 75 mg/day) or placebo was administered to 38 dysthymic men. They reported that treatment led to improvement in symptoms such as anxiety, lack of drive, lack of desire, and impaired satisfaction (Itil et al., 1978). Finally, they administered high dose mesterolone (i.e. 450 mg/day) or placebo in a 6-week randomized trial to 52 men (mean age 40 years) with dysthymia, unipolar depression, and bipolar depression (Itil et al., 1984). Both the mesterolone and placebo groups improved significantly, and there was no statistically significant difference demonstrable between the two. Mesterolone treatment led to a significant decrease in LH and testosterone levels – likely due to feedback inhibition at the hypothalamus and pituitary. Notably, of those patients who improved on mesterolone – initial drug responders, and placebo non-responders who were crossed over and responded – improvement in psychopathology was positively correlated with the decrease in testosterone levels during weeks 3 to 6 of treatment. Vogel, Klaiber, and Broverman (Vogel et al., 1985) administered mesterolone openly for 7 weeks to 13 eugonadal men (mean age 39 years) with refractory, chronic unipolar depression. Eleven responded, most by the second week, with a mean HAM-D decrease (in these 11) from 21.1 to 5.6 ($P < 0.001$). The same investigators, in a 12-week randomized, double blind trial, gave mesterolone or amitriptyline to 34 chronically depressed, eugonadal men aged 27 to 62 years (Vogel et al., 1978). Mesterolone was as effective as amitriptyline in reducing depressive symptoms: mean HAM-D score decreased by 8 in both groups.

Rabkin and colleagues (Rabkin et al., 1995) administered testosterone openly to 52 HIV-positive men who had testosterone levels below 450 ng/dl and a depressive disorder (42% with major depression, the remainder with a minor depressive syndrome). Twenty-eight patients (64%) improved, with mean HAM-D decrease from 13.6 to 4.1 at week 8. Notably, neither baseline nor final testosterone levels were associated with antidepressant response.

Rabkin and colleagues (Rabkin et al., 1997) administered testosterone openly for 12 weeks to 112 HIV-positive men who had testosterone levels below 500 ng/dl and clinical symptoms of hypogonadism (low libido, low mood, and/or low energy). Of the 102 (91%) whose sexual function improved, 77 completed a 6-week, randomized, double blind, placebo-controlled, discontinuation trial. Seventy eight percent of completers randomized to testosterone maintained their improved sexual function, compared to 13% randomized to placebo. Thirty-four patients with MDD or dysthymia completed 8 weeks of open testosterone treatment. Mean HAM-D decreased from 18.5 to 3.0 at week 8 ($P < 0.001$), as did symptom inventories for depressive, anxious, and somatic symptoms ($P < 0.001$). Notably, among men who had low mood at study entry but did not meet MDD or dysthymia criteria, mean HAM-D decreased from 11.9 to 2.7 by week 8 ($P < 0.001$).

Seidman and Rabkin (1998) administered testosterone openly to five men who had SSRI-refractory major depression and testosterone level below 350 ng/dl. In this 6-week trial, all five achieved remission, with a mean HAM-D decrease from 19.2 to 7.2 by week 2, and to 4.0 by week 8. Finally, in a recently completed study, our group enrolled 32 hypogonadal men (testosterone $<$ 350 ng/dl) with comorbid MDD in a randomized trial of physiologic testosterone replacement (i.e. 200 mg per week) vs. placebo. Preliminary data are striking for the high placebo response, and the apparently idiosyncratic mood-elevating effects of physiologic testosterone in a minority of subjects. Such variable effects of testosterone are in keeping with the growing experience of other investigators using exogenous testosterone, including Rabkin (1997), Pope (Pope Jr et al., in press), and Yates (Yates et al., 1999).

Treatment with exogenous testosterone

Treatment with testosterone should generally be done in consultation with an endocrinologist or urologist. Indications include morning total testosterone $<$ 250 ng/dl or bioavailable testosterone $<$ 70 ng/dl, especially when associated with sexual dysfunction. Testosterone is available in several forms: oral, injectable, transdermal patches (scrotal and nonscrotal), and implantable pellets (Sternbach, 1998).

A short course of physiologic or moderately supraphysiologic testosterone has few medically significant side effects. Of primary concern are the implications of testosterone's known effects on erythropoiesis, cholesterol profile, and prostate cancer. Exogenous androgen treatment stimulates erythropoiesis, reduces plasma HDL cholesterol, and stimulates the growth of established prostate adenocarcinoma. The theoretic risks of inducing polycythemia, worsening coronary artery disease, or promoting the development of precursor prostatic lesions into cancer have never been demonstrated (Rabkin et al., 1997; Snyder, 1996). Most clinicians consider the risk of prostate cancer the most worrisome possibility, and do not administer testosterone to men who have an abnormal digital rectal exam of the prostate, or an elevated PSA (>3.0 ng/ml) (Rabkin et al., 1997; Snyder, 1996). Other potential side effects include decreased sperm count, which may temporarily affect fertility, weight gain, acne, irritability, hair loss, reduction in testicular size, decreased ejaculate, worsening of sleep apnea, and worsening of asymptomatic BPH. These side effects are usually not medically serious, are entirely reversible, and generally evolve after more than 6 months of treatment. Gynecomastia, which probably results from testosterone's conversion to E_2, although rare, may not be entirely reversible. It is readily prevented by early detection of breast tenderness and discontinuation of exogenous testosterone.

Summary

In summary, androgens have psychoactive properties. There is limited, suggestive, evidence that exogenous androgen treatment has antidepressant effects in some male depressives. Such effects may be more prominent among men who are hypogonadal, although this is not well established. In general, the evidence is too limited to evaluate whether the presumed antidepressant efficacy is related to testosterone replacement, symptomatic improvement such as increased libido or energy, or non-specific placebo effects.

ACKNOWLEDGMENT

We thank B. Timothy Walsh and Donald F. Klein for their critical review.

REFERENCES

Altschule, M. D. & Tillotson, K. J. (1948). The use of testosterone in the treatment of depressions. *The New England Journal of Medicine.* **239**, 1036–8.

Amsterdam, J. D., Winokur, A., Caroff, S. & Snyder, P. (1981). Gonadotropin release after administration of GnRH in depressed patients and healthy volunteers. *Journal of Affective Disorders.* **3**(4), 367–80.

Anderson, R. A., Bancroft, J. & Wu, F. C. (1992). The effects of exogenous testosterone on sexuality and mood of normal men. *Journal of Clinical Endocrinology & Metabolism,* **75**(6), 1503–7.

Araujo, A. B., Durante, R., Feldman, H. A., Goldstein, I. & McKinlay, J. B. (1998). The relationship between depressive symptoms and male erectile dysfunction: cross sectional results from the Massachusetts Male Aging Study. *Psychosomatic Medicine,* **60**(4), 458–65.

Archer, J. (1991). The influence of testosterone on human aggression. [Review] [150 refs]. *British Journal of Psychology,* **82**(1), 1–28.

Bagatell, C. J. & Bremner, W. J. (1996). Androgens in men – uses and abuses. [Review] [91 refs]. *New England Journal of Medicine,* **334**(11), 707–14.

Bagatell, C. J., Heiman, J. R., Matsumoto, A. M., Rivier, J. E. & Bremner, W. J. (1994a). Metabolic and behavioral effects of high-dose, exogenous testosterone in healthy men. *Journal of Clinical Endocrinology and Metabolism,* **79**(2), 561–7.

Bagatell, C. J., Heiman, J. R., Rivier, J. E. & Bremner, W. J. (1994b). Effects of endogenous testosterone and estradiol on sexual behavior in normal young men [published erratum appears in *Journal of Clinical Endocrinology and Metabolism,* 1994 Jun; 78(6), 1520]. *Journal of Clinical Endocrinology and Metabolism,* **78**(3), 711–16.

Bancroft, J. & Wu, F. C. (1983). Changes in erectile responsiveness during androgen replacement therapy. *Archives of Sexual Behavior,* **12**(1), 59–66.

Benkert, O., Witt, W., Adam, W. & Leitz, A. (1979). Effects of testosterone undecanoate on sexual potency and the hypothalamic–pituitary–gonadal axis of impotent males. *Archives of Sexual Behavior,* **8**(6), 471–9.

Berenbaum, S. A. & Resnick, S. M. (1997). Early androgen effects on aggression in children and adults with congenital adrenal hyperplasia. *Psychoneuroendocrinology,* **22**(7), 505–15.

Bonson, K. R. & Winter, J. C. (1992). Reversal of testosterone-induced dominance by the serotonergic agonist quipazine. *Pharmacology, Biochemistry and Behavior,* **42**(4), 809–13.

Bouissou, M. F. (1983). Androgens, aggressive behaviour and social relationships in higher mammals. [Review] [107 refs]. *Hormone Research,* **18**(1–3), 43–61.

Brambilla, F., Maggioni, M., Ferrari, E., Scarone, S. & Catalano, M. (1990). Tonic and dynamic gonadotropin secretion in depressive and normothymic phases of affective disorders. *Psychiatry Research,* **32**, 229–39.

Brown-Sequard, C. E. (1889). The effects produced on man by subcutaneous injections of a liquid obtained from the testicles of animals. *Lancet,* **ii**, 105–7.

Burris, A. S., Banks, S. M., Carter, C. S., Davidson, J. M. & Sherins, R. J. (1992). A long-term, prospective study of the physiologic and behavioral effects of hormone replacement in untreated hypogonadal men. *Journal of Andrology,* **13**(4), 297–304.

Cappa, S. F., Guariglia, C., Papagno, C., Pizzamiglio, L., Vallar, G., Zoccolotti, Ambrosi, B. &

Santiemma, V. (1988). Patterns of lateralization and performance levels for verbal and spatial tasks in congenital androgen deficiency. *Behavioural Brain Research*, **31**(2), 177–83.

Carani, C., Granata, A. R., Bancroft, J. & Marrama, P. (1995). The effects of testosterone replacement on nocturnal penile tumescence and rigidity and erectile response to visual erotic stimuli in hypogonadal men. *Psychoneuroendocrinology*, **20**(7), 743–53.

Carani, C., Scuteri, A., Marrama, P. & Bancroft, J. (1990). The effects of testosterone administration and visual erotic stimuli on nocturnal penile tumescence in normal men. *Hormones and Behavior*, **24**(3), 435–41.

Chatterjee, B. & Roy, A. K. (1990). Changes in hepatic androgen sensitivity and gene expression during aging. *Journal of Steroid Biochemistry and Molecular Biology*, **37**(3), 437–45.

Christiansen, K. & Knussmann, R. (1987). Sex hormones and cognitive functioning in men. *Neuropsychobiology*, **18**, 27–36.

Cunningham, G. R., Hirshkowitz, M., Korenman, S. G. & Karacan, I. (1990). Testosterone replacement therapy and sleep-related erections in hypogonadal men. *Journal of Clinical Endocrinology and Metabolism*, **70**(3), 792–7.

Dabbs, J. M., Hargrove, M. F. & Heusel, C. (1996). Testosterone differences among college fraternities: well-behaved vs. rambunctious. *Personality and Individual Differences*, **20**, 157–61.

Dabbs, J. M., Hopper, C. H. & Jurkovic, G. J. (1990). Testosterone and personality among college students and military veterans. *Personality & Individual Differences*, **11**, 1263–9.

Dai, W. S., Kuller, L. H., LaPorte, R. E., Gutai, J. P., Falvo-Gerard, L. & Caggiula, A. (1981). The epidemiology of plasma testosterone levels in middle-aged men. *American Journal of Epidemiology*, **114**, 804–16.

Danziger, L., Schroeder, H. T. & Unger, A. A. (1944). Androgen therapy for involutional melancholia. *Archives of Neurology and Psychiatry*, **51**, 457–61.

Davidson, J. M., Camargo, C. A. & Smith, E. R. (1979). Effects of androgen on sexual behavior in hypogonadal men. *Journal of Clinical Endocrinology and Metabolism*, **48**(6), 955–8.

Davies, R. H., Harris, B., Thomas, D. R., Cook, N., Read, G. & Riad-Fahmy, D. (1992). Salivary testosterone levels and major depressive illness in men [see comments]. *British Journal of Psychiatry*, **161**, 629–32.

Ettigi, P. G., Brown, G. M. & Seggie, J. A. (1979). TSH and LH responses in subtypes of depression. *Psychosomatic Medicine*, **41**(3), 203–8.

Field, A. E., Colditz, G. A., Willett, W. C., Longcope, C. & McKinlay, J. B. (1994). The relation of smoking, age, relative weight, and dietary intake to serum adrenal steroids, sex hormones, and sex hormone-binding globulin in middle-aged men. *Journal of Clinical Endocrinology and Metabolism*, **79**(5), 1310–16.

Gonzalez, M. I., Farabollini, F., Albonetti, E. & Wilson, C. A. (1994). Interactions between 5-hydroxytryptamine (5–HT) and testosterone in the control of sexual and nonsexual behaviour in male and female rats. *Pharmacology, Biochemistry and Behavior*, **47**(3), 591–601.

Gordon, H. W. & Lee, P. A. (1986). A relationship between gonadotropins and visuospatial function. *Neuropsychologia*, **24**(4), 563–76.

Gouchie, C. & Kimura, D. (1991). The relationship between testosterone levels and cognitive ability patterns. *Psychoneuroendocrinology*, **16**(4), 323–34.

Grady, D., Rubin, S. M., Petitti, D. B., Fox, C. S., Black, D., Ettinger, B., Ernster, V. L. & Cummings,

S. R. (1992). Hormone therapy to prevent disease and prolong life in postmenopausal women [see comments]. [Review] [265 refs]. *Annals of Internal Medicine*, 117(12), 1016–37.

Gray, A., Berlin, J. A., McKinlay, J. B. & Longcope, C. (1991). An examination of research design effects on the association of testosterone and male aging: Results of a meta-analysis. *Journal of Clinical Epidemiology*, 7, 671–84.

Hamilton, D. (1986). *The Monkey Gland Affair*. London: Chatto and Windus.

Hampson, E. (1990). Estrogen-related variations in human spatial and articulatory–motor skills. *Psychoneuroendocrinology*, 15(2), 97–111.

Hampson, E. & Moffat, S. D. (1994). Is testosterone related to spatial cognition and hand preference in humans? *Brain and Cognition*, 26(2), 255–66.

Hannan, C. J. Jr, Friedl, K. E., Zold, A., Kettler, T. M. & Plymate, S. R. (1991). Psychological and serum homovanillic acid changes in men administered androgenic steroids. *Psychoneuroendocrinology*, 16(4), 335–43.

Heuser, I. (1998). Testosterone, gonadotropin and cortisol secretion in male patients with major depression [Abstract]. *The International Journal of Neuropsychopharmacology*, 19.

Horwath, E., Johnson, J. & Klerman, G. L. (1992). Depressive symptoms as relative and attributable risk factors for first-onset major depression. *Archives of General Psychiatry*, 49, 817–23.

Itil, T. M., Herrmann, W. M., Blasucci, D. & Freedman, A. (1978). Male hormones in the treatment of depression: effects of mesterolone. *Progress in Neuropsychopharmacology*, 2, 457–67.

Itil, T. M., Michael, S. T., Shapiro, D. M. & Itil, K. Z. (1984). The effects of mesterolone, a male sex hormone in depressed patients (a double blind controlled study). *Methods and Findings in Experimental and Clinical Pharmacology*, 6(6), 331–7.

Janowsky, J. S., Oviatt, S. K. & Orwoll, E. S. (1994). Testosterone influences spatial cognition in older men. *Behavioral Neuroscience*, 108(2), 325–32.

Kemper, T. D. (1990). *Social Structure and Testosterone*. New Brunswick: Rutgers University Press.

Kerman, E. F. (1943). Testosterone therapy of involutional psychosis. *Archives of Neurology and Psychiatry*, 49, 306–7.

Kertzman, C., Robinson, D. L., Sherins, R. J., Schwankhaus, J. D. & McClurkin, J. W. (1990). Abnormalities in visual spatial attention in men with mirror movements associated with isolated hypogonadotropic hypogonadism. *Neurology*, 40(7), 1057–63.

Klaiber, E. L., Broverman, D. M., Vogel, W. & Kobayashi, Y. (1979). Estrogen therapy for severe persistent depressions in women. *Archives of General Psychiatry*, 36(5), 550–4.

Kreuz, L. E., Rose, R. M. & Jennings, J. R. (1972). Suppression of plasma testosterone levels and psychological stress. *Archives of General Psychiatry*, 26, 479–82.

Kwan, M., Greenleaf, W. J., Mann, J., Crapo, L. & Davidson, J. M. (1983). The nature of androgen action on male sexuality: a combined laboratory-self-report study on hypogonadal men. *Journal of Clinical Endocrinology and Metabolism*, 57(3), 557–62.

Lamberts, S. W., van den Beld, A. W. & van der Lely, A. J. (1997). The endocrinology of aging [see comments]. [Review] [65 refs]. *Science*, 278(5337), 419–24.

Laycock, J. F. & Wise, P. H. (1996). Male reproductive endocrinology. In *Essential Endocrinology*, ed. Anonymous. New York: Oxford University Press.

Levitt, A. J. & Joffe, R. T. (1988). Total and free testosterone in depressed men. *Acta Psychiatrica Scandinavica*, 77(3), 346–8.

Lewinsohn, P. M., Seeley, J. R., Roberts, R. E. & Allen, N. B. (1997). Center for Epidemiologic Studies Depression Scale (CES-D) as a screening instrument for depression among community-residing older adults. *Psychology and Aging*, 12(2), 277–87.

Luisi, M. & Franchi, F. (1980). Double-blind group comparative study of testosterone undecanoate and mesterolone in hypogonadal male patients. *Journal of Endocrinological Investigation*, 3(3), 305–8.

Mason, J. W., Giller, E. L. & Kosten, T. R. (1988). Serum testosterone differences between patients with schizophrenia and those with affective disorder. *Biological Psychiatry*, 23(4), 357–66.

Matsumoto, A. M. (1990). Effects of chronic testosterone administration in normal men: safety and efficacy of high dosage testosterone and parallel dose-dependent suppression of luteinizing hormone, follicle-stimulating hormone, and sperm production. *Journal of Clinical Endocrinology and Metabolism*, 70(1), 282–7.

Mazur, A. (1995). Biosocial models of deviant behavior among male army veterans. *Biological Psychology*, 41(3), 271–93.

McEwen, B. S. (1998). Gonadal and adrenal steroids and the brain: Implications for depression. In *Hormones and Depression*. ed. U. Halbreich, pp. 239–53. New York: Raven Press.

Meehan, P. J., Saltzman, L. E. & Sattin, R. W. (1991). Suicide among older United States residents: epidemiologic characteristics and trends. *American Journal of Public Health*, 81, 1198–200.

Moffat, S. D. & Hampson, E. (1996). A curvilinear relationship between testosterone and spatial cognition in humans: possible influence of hand preference. *Psychoneuroendocrinology*, 21(3), 323–37.

Money, J., Schwartz, M. & Lewis, V. G. (1984). Adult erotosexual status and fetal hormonal masculinization and demasculinization: 46,XX congenital virilizing adrenal hyperplasia and 46,XY androgen-insensitivity syndrome compared. *Psychoneuroendocrinology*, 9(4), 405–14.

Morley, J. E., Kaiser, F. E., Sih, R., Hajjar, R. & Perry, H. M. (1997). Testosterone and frailty. *Clinics in Geriatric Medicine*, 13(4), 685–95.

Morley, J. E., Perry, H. M. 3rd, Kaiser, F. E., Kraenzle, D., Jensen, J., Houston, K., Mattammal, M. & Perry, H. M. Jr. (1993). Effects of testosterone replacement in old hypogonadal males: a preliminary study. *Journal of the American Geriatric Society*, 41, 149–52.

O'Carroll, R. & Bancroft, J. (1984). Testosterone therapy for low sexual interest and erectile dysfunction in men: a controlled study. *British Journal of Psychiatry*, 145, 146–51.

O'Carroll, R., Shapiro, C. & Bancroft, J. (1985). Androgens, behaviour and nocturnal erection in hypogonadal men: the effects of varying the replacement dose. *Clinical Endocrinology*, 23(5), 527–38.

Olweus, D., Mattsson, A., Schalling, D. & Low, H. (1988). Circulating testosterone levels and aggression in adolescent males: a causal analysis. *Psychosomatic Medicine*, 50(3), 261–72.

Paganini-Hill, A. & Henderson, V. W. (1994). Estrogen deficiency and risk of Alzheimer's disease in women. *American Journal of Epidemiology*, 140(3), 256–61.

Pardoll, D. H. & Belinson, L. (1941). Androgen therapy in psychosis: effect of testosterone propionate in male involutional psychotics. *Journal of Clinical Endocrinology*, 1, 138–41.

Plymate, S. (1994). Hypogonadism. *Endocrinology and Metabolism Clinics of North America*, 23, 749–72.

Pope, H. G., Jr & Katz, D. L. (1994). Psychiatric and medical effects of anabolic-androgenic steroid use. A controlled study of 160 athletes. *Archives of General Psychiatry*, 51(5), 375–82.

Pope, H. G., Jr, Kouri, E. M. & Hudson, J. I. (in press). The effects of supraphysiologic doses of testosterone on mood and aggression in normal men. A randomized controlled trial. *Biological Psychiatry*,

Popova, N. K. & Amstislavskaya, T. G. (1989). Effect of 5–HT1A receptor agonists on plasma testosterone and behavior in sexual arousal in male mice [Abstract]. *Pharmacology, Biochemistry and Behavior*, 35, 74–5.

Rabkin, J. G., Rabkin, R. & Wagner, G. (1995). Testosterone replacement therapy in HIV illness. *General Hospital Psychiatry*, 17(1), 37–42.

Rabkin, J. G., Rabkin, R. & Wagner, G. J. (1997). Testosterone treatment of clinical hypogonadism in patients with HIV/AIDS. [Review] [53 refs]. *International Journal of STD and AIDS*, 8(9), 537–545.

Reiter, T. (1965). Testosterone implantation: the method of choice for treatment of testosterone deficiency. *Journal of the American Geriatrics Society*, 13(12), 1003–12.

Rinieris, P. M., Malliaras, D. E., Batrinos, M. L. & Stefanis, C. N. (1979). Testosterone treatment of depression in two patients with Klinefelter's syndrome. *American Journal of Psychiatry*, 136(7), 986–8.

Roberts, R. E. & Vernon, S. W. (1983). The Center for Epidemiologic Studies Depression Scale: Its use in a community sample. *American Journal of Psychiatry*, 140, 41–6.

Robinson, D., Friedman, L., Marcus, R., Tinklenberg, J. & Yesavage, J. (1994). Estrogen replacement therapy and memory in older women. *Journal of the American Geriatrics Society*, 42(9), 919–22.

Rose, R. M., Bernstein, I. S. & Gordon, T. P. (1975). Consequences of social conflict on plasma testosterone levels in rhesus monkeys. *Psychosomatic Medicine*, 37, 50–61.

Rubin, R. T. (1981). Sex steroid hormone dynamics in endogenous depression: a review. *International Journal of Mental Health*, 10, 43–59.

Rubin, R. T., Poland, R. E. & Lesser, I. M. (1989). Neuroendocrine aspects of primary endogenous depression VIII. Pituitary–gonadal axis activity in male patients and matched control subjects. *Psychoneuroendocrinology*, 14, 217–29.

Rubinow, D. R. & Schmidt, P. J. (1996). Androgens, brain, and behavior. [Review] [179 refs]. *American Journal of Psychiatry*, 153(8), 974–84.

Rupprecht, R., Rupprecht, C., Rupprecht, M., Noder, M. & Schwarz, W. (1988). Different reactivity of the hypothalamo–pituitary–gonadal axis in depression and normal controls. *Pharmacopsychiatry*, 21(6), 438–9.

Sachar, E. J., Halpern, F., Rosenfeld, R. S., Galligher, T. F. & Hellman, L. (1973). Plasma and urinary testosterone levels in depressed men. *Archives of General Psychiatry*, 28(1), 15–18.

Schiavi, R. C., White, D. & Mandeli, J. (1992). Pituitary-gonadal function during sleep in healthy aging men. *Psychoneuroendocrinology*, 17(6), 599–609.

Schiavi, R. C., White, D., Mandeli, J. & Levine, A. C. (1997). Effect of testosterone administration on sexual behavior and mood in men with erectile dysfunction. *Archives of Sexual Behavior*, 26(3), 231–41.

Schmidt, P. J. & Rubinow, D. R. (1997). Neuroregulatory role of gonadal steroids in humans. *Psychopharmacology Bulletin*, 33(2), 219–20.

Schneider, L. S., Farlow, M. R., Henderson, V. W. & Pogoda, J. M. (1996). Effects of estrogen

S. N. Seidman and S. P. Roose

142

replacement therapy on response to tacrine in patients with Alzheimer's disease. *Neurology*, **46**(6), 1580–4.

Schneider, L. S., Small, G. W., Hamilton, S. H., Bystritsky, A., Nemeroff, C. B. & Meyers, B. S. (1997). Estrogen replacement and response to fluoxetine in a multicenter geriatric depression trial. Fluoxetine Collaborative Study Group. *American Journal of Geriatric Psychiatry*, **5**(2), 97–106.

Seidman, S. N. & Rabkin, J. G. (1998). Testosterone replacement therapy for hypogonadal men with SSRI-refractory depression. *Journal of Affective Disorders*, **48**, 157–61.

Shain, S. A. & Boesel, R. W. (1977). Aging-associated diminished rat prostate androgen receptor content concurrent with decreased androgen dependence. *Mechanisms of Aging and Development*, **6**(3), 219–32.

Siegel, A. & Demetrikopoulos, M. K. (1998). Hormones and aggression. In *Hormonally Induced Changes in the Mind and Brain*, ed. Anonymous, pp. 99–127. New York: Academic Press Inc.

Sih, R., Morley, J. E., Kaiser, F. E., Perry, H. M., Patrick, P. & Ross, C. (1997). Testosterone replacement in older hypogonadal men: a 12-month randomized controlled trial [see comments]. *Journal of Clinical Endocrinology and Metabolism*, **82**(6), 1661–7.

Snyder, P. J. (1996). Development of criteria to monitor the occurrence of prostate cancer in testosterone clinical trials. In *Pharmacology, Biology and Clinical Applications of Androgens*, ed. S. Bhasin, J. Spieler, R. Swerdloff, C. Wang, C. Kelly & H. Grabelnick, pp. 143–50. New York: Wiley.

Steiger, A., von Bardeleben, U., Guldner, J., Lauer, C., Rothe, B. & Holsboer, F. (1993). The sleep EEG and nocturnal hormonal secretion studies on changes during the course of depression and on effects of CNS-active drugs. *Progress in Neuro-Psychopharmacology and Biological Psychiatry*, **17**(1), 125–37.

Sternbach, H. (1998). Age-associated testosterone decline in men. *American Journal of Psychiatry*, **155**(10), 1310–18.

Su, T. P., Pagliaro, M., Schmidt, P. J., Pickar, D., Wolkowitz, O. & Rubinow, D. R. (1993). Neuropsychiatric effects of anabolic steroids in male normal volunteers. *Journal of the American Medical Association*, **269**(21), 2760–4.

Swerdloff, R. S. & Wang, C. (1993). Androgen deficiency and aging in men [see comments]. [Review] [102 refs]. *Western Journal of Medicine*, **159**(5), 579–85.

Tang, M. X., Jacobs, D., Stern, Y., Marder, K., Schofield, P., Gurland, B., Andrews, H. & Mayeux, R. (1996). Effect of oestrogen during menopause on risk and age at onset of Alzheimer's disease [see comments]. *Lancet*, **348**(9025), 429–32.

Tenover, J. L. (1997). Testosterone and the aging male. [Review] [14 refs]. *Journal of Andrology*, **18**(2), 103–6.

Tenover, J. S. (1992). Effects of testosterone supplementation in the aging male. *Journal of Clinical Endocrinology and Metabolism*, **75**, 1092–8.

Tricker, R., Casaburi, R., Storer, T. W., Clevenger, B., Berman, N., Shirazi, A. & Bhasin, S. (1996). The effects of supraphysiological doses of testosterone on angry behavior in healthy eugonadal men: a clinical research center study. *Journal of Clinical Endocrinology and Metabolism*, **81**(10), 3754–8.

Unden, F., Ljunggren, J. G., Beck-Friis, J., Kjellman, B. F. & Wetterberg, L. (1988).

Hypothalamic–pituitary–gonadal axis in major depressive disorders. *Acta Psychiatrica Scandinavica*, **78**(2), 138–46.

Uzych, L. (1992). Anabolic-androgenic steroids and psychiatric-related effects: a review. [Review] [28 refs]. *Canadian Journal of Psychiatry – Revue Canadienne de Psychiatrie*, **37**(1), 23–8.

Vermeulen, A., Kaufman, J. M. & Giagulli, V. A. (1998). Influence of some biological indexes on sex hormone binding globulin and androgen levels in aging or obese males. *Journal of Clinical Endocrinology and Metabolism*, **81**, 1821–6.

Villareal, D. T. & Morley, J. E. (1994). Trophic factors in aging. *Drugs and Aging*, **4**, 492–509.

Vogel, W., Broverman, D. M., Klaiber, E. L., Abraham, G. & Cone, F. L. (1971). Effects of testosterone infusions upon EEGs of normal male adults. *Electroencephalography and Clinical Neurophysiology*, **31**(4), 400–3.

Vogel, W., Klaiber, E. L. & Broverman, D. M. (1978). Roles of the gonadal steroid hormones in psychiatric depression in men and women. *Progress in Neuro-Psychopharmacology*, **2**, 487–503.

Vogel, W., Klaiber, E. L. & Broverman, D. M. (1985). A comparison of the antidepressant effects of a synthetic androgen (mesterolone) and amitriptyline in depressed men. *Journal of Clinical Psychiatry*, **46**(1), 6–8.

Wallen, K., Eisler, J. A., Tannenbaum, P. L., Nagell, K. M. & Mann, D. R. (1991). Antide (Nal–Lys GnRH antagonist) suppression of pituitary–testicular function and sexual behavior in group-living rhesus monkeys A1. *Physiology and Behavior*, **50**(2), 429–35.

Wang, C., Alexander, G., Berman, N., Salehian, B., Davidson, T., McDonald, V., Steiner, B., Hull, L., Callegari, C. & Swerdloff, R. S. (1996). Testosterone replacement therapy improves mood in hypogonadal men: a clinical research center study. *Journal of Clinical Endocrinology and Metabolism*, **81**(10), 3578–3.

Weinbauer, G. F., Gromoll, J., Simoni, M. & Nieschlag, E. (1997). Physiology of testicular function. In *Andrology: Male Reproductive Health and Dysfunction*, ed. E. Nieschlag & H. Behre, pp. 25–60. Berlin: Springer-Verlag.

Wexler, B. E., Mason, J. W. & Giller, E. L. (1989). Possible subtypes of affective disorder suggested by differences in cerebral laterality and testosterone. A preliminary report. *Archives of General Psychiatry*, **46**(5), 429–33.

Woodman, C. L. & Williams, W. R. (1996). Testosterone, mood and psychotropic medication [Abstract]. American Psychiatric Association, 149th Annual Meeting.

World Health Organization Task Force on Methods for the Regulation of Male Fertility. (1990). Contraceptive efficacy of testosterone-induced azoospermia in normal men. *Lancet*, **336**, 955–9.

Yaffe, K., Sawaya, G., Lieberburg, I. & Grady, D. (1998). Estrogen therapy in postmenopausal women: effects on cognitive function and dementia. *Journal of the American Medical Association*, **279**(9), 688–95.

Yates, W. R., Perry, P., Macindoe, J., Holman, T. & Ellingrad, V. (1999). Psychosexual effects of three doses of testosterone in cycling and normal men. *Biological Psychiatry*, **45**(3), 254–60.

Yesavage, J. A., Davidson, J., Widrow, L. & Berger, P. A. (1985). Plasma testosterone levels, depression, sexuality, and age. *Biological Psychiatry*, **20**(2), 222–5.

7

Dehydroepiandrosterone in aging and mental health

Owen M. Wolkowitz, Patricia D. Kroboth, Victor I. Reus and Tanya J. Fabian

Introduction

Dehydroepiandrosterone (DHEA) and its sulfated metabolite, DHEA-S (together abbreviated DHEA(S)), are quantitatively the most important adrenal corticosteroids in man, although their physiological roles are unknown. These steroids have captured widespread scientific and public attention in recent years due to three key observations. First, circulating levels of these steroids progressively decline from young adulthood through the end of the lifespan; they also decrease in response to chronic stress or illness. Second, preclinical studies suggest that DHEA(S) protects against certain pathological processes seen in illness and with aging. Third, some epidemiological studies in man suggest that relatively higher DHEA(S) levels are associated with enhanced physical and mental well-being. Such findings have raised hope that replacement dosing with pharmaceutical DHEA may enhance and prolong life, although very limited clinical data exist to support this. This chapter will review preclinical and clinical data regarding the effects of DHEA(S) in the central nervous system, its biological role in aging and mental health and its possible efficacy in treating neuropsychiatric illness in the middle-aged and elderly.

DHEA(S) as a neurosteroid

DHEA(S) is synthesized in situ in brain, with glial cells playing a major role in its formation and metabolism; it has therefore, been termed a neurosteroid (Baulieu, 1997). Accumulation of DHEA(S) in rat brain is largely independent of adrenal and gonadal synthesis, remaining constant after orchiectomy, adrenalectomy and dexamethasone administration (Robel & Baulieu, 1995; Corpechot et al., 1981). In contrast, brain levels of DHEA-S significantly rise following stress, even in the adrenalectomized and orchiectomized rat, irrespective of changes in corresponding plasma samples.

DHEA and DHEA-S are widely distributed throughout the body, with DHEA concentrations highest in brain, then plasma, spleen, kidneys, and liver based on data from male rats (Corpechot et al., 1981). The amounts of DHEA-S in the brain also exceed those in adrenals, spleen, kidneys, testes, liver, and plasma (in descending order; Corpechot et al., 1981). In human brain tissue, concentrations of DHEA have been noted to be 6.5 times higher than in plasma (LaCroix et al., 1987). Although there is a linear relationship between blood and cerebrospinal fluid (CSF) concentrations of DHEA and DHEA-S in humans, CSF concentrations are only 5.4% and 0.15% of those in plasma for DHEA and DHEA-S, respectively (Guazzo et al., 1996).

DHEA(S) levels decrease as a function of aging, chronic stress and illness

Perhaps the most remarkable and well-replicated observation about DHEA(S) is that its circulating levels in men and women peak in the mid-20s and then progressively decrease with age, approaching a nadir (~20% of peak levels) at approximately 65 to 70 years, the age at which the incidence of many age-related illnesses steeply increases (Regelson & Kalimi, 1994). CSF levels similarly decrease with aging (in men: Azuma et al., 1993; in both genders: Guazzo et al., 1996). Levels of DHEA(S) also decrease with chronic stress and medical illness (Spratt et al., 1993; Parker et al., 1985b; Nishikaze, 1998; Ozasa et al., 1990). The age-, stress- and illness-related declines in levels of DHEA(S) are unique among adrenocortical hormones, although in males, the decrease in plasma DHEA(S) levels is paralleled by decreases in levels of bioavailable testosterone (Morley et al., 1997). Glucocorticoids fail to show a similar pattern of decrease with age, illness or stress. Cortisol levels typically rise or do not change in these conditions, and there is a highly significant decrease in plasma ratios of DHEA(S)-to-cortisol with age and chronic stress in both men and women (Leblhuber et al., 1993; Reus et al., 1993; Guazzo et al., 1996). Several authors have suggested that these ratios are more meaningful than are levels of DHEA(S) or cortisol alone (Leblhuber et al., 1992; Wolkowitz et al., 1992; Hechter et al., 1997; McKenna et al., 1997; Goodyer et al., 1998; Oberbeck et al., 1998; Fava et al., 1989; Nishikaze, 1998; Ozasa et al., 1990; Parker et al., 1985b).

An important but frequently overlooked observation is that there is a high degree of interindividual variability in DHEA(S) levels. Whereas levels over time are highly correlated within individuals – suggesting their possible utility as individual markers (Thomas et al., 1994) – cross-sectional levels among age- and gender-matched individuals vary up to 6.5-fold (Orentreich et al., 1984, 1992; Thomas et al., 1994). Further, whereas studies uniformly confirm age-related decreases in mean DHEA(S) levels, 15% of individual male subjects have been reported to show increasing DHEA(S) levels over time (Orentreich et al., 1992). The causes of such interindividual variability, and its functional significance are unknown. It is tempting to theorize that greater rates of decline in DHEA(S) levels over time are associated with less successful aging and with deteriorating memory function. Lupien et al. (1995) noted greater cognitive deterioration in elderly men and women who showed greater decreases in DHEA-S-to-cortisol ratios over a 2-year period; changes in DHEA-S levels alone, however, were not significantly correlated with cognitive change.

As mentioned, DHEA(S) levels also decrease in response to chronic stress or illness (Parker et al., 1985b). Following an acute stressor, generalized hypothalamic–pituitary–adrenal (HPA) axis responses include increased secretion of both cortisol and DHEA(S) in humans. With continued stress, however, DHEA(S) levels and/or DHEA(S)-to-cortisol ratios decrease to below baseline while cortisol levels remain elevated (Parker et al., 1985b; Bernton et al., 1995; Ozasa et al., 1990); this suggests independent regulation of these two stress-responsive hormones (Parker et al., 1985a; McKenna et al., 1997; Osran et al., 1993).

Although there is no direct evidence that age-related or illness- and stress-related decreases in DHEA(S) levels are causally related to the onset of various diseases, several preclinical and clinical studies reviewed below raise the possibility that decreased DHEA(S) levels (or decreased DHEA(S)-to-cortisol ratios) contribute to the development or progression of cognitive decline as well as to affective disturbances and impaired physical and emotional well-being in the aged or chronically ill.

DHEA(S) improves learning and memory in animals

DHEA and DHEA-S generally have memory-enhancing effects in animals. Administered intracerebroventricularly (i.c.v.) immediately following training, DHEA and DHEA-S improve long-term memory and diminish amnesia in male mice (Flood et al., 1988, 1992; Flood & Roberts, 1988). DHEA, administered orally in drinking water, also significantly enhances retention in long-term memory (Flood & Roberts, 1988; Flood et al., 1988). Untreated middle-aged and old mice perform more poorly than do young mice in certain memory tasks such as foot-shock active avoidance training. However, post-trial subcutaneous injection of DHEA in old male mice (Flood & Roberts, 1988), as well as oral administration of DHEA-S to old rats (Tejkalova et al., 1998), improves memory retention to the high levels seen in younger animals. In certain paradigms, however, DHEA-S impairs memory. Fleshner and colleagues (1997), for example, reported that chronic exposure of animals to high levels of DHEA-S interfered with contextual fear conditioning in a manner similar to that seen post-adrenalectomy. They interpreted this as evidence of a functional antiglucocorticoid effect of DHEA-S.

DHEA(S) significantly reverses pharmacologically induced amnesia in mice. Dimethylsulfoxide (DMSO), a membrane perturbant, doubles the number of training trials that mice require to learn to actively avoid foot shock; i.c.v. administration of DHEA fully prevents this effect (Roberts, 1990). DHEA and DHEA-S also block the memory-impairing effect of ethanol in mice (Melchior & Ritzmann, 1996). Anisomycin, a protein synthesis-inhibitor, decreases active avoidance recall from 80% correct to 13%, but adding DHEA-S to the anisomycin restores recall to 80%. Similarly, scopolamine, an anticholinergic drug, decreases active avoidance recall from 80% to 7%. Adding DHEA-S to scopolamine restores recall to 80% (Flood et al., 1988; Roberts, 1990). Rhodes and colleagues (1996) demonstrated that DHEA-S, administered intraperitoneally to anesthetized rats, significantly increases hippocampal release of acetylcholine; this may account for the ability of DHEA-S to counter scopolamine's effects. DHEA-S, as opposed to DHEA, may be more important in antagonizing scopolamine-amnesia, since both the memory effect (Li et al., 1997), as well as the hippocampal acetylcholine release effect (Rhodes et al., 1997), are potentiated by co-administration of a steroid sulfatase inhibitor, which decreases the conversion of DHEA-S to DHEA. These data suggest that DHEA and DHEA-S administration, either i.c.v., subcutaneously or orally, can have significant promemory effects (i.e. improved long-term memory and retention) in vivo. Further, certain age-related memory deficits are pharmacologically reversible, and specific amnestic effects are attenuated by DHEA and DHEA-S. The reversal of scopolamine amnesia is particularly noteworthy as it has been proposed as a pharmacologic model in normal humans of the cognitive deficits seen in Alzheimer's disease (Christensen et al., 1992; Sunderland et al., 1990).

Antidepressant and anti-anxiety effects in animals

DHEA-S has antidepressant-like effects in mice tested in the Porsolt forced swim test. In this test, DHEA-S significantly decreases immobility time (consistent with antidepressant effects) without non-specifically changing ambulation or open field activity (Reddy et al., 1998). This effect is related to DHEA-S's functioning as an agonist at the sigma-1 receptor, since it is blocked by pre-treatment with specific sigma-1 antagonists (Reddy et al., 1998). DHEA (non-sulfated) also has antidepressant effects in the Porsolt forced swim test, but interestingly, only in high anxiety rats (Prasad et al., 1997).

DHEA and DHEA-S also have antianxiety-like effects in mice in the elevated-plus-maze test (Melchior & Ritzmann, 1994). However, whereas DHEA augments the anxiolytic effect of ethanol in this model, DHEA-S blocks it (Melchior & Ritzmann, 1994). Consistent with possibly different effects of DHEA and DHEA-S in animal models of anxiety, DHEA-S has been found to be anxiogenic in the 'mirrored chamber' test, another test of anxiety in mice (Reddy & Kulkarni, 1997).

Neurotrophic potential of DHEA(S)

Several studies also suggest that DHEA(S) has neurotrophic potential. DHEA and DHEA-S, for example, enhance neuronal and glial survival, and differentiation in dissociated cultures of mouse embryo brain (Bologa et al., 1987; Roberts et al., 1987). DHEA also increases the length of neurites with the Tau-1 axonal marker in primary cultures of mouse embyonic neocortical neurons, while DHEA-S increases the length of a different subclass of neurite extension (Compagnone & Mellon 1998). Del Cerro et al. (1995) reported that both DHEA and DHEA-S (in contrast to other neurosteroids, pregnenolone and pregnenolone sulfate) induced the formation of hypertrophic, highly glial fibrillary acidic protein (GFAP)-reactive cells in hippocampal slice cultures derived from orchiectomized adult male rats. These cells appeared similar to the reactive astroglia that may be involved in restorative events following brain injury. DHEA and DHEA-S have also been shown to prevent or reduce the hippocampal neurotoxic actions of the glutamate agonist, N-methyl-D-aspartic acid (NMDA), both in vitro and in vivo (Kimonides et al., 1998). In vivo administration of DHEA to animals, resulting in plasma levels comparable to those seen in young adult humans, protected neurons against NMDA infused directly into the hippocampus (Kimonides et al., 1998). Because glutamate release has been implicated in neural damage resulting from cerebral ischemia and other neuronal insults, these data raise the possibility that decreased DHEA(S) levels contribute to the increased vulnerability of the aging or stressed human brain to such damage (Kimonides et al., 1998). These investigators have also found that DHEA protects against corticosterone-induced neurotoxicity in rat hippocampal neurons (Kimonides et al., 1999), consistent with DHEA's reputed antiglucocorticoid actions in brain.

DHEA(S) levels correlate with mood, memory and functional abilities in humans

Mood

Many, but not all, studies have reported lowered levels of DHEA(S) in depressed individuals. Among 622 community-based French subjects followed over 4 years, significantly lower DHEA-S levels were recorded in women with depression, poor life satisfaction and functional limitations; men showed trends in the same directions (Berr et al., 1996). Yaffe et al. (1998a) also reported that healthy, community-dwelling elderly women with undetectable serum DHEA-S levels had higher depression ratings compared to women with detectable levels. Further, Legrain et al. (1995) noted that, among aged long-term care patients (largely with dementia, treated depression, hypertension, cardiac arrhythmias, or Parkinson's Disease), DHEA-S levels were lower in those being treated for depression. A recent Japanese report also found low levels of 17-ketosteroid sulfates (e.g. DHEA-S) in conditions of psychosocial stress, severe depression and spousal bereavement (Furuya et al., 1998). Osran and colleagues (1993) and Ferrari and colleagues (1997) found that DHEA-to-cortisol ratios more accurately discriminated depressed from non-depressed individuals than did levels of either hormone alone, with lower morning ratios seen in the depressives (Osran et al., 1993). In that study, circadian rhythms of DHEA production were also altered; DHEA levels in the depressed patients increased from 8 am to 4 pm, whereas normals showed a decrease over that time period (Osran et al., 1993). Michael and colleagues (in press) also recently reported low morning (but not evening) salivary DHEA levels in adult depressives; morning DHEA levels were inversely correlated with depression severity ratings (Michael et al., in press). This study replicated their prior findings in adolescents (Goodyer et al., 1996). Together with the findings of Osran et al. (1993), these studies suggest that not only may absolute levels of DHEA be altered in depression, but also that their circadian variability may differ from that seen in normals.

The remaining literature examining endogenous serum or urinary DHEA(S) levels in depression is inconsistent, with reports of increased (Tollefson et al., 1990; Hansen et al., 1982; Heuser et al., 1998b; Takebayashi et al., 1998), decreased (Ferguson et al., 1964; Buckwalter et al., 1999) or unaltered (Reus et al., 1993; Fava et al., 1989; Shulman et al., 1992) levels. In one of these studies, DHEA-S-to-cortisol ratios were lower in patients with depression compared to patients with panic disorder, but did not differ between depressives and controls (Fava et al., 1989). The study by Heuser and colleagues (1998b), which showed increased plasma DHEA levels in depression, was particularly detailed and involved plasma sampling every 30 minutes for 24 hours. However, their subject sample may not be comparable to some of those used in other studies since their subjects were severely depressed and hypercortisolemic and were allowed to receive chloral hydrate during the study. In one of the other studies showing high DHEA-S levels in depressed patients, the levels were positively correlated with depression severity ratings (Tollefson et al., 1990); hormone levels, however, tended to be inversely correlated with depression severity ratings ($P<0.10$) in another (Takebayashi et al., 1998).

Response to antidepressant and antianxiety medication

DHEA(S)'s responsiveness to antidepressant and antianxiety medication has also been examined, with some, but not all studies showing treatment-associated increases in levels of these hormones. In two of the studies in major depression reviewed above, electroconvulsive therapy was found to increase DHEA-S levels (Ferguson et al., 1964), but the tricyclic antidepressant, imipramine, was found to lower urinary DHEA-S levels (Tollefson et al., 1990). Similarly, Takebayashi and colleagues (1998) recently determined that another tricyclic antidepressant, clomipramine, lowered plasma DHEA-S levels. Romeo and colleagues (1998) found no significant effect of antidepressant treatment (mainly tricyclic antidepressants) on plasma DHEA levels; DHEA-S levels were not assessed. Similarly, Uzunova and colleagues (1998) found no significant effect of the serotonin specific reuptake inhibitor (SSRI) antidepressants, fluoxetine and paroxetine, on CSF DHEA(S) levels in depressed patients, confirming a prior preclinical study showing no effect of fluoxetine on brain DHEA levels in rats (Uzunov et al., 1996). Despite these negative results with tricyclic or SSRI antidepressants, bupropion, a dopamine and norepinephrine reuptake blocking antidepressant, has been shown to increase DHEA-S levels in women with sexual dysfunction (Crenshaw & Goldberg, 1996). Levels of other sex hormones did not change, and the bupropion-induced increases in DHEA-S levels were positively correlated with recovery from sexual dysfunction (Crenshaw & Goldberg, 1996).

Only one study to date has examined the effects of anti-anxiety medication on DHEA(S) levels. Kroboth and colleagues (1999) found that the acute administration of alprazolam (a triazolo-benzodiazepine with antianxiety and mild antidepressant effects) significantly increased plasma DHEA levels in healthy young and elderly men; DHEA-S levels were unaffected. The increase in DHEA levels is especially noteworthy since cortisol levels were significantly decreased in these subjects, in accord with alprazolam's ability to inhibit hypothalamic corticotropin-releasing hormone (CRH) release (Kalogeras et al., 1990). Interestingly, subjects who responded to alprazolam with greater increases in DHEA levels were better able to counteract alprazolam's psychomotor impairing effects, although at the highest DHEA levels, a u-shaped function became apparent. The lowest and highest concentrations were associated with the greatest decrement, while concentrations between 10 and 16 ng/ml were associated with the least decrement (Kroboth et al., 1999). The authors suggested that the increased production of DHEA, a mild GABA–A receptor antagonist, represented a homeostatic mechanism, functioning to buffer alprazolam's acute GABA–A receptor stimulation. At the highest plasma DHEA levels, however, there may have been greater conversion of DHEA to androsterone or other GABA–A receptor agonists, augmenting alprazolam's psychomotor effects.

General functional abilities and sense of well-being

In most population-based studies in the elderly, cognitive and general functional abilities have been shown to be positively correlated with DHEA(S) levels, but demonstration of differences between demented individuals and controls has been inconsistent. One large epidemiological study involving 4030 elderly men and women found DHEA-S levels to vary directly with cognitive and physical performance (Berkman et al., 1993). Another study found that men, but not women, with higher serum DHEA-S levels were significantly younger, leaner, more fit, and had more favorable lipid profiles (Abbasi et al., 1998). A prospective French study found, among 622 elderly subjects, significantly lower DHEA-S levels in women with functional limitations; men showed trends in the same direction (Berr et al., 1996). In both genders, lower DHEA-S levels were associated with poorer subjective ratings of overall health (Berr et al., 1996). Morrison and colleagues also noted, in a convenience sample selected from a nursing home population, that low DHEA-S levels were correlated with self-rated disability and insomnia and, in women, with increased number of pain sites (Morrison et al., 1998). Cawood and colleagues (1996) assessed 'sense of well-being' in 145 healthy community-living women, aged 40 to 60 years, who were not taking estrogen replacement. Among the hormones, estradiol, estrone, DHEA, DHEA-S, and androstenedione, only DHEA (but not DHEA-S) was significantly and positively related to ratings of well-being, positive affect, and sensation seeking.

In a study directly assessing plasma DHEA-S levels in relation to functional abilities (independent of diagnosis), Rudman et al. (1990) reported significantly lower DHEA-S levels in elderly men living in nursing homes compared to age-matched men living in the community. The prevalence of low DHEA-S levels was 41% in the nursing home men compared to 6% in the community men. In the nursing home sample, plasma DHEA-S levels were significantly and inversely correlated with severity scores on measures of activities of daily living (e.g., eating, transferring, mobility, toileting) and with the principal diagnosis of organic brain syndrome. Nursing home men with the least functional impairment had a mean DHEA-S level of 176 mcg/dl; those with the greatest functional impairment had a mean level of 18 mcg/dl. Similarly, Ravaglia et al. (1996, 1997) reported that DHEA-S levels in very old healthy men (90 to 106 years old) were significantly and directly correlated with ability to successfully perform activities of daily living. The same relationship, albeit non-significant, was seen in women. Based on these data, the authors proposed that DHEA(S) plays a role in successful aging (Ravaglia et al., 1996, 1997).

Cognitive function

Kalmijn and colleagues (1998), studying healthy middle-aged to elderly adults in a prospective design, reported a statistically significant inverse relationship between DHEA-S-to-cortisol ratios and cognitive impairment and a trend towards a significant inverse relationship between DHEA-S levels alone and cognitive impairment (odds ratio = 0.5). In another study (Reus et al., 1993), normal controls as well as depressed patients, between the ages of 24 and 70, showed decreasing ratios of DHEA-to-cortisol and DHEA-S-to-cortisol with age; these ratios were directly correlated with performance on cognitive tests involving automatic processing and access to semantic (or knowledge) memory. Specifically, greater ratios of DHEA or DHEA-S-to-cortisol were associated with better performance in these cognitive measures. In a study of hormonal correlates of cognitive function in pregnant women, Buckwalter and colleagues (1999) found that plasma DHEA levels were significantly correlated with better visuoperceptual skills, executive control processes, and free recall. After delivery, maternal DHEA levels remained significantly correlated with better executive control processes and free recall. In another study, however, cognitive impairment in female (but not male) nursing home residents was associated with higher DHEA-S levels (Morrison et al., 1998), leading the authors to conclude that contradictory relationships exist between DHEA-S levels and neuropsychiatric function, and that these relationships may be gender- (and perhaps, age-) specific.

Some but not all studies have noted markedly decreased serum DHEA(S) levels in patients with Alzheimer's disease or other dementias. Sunderland et al. (1989) first reported, in a small group of Alzheimer's disease patients, that plasma DHEA-S levels averaged 48% lower than those in age- and sex-matched normals. This finding was replicated in two larger-scale studies comparing Alzheimer's disease and multi-infarct dementia patients with healthy elderly controls (Nasman et al., 1991; Yanase et al., 1996), although the fact that Alzheimer's disease patients and multi-infarct dementia patients had similarly low levels calls into question the specificity of this finding. Solerte and colleagues (1999) recently assessed 24-hour DHEA-S levels in Alzheimer's disease patients and elderly controls and found decreased DHEA-S levels in the patient group. In addition, a trend towards lower DHEA-S-to-cortisol ratios in Alzheimer's disease patients, compared to healthy age-matched controls, was reported by Leblhuber et al. (1993), supporting the utility of examining these hormones in ratio form (Leblhuber et al., 1992; Wolkowitz et al., 1992). Leblhuber et al. (1995) also reported low serum DHEA-S levels and DHEA-S-to-cortisol ratios in patients with Huntington's disease, another dementing illness, but this differs from a prior report in this population (Bruyn & de Jong, 1973).

Further raising the possibility of dysregulation of both cortisol and DHEA(S) in Alzheimer's disease, Heuser and colleagues (1998a) noted significantly increased plasma cortisol levels in Alzheimer's disease patients (57% of whom had probable Alzheimer's disease diagnoses) along with a near-significant decrease in plasma DHEA-S levels ($P<0.07$). Hippocampal volume and cognitive test performance, however, were not significantly correlated with plasma DHEA-S levels.

Several other studies, however, have failed to demonstrate lowered DHEA(S) levels in patients with dementia (Cuckle et al., 1990; Spath-Schwalbe et al., 1990; Schneider & Hinsey, 1992; Legrain et al., 1995; Birkenhager-Gillesse et al., 1994; Berr et al., 1996), and another found lowered levels ($P < 0.05$, one tailed) of DHEA, but these were not significantly correlated with dementia severity (Merril et al., 1990). Unexpectedly, Miller and colleagues found that, in patients with Alzheimer's disease, higher DHEA levels were associated with poorer performance on cognitive tests (Miller et al., 1998). This seems consistent with the findings of Morrison and colleagues (1998), cited above, but the results are not directly comparable since, in the Miller et al. study, DHEA but not DHEA-S levels were assayed, data were not reported separately for men vs. women, and some of the female subjects were receiving estrogen replacement therapy. This latter point renders the DHEA/cognition correlations difficult to interpret, since estrogen treatment itself may lower DHEA levels (Casson et al., 1997) and enhance cognitive performance (Yaffe et al., 1998b).

In addition to assessing cross-sectional differences in DHEA(S) levels in demented patients vs. controls, several studies have evaluated whether low DHEA(S) levels at an index time point predict the subsequent development or progression of dementia or cognitive decline. Yaffe and colleagues (1998a) found that baseline serum levels of DHEA-S did not significantly predict change in cognitive function four to six years later in healthy females. Similarly, Barrett-Connor and Edelstein (1994) prospectively evaluated the ability of plasma DHEA-S levels obtained in 1972–74 to predict dementia ratings obtained in 1988–91. No significant correlations between these measures were found, except for low DHEA-S levels predicting impaired memory performance on the Buschke Selective Reminding Test in females. Contemporaneous (i.e. 1988–91) DHEA-S levels were not examined, however, and several of the male subjects with the lowest DHEA-S levels in 1972–74 died before cognitive testing could be performed in 1988–91, thus truncating the most informative subgroup of the sample. Finally, Miller and colleagues (1998) found that initial DHEA levels did not predict decline in cognitive function over time in patients with Alzheimer's disease, although, as noted above, the inclusion of women receiving estrogen replacement renders these results difficult to interpret.

Cumulatively, then, the descriptive and epidemiological data in humans raise the possibility of a direct relationship between DHEA(S) levels and functional abilities, memory, mood, and sense of well-being, although many inconsistencies exist in the literature, and abnormalities in depression and dementia per se have not been uniformly replicated. Nonetheless, even if endogenous DHEA(S) levels are not decreased in depression and dementia, it is possible that pharmacologic increases in their levels may have mood and memory-enhancing effects. This possibility is reviewed in the following section.

DHEA Treatment effects on well-being, mood, and memory in humans

Well-being and general functioning

DHEA was first used in clinical trials in 1952 by Strauss and Sands and colleagues (Strauss et al., 1952; Strauss & Stevenson 1955; Sands 1954; Sands & Chamberlain, 1952). Patients with inadequate personality or emotional immaturity, when treated openly with low doses of DHEA, showed rapid and impressive improvements in energy, insight, self-confidence, emotionality, vitality, adjustment to the environment, school and occupational performance, and decreases in anxiety, depression, apathy, and withdrawal.

Forty years after these early trials, DHEA was administered openly to patients with multiple sclerosis or systemic lupus erythematosus; many of these patients also showed increased energy, libido, and sense of well-being (Calabrese et al., 1990; Roberts & Fauble, 1990; van Vollenhoven et al., 1994). More recently, DHEA was administered to normal middle-aged and elderly subjects in a randomized, placebo-controlled, double-blind, cross-over study (Morales et al., 1994). Healthy subjects, aged 40 to 70 years old, received DHEA, 50 mg or placebo every evening for 3 months. This dosing schedule restored DHEA(S) levels to youthful levels within 2 weeks, and levels were sustained for the entire 3-month period. During DHEA treatment, subjects showed significant increases in perceived physical and psychological well-being, with no change in libido. Subjects reported improvements such as increased energy, deeper sleep, and improved mood; they also reported feeling more relaxed and having enhanced ability to handle stressful events. These behavioral results from a double blind trial of DHEA are intriguing, but the global subjective measure used to assess behavioral change (a single visual analog scale measuring sense of well-being) was relatively crude, and memory function was not assessed at all. Labrie and Diamond and colleagues treated 60- to 70-year-old women with daily percutaneous applications of a 10% DHEA cream for 12 months (Diamond et al., 1996; Labrie et al., 1997). This was preceded or followed by 6 months of placebo cream, although it is not stated if this was open-label, single-blind or double-blind. They noted, as did Morales and colleagues (1994), that 80% of the women reported well-being and an increase in energy during DHEA treatment. Unfortunately, these behavioral changes were also assessed via non-standardized daily diaries. An additional double blind study recently examined the effects of 2 weeks' treatment with DHEA, 50 mg/day, compared to 2 weeks of placebo in healthy elderly men and women (Wolf et al., 1997b; Kudielka et al.,

1998). Only women tended to report an increase in well-being ($P=0.11$) and mood ($P=0.10$), as assessed with questionnaires. They also showed better performance in one of six cognitive tests (picture memory) after DHEA. However, after post-hoc correction for multiple comparisons, this difference was no longer significant. No such trends were observed in the male subjects ($P>0.20$). This study employed reliable neuropsychological test instruments and had an adequate sample size, but the duration of treatment may have been too short for behavioral changes to become manifest (Polleri et al., 1998).

Mood

Wolkowitz and colleagues have reported antidepressant effects of DHEA in middle-aged-to-elderly patients with major depression. In an initial small-scale, open-label pilot study (Wolkowitz et al., 1997), six patients with major depression, aged 51 to 72 years and with low baseline serum levels of DHEA(S), were orally administered DHEA, 30 to 90 mg/d, for 4 weeks. Doses of DHEA were individually adjusted to achieve circulating DHEA(S) levels in the mid-to-high normal range for healthy young adults. Subjects demonstrated highly significant improvements in Hamilton Depression Ratings and Symptom Checklist-90 ratings. On memory testing, frequency monitoring (a test of automatic processing) showed a significant improvement at Week 3 of DHEA treatment. Mood improvements were significantly related to increases in circulating levels of DHEA and DHEA-S and to their ratios with cortisol; changes in cortisol concentrations were not correlated with behavioral changes. Improvements in specific symptoms of sadness, guilt, discouragement, and tiredness were most closely associated with increases in circulating DHEA and DHEA-S concentrations and with increases in the ratios of these hormones with cortisol (all: $P<0.05$). One subject from this study, a previously treatment-resistant elderly depressed woman, received extended open-label treatment with DHEA (60 mg/d for 4 months followed by 90 mg/d for an additional 2 months). Her depression ratings improved approximately 50% and her access to semantic memory improved 63% during DHEA treatment and returned to pretreatment levels after DHEA discontinuation. Increases in DHEA-S levels over time in this patient were also directly correlated with improvements in depression ratings and with improvements in recognition memory. Although these pilot trials were open label and very small scale, the strong correlations between changes in mood and memory and changes in hormone levels argue somewhat against a pure placebo effect.

This study was followed by a double blind placebo-controlled trial in which 22 depressed patients (age range 33 to 53 years old) received either DHEA (60 to 90 mg/d) or placebo for 4 weeks (Wolkowitz et al., 1999a, b). Some patients were medication-free at the time of entering the study; others were significantly depressed despite being on prestabilized (>6 weeks) antidepressant medication. In the former group, DHEA or placebo was used alone; in the latter group, DHEA or placebo was added to the stabilized antidepressant regimen. DHEA, compared to placebo, was associated with significant antidepressant responses; 5 of 11 DHEA-treated patients showed >50% improvement in depression ratings and had end-point Hamilton Depression Rating Scale ratings <10, compared none of the 11 placebo-treated ones. These results remain to be replicated in larger studies, but they raise the possibility that DHEA, used alone or as an antidepressant adjunct in refractory patients, has significant antidepressant effects in some patients.

Bloch and colleagues (Bloch et al., 1999) recently concluded a 12-week double blind placebo-controlled study in patients with mid-life dysthymia (one patient concurrently had major depression). Subjects received, in randomized order, DHEA (90 mg/day for 3 weeks, followed by 450 mg/day for 3 weeks) or placebo for 6 weeks. DHEA produced a robust antidepressant response at both doses.

Memory

In one of the first clinical reports of DHEA effects on memory, a single case was reported of a 47-year-old woman with a 20-year history of treatment-refractory learning and memory dysfunction and with low baseline DHEA(S) levels (Bonnet & Brown, 1990). She was treated openly with high oral daily doses of DHEA ranging from 12.5 mg/kg to 37 mg/kg for 2 years, and demonstrated improved verbal recall and recognition along with a normalization in EEG and P300 brain electrophysiology.

Recent studies by Wolf and others in Germany (Kudielka et al., 1998; Wolf et al., 1997a, b, 1998a, b) have failed to detect major cognitive effects of short-term DHEA administration in normal volunteers, although conclusions are limited by the short duration of DHEA administration in those studies (Polleri et al., 1998). Single-dose DHEA administration (300 mg dissolved in 5 cm^3 of ethanol) to healthy young adults failed to alter memory performance, despite significantly lowering cortisol levels (Wolf et al., 1997a). In another study (Wolf et al., 1997b; described above), 2 weeks of double blind DHEA administration to healthy elderly controls, showed only a trend towards improvement in picture memory in females, but this was not significant after adjusting for the number of tests administered. Event-related potentials (ERPs) were assessed in the male, but not the female subjects in this treatment paradigm (Wolf et al., 1998b). Certain significant ERP changes were induced by DHEA treatment, indicating changes in central nervous system stimulus processing, but these changes were apparently insufficient to significantly alter memory performance in these men (Wolf et al., 1998b). If DHEA exerts memory-enhancing effects via antiglucocorticoid actions (e.g. blocking the actions of cortisol), such benefits might only be apparent under conditions of hypercortisolemia or stress. To test this hypothesis, the same group of investigators tested cognitive performance before and after a laboratory stressor in DHEA vs. placebo-treated subjects. DHEA treatment yielded opposing effects on memory performance: It decreased the post-stress recall of visual material learned prior to the stressor, but enhanced post-stress attentional performance (Wolf et al., 1998a).

A great deal of excitement followed the initial reports of low serum DHEA(S) levels in patients with Alzheimer's disease (Sunderland et al., 1989). Although these reports were not universally replicated (as reviewed above), they raised the possibility that increasing DHEA(S) levels in such patients to the physiologic levels seen in healthy young adults might have salutary cognitive effects. An initial small-scale study addressing this possibility yielded unremarkable findings (Dukoff et al., 1998). Dukoff et al. (1998) recently reported that DHEA, 1600 mg. p.o. daily for 4 weeks, had no significant cognitive or mood effects in demented or non-demented elderly individuals. This negative report should be interpreted cautiously, however, since the sample size was small, the demented population was heterogeneous and the trial duration may have been too short to see cognitive change in this population. This study also employed very high (pharmacologic) doses of DHEA, which may be beyond a therapeutic window, as suggested by prior preclinical and clinical data (Roberts et al., 1987; Roberts & Fauble, 1990; Bologa et al., 1987; Lynda Lee et al., 1994; Svec & Porter, 1998).

Wolkowitz and colleagues (in review) recently treated 58 patients with Alzheimer's disease with either DHEA (formulation name: NPI-34133), 50 mg. p.o. BID, or placebo for 6 months in a between-groups design. At these doses, DHEA treatment restored serum DHEA(S) levels to, or slightly above, those seen in young adults. DHEA treatment, relative to placebo, was associated with significant improvement in cognitive performance at Month 3 ($P < 0.02$) and a trend towards significant improvement at Month 6 ($P = 0.062$). When clinically significant degrees of change were assessed, significantly more DHEA-treated subjects showed significant improvement at Month 6 than did placebo-treated ones ($P < 0.02$). No significant difference between treatments was seen on a global rating measure, however.

Review of the DHEA treatment literature in depression and dementia cumulatively suggests that, in certain situations, DHEA administration enhances mood, energy, sleep, sense of well-being, functional capabilities and memory. Such effects may be more likely in elderly or infirm patients than in young, healthy individuals. They may also be more likely to emerge after one or more months of treatment, and they may continue to evolve over 6 to 12 months or longer (Wolkowitz et al., 1999a, b; van Vollenhoven et al., 1998). Cognitive and mood effects in normals following short duration treatment (2 weeks or less) seem unlikely or else are quite mild.

Summary

Age-related declines in DHEA(S) are among the most reliable biomarkers of aging, although whether this marker is also pathophysiologic in the aging process is unknown. Elucidating the role of declining levels of gonadal steroids and precursor hormones such as DHEA in the aging process is among the most important issues in current gerontological research and in the study of the psychoneuroendocrinology of aging. If declining hormone levels are pathophysiologically related to the development of diseases of aging, simple, physiological and, hopefully, non-toxic treatments, aimed at restoring youthful hormone levels, might enter into clinical practice.

Despite the meteoric rise in research in DHEA(S) in recent years, its role in human neuropsychiatric diseases, and its possible place in clinical therapeutics, remain uncertain. This situation will hopefully be remedied in coming years. Unfortunate consequences of DHEA's ready, and inexpensive, availability to consumers in the United States have been the lack of interest on the part of pharmaceutical companies in developing this hormone as a drug, and the susceptibility of DHEA to overblown and faddish uses, which has cast it in an unfavorable scientific light. The provocative clinical and preclinical leads reviewed in this chapter, however, should bolster enthusiasm for systematically exploring the neuropsychotropic potential of DHEA(S).

The following tentative conclusions may be drawn from the existing literature:

Average DHEA(S) levels decrease with age from about the mid-20s until the end of the life span. There is large individual variability, however, and some people appear to show increases over time. It is unknown if the rate and direction of change in these hormones over time relates to 'successful' vs. unsuccessful aging.

DHEA(S) levels decline with chronic stress and chronic illness. It has been proposed, but not yet adequately tested, that these decreases further compromise host resistance to illness and to the deleterious effects of chronic stress, and that they lower energy, libido and mood. It remains to be seen if DHEA supplementation in stressed or medically ill patients improves physical outcome (van Vollenhoven 1997).

Low levels of DHEA(S) have been reported in several studies in patients with depression, but these findings have not been universally replicated. Group mean alterations in DHEA(S) levels have also not been consistently established in demented individuals, although exciting preclinical data suggest that low ambient DHEA(S) levels may impair the brain's ability to withstand neurotoxic insult. Thus, low DHEA(S) levels may play a permissive, rather than a direct causal role in dementing illnesses.

DHEA supplementation has been demonstrated in preliminary double blind trials to enhance sense of well-being in healthy middle-aged-to-elderly men and women, to have antidepressant effects in depressed and dysthymic patients, and to enhance cognitive function in patients with Alzheimer's disease. The clinical significance of these effects, their magnitude compared to existing treatments, and their long-term tolerability and side effect profiles remain to be established in larger and longer-term trials.

In our opinion, DHEA supplementation is not yet ready for broad clinical use, since its benefits and safety with long-term use have yet to be clearly established (van Vollenhoven, 1997; Katz & Morales, 1998). Individuals wishing to undertake DHEA supplementation nonetheless, should obtain DHEA from a reputable source (Parasrampuria et al., 1998) and take it under medical supervision, with appropriate laboratory and clinical monitoring (van Vollenhoven, 1997).

ACKNOWLEDGMENT

We gratefully acknowledge the collaboration and assistance of the individuals who wrote material from which parts of this article were adapted (Amy L. Pittenger, PharmD, MS and Reginald F. Frye, PharmD, PhD), collaborated in research investigating the neuropsychiatric effects of DHEA (Louann Brizendine, MD and Errol De Souza, MD, PhD), or provided stimulating discussions and ideas about the role of DHEA in human illness (Eugene Roberts, PhD and Steven M. Paul, MD). This research was partially funded by grants to OMW from the National Alliance for Research in Schizophrenia and Affective Disorders, the Stanley Foundation, the Alzheimer's Association, and the National Institute on Aging. We also gratefully acknowledge the support of NIH Grant MH-55756 and NIH/NCRR/GCRC Grant 5M01RR00056.

REFERENCES

Abbasi, A., Duthie, E. H. Jr., Sheldahl, L., Wilson, C., Sasse, E., Rudman, I. & Mattson, D. E. (1998). Association of dehydroepiandrosterone sulfate, body composition, and physical fitness in independent community-dwelling older men and women. *Journal of the American Geriatrics Society*, 46, 263–73.

Azuma, T., Matsubara, T., Shima, Y., Haeno, S., Fugimoto, T., Tone, K., Shiboda, N. & Sakoda, S. (1993). Neurosteroids in cerebrospinal fluid in neurologic disorders. *Journal of Neurological Sciences*, 120, 87–92.

Barrett-Connor, E. & Edelstein, S. L. (1994). A prospective study of dehydroepiandrosterone sulfate and cognitive function in an older population: the Rancho Bernardo Study. *Journal of the American Geriatrics Society*, 42, 420–3.

Baulieu, E. E. (1997). Neurosteroids: of the nervous system, by the nervous system, for the nervous system. *Recent Progress in Hormone Research*, 52, 1–32.

Berkman, L. F., Seeman, T. E., Albert, M., Blazer, D., Kahn, R., Mohs, R., Finch, C., Schneider, E.,

Cotman, C., McClearn, G. et al. (1993). High, usual and impaired functioning in community-dwelling older men and women: findings from the MacArthur Foundation Research Network on Successful Aging. *Journal of Clinical Epidemiology*, **46**, 1129–40.

Bernton, E., Hoover, D., Galloway, R. & Popp, K. (1995). Adaptation to chronic stress in military trainees. Adrenal androgens, testosterone, glucocorticoids, IGF-1, and immune function. *Annals of the New York Academy of Sciences*, **774**, 217–31.

Berr, C., Lafont, S., Debuire, B., Dartigues, J. F. & Baulieu, E. E. (1996). Relationships of dehydroepiandrosterone sulfate in the elderly with functional, psychological, and mental status, and short-term mortality: a French community-based study. *Proceedings of the National Academy of Sciences*, USA, **93**, 13410–15.

Birkenhager-Gillesse, E. G., Derksen, J., Lagaay, A. M. (1994). Dehydroepiandrosterone sulphate (DHEAS) in the oldest old, aged 85 and over. *Annals of the New York Academy of Sciences*, **719**, 543–52.

Bloch, M., Schmidt, P. J., Danaceau, M. A., Adams, L. F. & Rubinow, D. R. (1999). Dehydroepiandrosterone treatment of mid-life dysthymia. *Biological Psychiatry*, 45, 1533–41.

Bologa, L., Sharma, J. & Roberts, E. (1987). Dehydroepiandrosterone and its sulfate derivative reduce neuronal death and enhance astrocytic differentiation in brain cell cultures. *Journal of Neuroscience Research*, **17**, 225–34.

Bonnet, K. A. & Brown, R. P. (1990). Cognitive effects of DHEA replacement therapy. In *The Biologic Role of Dehydroepiandrosterone (DHEA)*, ed. M. Kalimi & W. Regelson, pp. 65–79. New York: Walter de Gruyter.

Bruyn, G. W. & de Jong, F. H. (1973). Dehydroepiandrosterone sulfate and Huntington's chorea. *Advances in Neurology*, **1**, 553–5.

Buckwalter, J. G., Stanczyc, F. Z., McCleary, C. A., Bluestein, B. W., Buckwalter, D. K., Rankin, K. P., Change, L. & Goodwin, T. M. (1999): Pregnancy, the postpartum, and steroid hormones: effects on cognition and mood. *Psychoneuroendocrinology*, **24**, 69–84.

Calabrese, V. P., Isaacs, E. R. & Regelson, W. (1990). Dehydroepiandosterone in multiple sclerosis: positive effects on the fatigue syndrome in a non-randomized study. In *The Biologic Role of Dehydroepiandrosterone (DHEA)*, ed. M. Kalimi & W. Regelson, pp. 95–100. New York: Walter de Gruyter.

Casson, P. R., Elkind-Hirsch, K. E., Buster, J. E., Hornsby, P. J., Carson, S. A. & Snabes, M. C. (1997). Effect of postmenopausal estrogen replacement on circulating androgens. *Obstetrics and Gynecology*, **90**, 995–8.

Cawood, E. H. & Bancroft, J. (1996). Steroid hormones, the menopause, sexuality and well-being of women. *Psychological Medicine*, **26**, 925–36.

Christensen, H., Maltby, N., Jorm, A. F., Creasey, H. Y. & Broe, G. A. (1992). Cholinergic blockade as a model of the cognitive deficits in Alzheimer's disease. Brain, 115, 1681–99.

Compagnone, N. A. & Mellon, S. H. (1998). Dehydroepiandrosterone: a potential signalling molecule for neocortical organization during development [see comments]. *Proceedings of the National Academy of Sciences*, USA, **95**, 4678–83.

Corpechot, C., Robel, P., Axelson, M., Sjovall, J. & Baulieu, E. E. (1981). Characterization and measurement of dehydroepiandrosterone sulfate in rat brain. *Proceedings of the National Academy of Sciences*, **78**, 4704–7.

Crenshaw, T. L. & Goldberg, J. P. (1996). Dehydroepiandrosterone (DHEA/DHEAS). In *Sexual*

Pharmacology: Drugs that Affect Sexual Functioning, ed. T. L. Crenshaw & J. P. Goldberg, pp. 129–50. New York: W.W. Norton and Co.

Cuckle, H., Stone, R., Smith, D., Wald, N., Brammer, M., Hajimohammedreza, I., Levy, R., Chard, T. & Perry, L. (1990). Dehydroepiandrosterone sulphate in Alzheimer's disease. *Lancet*, ii, 449–50.

Del Cerro, S., Garcia-Estrada, J. & Garcia-Segura, L. M. (1995). Neuroactive steroids regulate astroglia morphology in hippocampal cultures from adult rats. *Glia*, 14, 65–71.

Diamond, P., Cusan, L., Gomez, J. L., Belanger, A. & Labrie, F. (1996). Metabolic effects of 12-month percutaneous dehydroepiandrosterone replacement therapy in postmenopausal women. *Journal of Endocrinology*, 150(Suppl), S43–50.

Dukoff, R., Molchan, S., Putnam, K., Lai, J. & Sunderland, T. (1998). Dehydroepiandrosterone administration in demented patients and non-demented elderly volunteers (Abstract). *Biological Psychiatry*, 43, 55S.

Fava, M., Rosenbaum, J. F., MacLaughlin, R. A., Tesar, G. E., Pollack, M. H., Cohen, L. S. & Hirsch, M. (1989). Dehydroepiandrosterone-sulfate/cortisol ratio in panic disorder. *Psychiatry Research*, 28, 345–50.

Ferguson, H. C., Bartram, A. C. G., Fowlie, H. C., Cathro, D. M., Birchall, K. & Mitchell, F. L. (1964). A preliminary investigation of steroid excretion in depressed patients before and after electroconvulsive therapy. *Acta Endocrinologica*, 47, 58–66.

Ferrari, E., Borri, R., Casarotti, D., Giacchero, R., Trecate, L., Fioravanti, M., Solerte, S. B., Pezza, N. & Magri, F. (1997). Major depression in elderly patients: a chrono-neuroendocrine study. *Aging Clinical Experimental Research*, 9, 83.

Fleshner, M., Pugh, C. R., Tremblay, D. & Rudy, J. W. (1997). DHEA-S selectively impairs contextual-fear conditioning: support for the antiglucocorticoid hypothesis. *Behavioral Neuroscience*, 111, 512–17.

Flood, J. F. & Roberts, E. (1988). Dehydroepiandrosterone sulfate improves memory in aging mice. *Brain Research*, 448, 178–81.

Flood, J. F., Morley, J. E. & Roberts, E. (1992). Memory-enhancing effects in male mice of pregnenolone and steroids metabolically derived from it. *Proceedings of the National Academy of Sciences*, 89, USA, 1567–71.

Flood, J. F., Smith, G. E. & Roberts, E. (1988). Dehydroepiandrosterone and its sulfate enhance memory retention in mice. *Brain Research*, 447, 269–78.

Furuya, E., Maezawa, M. & Nishikaze, O. (1998). [17–KS sulfate as a biomarker in psychosocial stress]. *Rinsho Byori*, 46, 529–37.

Goodyer, I. M., Herbert, J. & Altham, P. M. (1998). Adrenal steroid secretion and major depression in 8- to 16-year-olds, III. Influence of cortisol/DHEA ratio at presentation on subsequent rates of disappointing life events and persistent major depression. *Psychological Medicine*, 28, 265–73.

Goodyer, I. M., Herbert, J., Altham, P. M., Pearson, J., Secher, S. M. & Shiers, H. M. (1996). Adrenal secretion during major depression in 8- to 16-year-olds, I. Altered diurnal rhythms in salivary cortisol and dehydroepiandrosterone (DHEA) at presentation. *Psychological Medicine*, 26, 245–56.

Guazzo, E. P., Kirkpatrick, P. J., Goodyer, I. M., Shiers, H. M. & Herbert, J. (1996). Cortisol, dehydroepiandrosterone (DHEA), and DHEA sulfate in the cerebrospinal fluid of man: relation to blood levels and the effects of age. *Journal of Clinical Endocrinology and Metabolism*, 81, 3951–60.

Hansen, C. R. Jr., Kroll, J. & Mackenzie,T. B. (1982). Dehydroepiandrosterone and affective disorders [letter]. *American Journal of Psychiatry*, 139, 386–7.

Hechter, O., Grossman, A. & Chatterton, R. T. Jr. (1997). Relationship of dehydroepiandrosterone and cortisol in disease. *Medical Hypotheses*, 49, 85–91.

Heuser, I., Colla, M., Deuschle, M. & Weber, B. (1998a). Adrenal steroid secretion, cognitive status and hippocampal atrophy in Alzheimer's disease, 37th Annual Meeting, American College of Neuro-Psychopharmacology. Puerto Rico, Poster Session III, Board No. 41.

Heuser, I., Deuschle, M., Luppa, P., Schweiger, U., Standhardt, H. & Weber, B. (1998b). Increased diurnal plasma concentrations of dehydroepiandrosterone in depressed patients. *Journal of Clinical Endocrinology and Metabolism*, 83, 3130–3.

Kalmijn, S., Launer, L. J., Stolk, R. P., deJong, F. H., Pols, H. A., Hofman, A., Breteler, M. M. & Lamberts, S. W. (1998). A prospective study on cortisol, dehydroepiandrosterone sulfate, and cognitive function in the elderly. *Jounal of Clinical Endocrinology and Metabolism*, 83, 3487–92.

Kalogeras, K. T., Calogero, A. E., Kuribayiashi, T., Khan, I., Gallucci, W. T., Kling, M. A., Chrousos, G. P. & Gold, P. W. (1990). *In vitro* and *in vivo* effects of the triazolobenzodiazepine alprazolam on hypothalamic–pituitary–adrenal function: pharmacological and clinical implications. *Journal of Clinical Endocrinology Metabolism*, 70, 1462–71.

Katz, S. & Morales, A. J. (1998), Dehydroepiandrosterone (DHEA) and DHEA-sulfate (DS) as therapeutic options in menopause. *Seminars in Reproductive Endocrinology*, 16, 161–70.

Kimonides, V. G., Khatibi, N. H., Svendsen, C. N., Sofroniew, M. V. & Herbert, J. (1998). Dehydroepiandrosterone (DHEA) and DHEA-sulfate (DHEAS) protect hippocampal neurons against excitatory amino acid-induced neurotoxicity. *Proceedings of the National Academy of Sciences, USA*, 95, 1852–7.

Kimonides, V. G., Spillantini, M. G., Sofroniew, M. V., Fawcett, J. W. & Herbert, J. (1999). Dehydroepiandrosterone (DHEA) antagonizes the neurotoxic effects of corticosterone and translocation of stress-activated protein kinase 3 (SAPK3) in hippocampal primary cultures. *Neuroscience*, 89, 429–36.

Kroboth, P. D., Salek, F. S., Stone, R. A., Bertz, R. J. & Kroboth, III. F. J. (1999). Alprazolam increases DHEA concentrations. *Journal of Clinical Psychopharmacology*, 19, 114–24.

Kudielka, B. M., Hellhammer, J., Hellhammer, D. H., Wolf, O. T., Pirke, K. M., Varadi, E., Pilz, J. & Kirschbaum, C. (1998). Sex differences in endocrine and psychological responses to psychosocial stress in healthy elderly subjects and the impact of a 2-week dehydroepiandrosterone treatment. *Journal of Clinical Endocrinology and Metabolism*, 83, 1756–61.

Labrie, F., Diamond, P., Cusan, L., Gomez, J. L., Belanger, A. & Candas, B. (1997). Effect of 12-month dehydroepiandrosterone replacement therapy on bone, vagina, and endometrium in postmenopausal women. *Journal of Clinical Endocrinology and Metabolism*, 82, 3498–505.

LaCroix, C., Fiet, J., Benais, J. P., Gueux, B., Bonete, R., Villette, J. M., Gourmel, B. & Dreux, C. (1987). Simultaneous radioimmunoassay of progesterone, androstenedione, pregnenolone, dehydroepiandrosterone and 17-hydroxyprogesterone in specific regions of human brain. *Journal of Steroid Biochemistry*, 28, 317–25.

Leblhuber, F., Neubauer, C., Peichl, M., Reisecker, F., Steinparz, F. X., Windhager, E. & Dienstl, E. (1993). Age and sex differences of dehydroepiandrosterone sulfate (DHEAS) and cortisol

(CRT) plasma levels in normal controls and Alzheimer's disease (AD). *Psychopharmacology*, 111, 23–6.

Leblhuber, F., Peichl, M., Neubauer, C., Reisecker, F., Steinparz, F. X., Windhager, E. & Maschek, W. (1995). Serum dehydroepiandrosterone and cortisol measurements in Huntington's chorea. *Journal of Neurological Sciences*, 132, 76–9.

Leblhuber, F., Windhager, E., Neubauer, C., Weber, J., Reisecker, F. & Dienstl, E. (1992). Antiglucocorticoid effects of DHEA-S in Alzheimer's disease [letter] [published erratum appears in *American Journal of Psychiatry*, 1992, 149(11), 1622]. *American Journal of Psychiatry*, 149, 1125–6.

Legrain, S., Berr, C., Frenoy, N., Gourlet, V., Debuire, B. & Baulieu, E. E. (1995). Dehydroepiandrosterone sulfate in a long-term care aged population. *Gerontology*, 41, 343–51.

Li, P. K., Rhodes, M. E., Burke, A. M. & Johnson, D. A. (1997). Memory enhancement mediated by the steroid sulfatase inhibitor (*p*-sulfamoyl)-*N*-tetradecanoyl tyramine. *Life Sciences*, 60, L45–51.

Lupien, S., Sharma, S., Arcand, J. F., Schwartz, G., Nair, N. P. V., Meaney, M. J. & Hauger, R. L. (1995). Dehydroepiandrosterone-sulfate (DHEA-S) levels, cortisol levels and cognitive function in elderly human subjects. *International Society of Psychoneuroendocrinology*, p. 24.

Lynda Lee, Y. S., Kohlmeier, L., van Vollenhoven, R. F., Marcus, R. & McGuire, J. (1994). The effects of dehydroepiandrosterone (DHEA) on bone metabolism in healthy post-menopausal women. *Arthritis and Rheumatism*, 37:S182.

McKenna, T. J., Fearon, U., Clarke, D. & Cunningham, S. K. (1997). A critical review of the origin and control of adrenal androgens. *Baillieres Clinical Obstetrics and Gynaecology*, 11, 229–48.

Melchior, C. L. & Ritzmann, R. F. (1994). Dehydroepiandrosterone is an anxiolytic in mice on the plus maze. *Pharmacology, Biochemistry and Behavior*, 47, 437–41.

Melchior, C. L. & Ritzmann, R. F. (1996). Neurosteroids block the memory-impairing effects of ethanol in mice. *Pharmacology, Biochemistry and Behavior*, 53, 51–6.

Merril, C. R., Harrington, M. G. & Sunderland, T. (1990). Reduced plasma dehydroepiandrosterone concentrations in HIV infection and Alzheimer's disease. In *The Biologic Role of Dehydroepiandrosterone (DHEA)*, ed. M. Kalimi & W. Regelson, pp. 101–5. Berlin: Walter de Gruyter.

Michael, A., Jenaway, A., Paykel, E. S. & Herbert, J. (in press). Altered salivary DHEA levels in major depression in adults.

Miller, T. P., Taylor, J., Rogerson, S., Mauricio, M., Kennedy, Q., Schatzberg, A., Tinklenberg, J. & Yesaavage, J. (1998). Cognitive and noncognitive symptoms in dementia patients: relationship to cortisol and dehydroepiandrosterone. *International Psychogeriatrics*, 10, 85–96.

Morales, A. J., Nolan, J. J., Nelson, J. C. & Yen, S.S. (1994). Effects of replacement dose of dehydroepiandrosterone in men and women of advancing age [published erratum appears in *Journal of Clinical Endocrinology and Metabolism*, 1995, 80(9):2799]. *Journal of Clinical Endocrinology and Metabolism*, 78, 1360–7.

Morley, J. E., Kaiser, F., Raum, W. J., Perry, H. M. 3rd, Flood, J. F., Jensen, J., Silver, A. J. & Roberts, E. (1997). Potentially predictive and manipulable blood serum correlates of aging in the healthy human male: progressive decreases in bioavailable testosterone, dehydroepiandrosterone sulfate, and the ratio of insulin-like growth factor 1 to growth hormone. *Proceedings of the National Academy of Sciences*, 94, USA, 7537–42.

Morrison, M. F., Katz, I. R., Parmelee, P., Boyce, A. A. & TenHave, T. (1998). Dehydroepiandrosterone sulfate (DHEA-S) and psychiatric and laboratory measures of frailty in a residential care population. *American Journal of Geriatrics Psychiatry*, 6, 277–84.

Nasman, B., Olsson, T., Backstrom, T., eriksson, S., Grankvist, K., Viitanen, M. & Bucht, G. (1991). Serum dehydroepiandrosterone sulfate in Alzheimer's disease and in multi-infarct dementia. *Biological Psychiatry*, 30, 684–90.

Nishikaze, O. (1998). [17–KS sulfate as a biomarker in health and disease]. *Rinsho Byori, Japanese Journal of Clinical Pathology*, 46, 520–8.

Oberbeck, R., Benschop, R. J., Jacobs, R., Hosch, W., Jetschmann, J. U., Schurmeyer, T. H., Schmidt, R. E. & Schedlowski, M. (1998). Endocrine mechanisms of stress-induced DHEA-secretion. *Journal of Endocrinology Investigation*, 21, 148–53.

Orentreich, N., Brind, J. L., Rizer, R. L. & Vogelman. J. H. (1984). Age changes and sex differences in serum dehydroepiandrosterone sulfate concentrations throughout adulthood. *Journal of Clinical Endocrinology and Metabolism*, 59, 551–5.

Orentreich, N., Brind, J. L., Vogelman, J. H., Andres, R. & Baldwin, H. (1992). Long-term longitudinal measurements of plasma dehydroepiandrosterone sulfate in normal men. *Journal of Clinical Endocrinology and Metabolism*, 75, 1002–4.

Osran, H., Reist, C., Chen, C. C., Lifrak, E. T., Chicz-DeMet, A. & Parker, L. N. (1993). Adrenal androgens and cortisol in major depression. *American Journal of Psychiatry*, 150, 806–9.

Ozasa, H., Kita, M., Inoue, T. & Mori, T. (1990). Plasma dehydroepiandrosterone-to-cortisol ratios as an indicator of stress in gynecologic patients. *Gynecologic Oncology*, 37, 178–82.

Parasrampuria, J., Schwartz, K. & Petesch, R. (1998). Quality control of dehydroepiandrosterone dietary supplement products. *Journal of the American Medical Association*, 280, 1565.

Parker, L., Eugene, J., Farber, D., Lifrak, E., Lai, M. & Juler, G. (1985a). Dissociation of adrenal androgen and cortisol levels in acute stress. *Hormones and Metabolism Research*, 17, 209–12.

Parker, L. N., Levin, E. R. & Lifrak, E. T. (1985b). Evidence for adrenocortical adaptation to severe illness. *Journal of Clinical Endocrinology and Metabolism*, 60, 947–52.

Polleri, A., Gianelli, M. V. & Murialdo, G. (1998). Dehydroepiandrosterone: dream or nightmare? *Journal of Endocrinology Investigation*, 21(8), 544.

Prasad, A., Imamura, M. & Prasad, C. (1997). Dehydroepiandrosterone decreases behavioral despair in high- but not low-anxiety rats. *Physiology and Behavior*, 62, 1053–7.

Ravaglia, G., Forti, P., Maioli, F., Boschi, F., Cicognani, A., Bernardi, M., Pratelli, L., Pizzoferrato, A., Porcu, S. & Gasbarrini, G. (1996). The relationship of dehydroepiandrosterone sulfate (DHEAS) to endocrine–metabolic parameters and functional status in the oldest-old. Results from an Italian study on healthy free-living over-ninety-year-olds. *Journal of Clinical Endocrinology and Metabolism*, 81, 1173–8.

Ravaglia, G., Forti, P., Maioli, F., Boschi, F., Cicognani, A., Bernardi, M., Pratelli, L., Pizzoferrato, A., Porcu, S, & Gasbarrini, G. (1997). Determinants of functional status in healthy Italian nonagenarians and centenarians: a comprehensive functional assessment by the instruments of geriatric practice. *Journal of the American Geriatric Society*, 45, 1196–202.

Reddy, D. S. & Kulkarni, S. K. (1997). Differential anxiolytic effects of neurosteroids in the mirrored chamber behavior test in mice. *Brain Research*, 752, 61–71.

Reddy, D. S., Kaur, G. & Kulkarni, S. K. (1998). Sigma (sigma1) receptor mediated antidepressant-like effects of neurosteroids in the Porsolt forced swim test [In Process Citation]. *Neuroreport*, 9, 3069–73.

Regelson, W. & Kalimi, M. (1994). Dehydroepiandrosterone (DHEA) – the multifunctional steroid. II. Effects on the CNS, cell proliferation, metabolic and vascular, clinical and other effects. Mechanism of action? *Annals of the New York Academy of Sciences*, 719, 564–75.

Reus, V. I., Wolkowitz, O. M., Roberts, E., Chan, T., Turestcky, N., Manfredi, F. & Weingartner, H. (1993). Dehydroepiandrosterone (DHEA) and memory in depressed patients. *Neuropsychopharmacology*, 9, 66S.

Rhodes, M. E., Li, P. K., Burke, A. M. & Johnson, D. A. (1997). Enhanced plasma DHEAS, brain acetylcholine and memory mediated by steroid sulfatase inhibition. *Brain Research*, 773, 28–32.

Rhodes, M. E., Li, P. K., Flood, J. F. & Johnson, D. A. (1996). Enhancement of hippocampal acetylcholine release by the neurosteroid dehydroepiandrosterone sulfate: an *in vivo* microdialysis study. *Brain Research*, 733, 284–6.

Robel, P. & Baulieu, E. E. (1995). Dehydroepiandrosterone (DHEA) is a neuroactive neurosteroid. *Annals of the New York Academy of Sciences*, 774, 82–110.

Roberts, E. (1990). Dehydroepiandrosterone (DHEA) and its sulfate (DHEAS) as neural facilitators: effects on brain tissue in culture and on memory in young and old mice. A cyclic GMP hypothsis of action of DHEA and DHEAS in nervous system and other tissues. In *The Biologic Role of Dehydroepiandrosterone (DHEA)*, ed. M. Kalimi & W. Regelson, pp. 13–42. Berlin: Walter de Gruyter.

Roberts, E. & Fauble, T. (1990). Oral dehydroepiandrosterone in multiple sclerosis. Results of a phase one, open study. In *The Biologic Role of Dehydroepiandrosterone (DHEA)*, ed. M. Kalimi & W. Regelson, pp. 81–94. Berlin: Walter de Gruyter.

Roberts, E., Bologa, L., Flood, J. F. & Smith, G. E. (1987). Effects of dehydroepiandrosterone and its sulfate on brain tissue in culture and on memory in mice. *Brain Research*, 406, 357–62.

Romeo, E., Strohle, A., Spalletta, G., diMichele, F., Hermann, B., Holsboer, F., Pasini, A. & Rupprecht, R. (1998). Effects of antidepressant treatment on neuroactive steroids in major depression. *American Journal of Psychiatry*, 155, 910–13.

Rudman, D., Shetty, K. R. & Mattson, D. E. (1990). Plasma dehydroepiandrosterone sulfate in nursing home men. *Journal of the American Geriatrics Society*, 38, 421–7.

Sands, D. (1954). Further studies on endocrine treatment in adolescence and early adult life. *Journal of the Mental Sciences*, 100, 211–19.

Sands, D. E. & Chamberlain, G. H. A. (1952). Treatment of inadequate personality in juveniles by dehydroisoandrosterone. *British Medical Journal*, 2, 66.

Schneider, L. S. & Hinsey, M. S. L. (1992). Plasma dehydroepiandrosterone sulfate in Alzheimer's disease. *Biological Psychiatry*, 31, 205–8.

Shulman, L. H., DeRogatis, L., Spielvogel, R., Miller, J. L. & Rose, L. I. (1992). Serum androgens and depression in women with facial hirsutism. *Journal of the American Academy of Dermatology*, 27, 178–81.

Solerte, S. B., Fioravanti, M., Schifino, N., Cuzzoni, G., Fontana, I., Vignati, G., Govoni, S., & Ferrari, E. (1999). Dehydroepiandrosterone sulfate decreases the interleukin-2-mediated overactivity of the natural killer cell compartment in senile dementia of the Alzheimer type. *Dementia and Geriatric Cognition Disorder*, 10, 21–7.

Spath-Schwalbe, E., Dodt, C., Dittmann, J., Schuttler, R. & Fehm, H. L. (1990). Dehydroepiandrosterone sulfate in Alzheimer's disease. *Lancet*, 335, 1412.

Spratt, D. I., Longcope, C., Cox, P. M., Bigos, S. T. & Wilbur-Welling, C. (1993). Differential changes in serum concentrations of androgens and estrogens (in relation with cortisol) in postmenopausal women with acute illness. *Journal of Clinical Endocrinology and Metabolism*, 76, 1542–7.

Strauss, E. B. & Stevenson, W. A. H. (1955). Use of dehydroisoandrosterone in psychiatric practice. *Journal of Neurology, Neurosurgery and Psychiatry*, 18, 137–44.

Strauss, E. B., Sands, D. E., Robinson, A. M., Tindall, W. J. & Stevenson, W. A. H. (1952). Use of dehydroisoandrosterone in psychiatric treatment: a preliminary survey. *British Medical Journal*, 2, 64–6.

Sunderland, T., Merril, C. R., Harrington, M., Lawlor, B. A., Molchan, S. E., Martinez, R. & Murphy, D. L. (1989). Reduced plasma dehydroepiandrosterone concentrations in Alzheimer's disease. *Lancet*, 570.

Sunderland, T., Molchan, S., Martinez, R., Vitiello, B. & Martin, P. (1990). Drug challenge strategies in Alzheimer's disease: a focus on the scopolamine model. In *Alzheimer Disease: Current Research in Early Diagnosis*, ed. R. E. Becker & E. Giaciboni, pp. 173–91. New York: Taylor & Francis.

Svec, F. & Porter, J. R. (1998). The actions of exogenous dehydroepiandrosterone in experimental animals and humans. *Proceedings of the Society for Experimental Biology and Medicine*, 218, 174–91.

Takebayashi, M., Kagaya, A., Uchitomi, Y., Kugaya, A., Muraoka, M., Yokota, N., Horiguchi, J. & Yamawaki, S. (1998). Plasma dehydroepiandrosterone sulfate in unipolar major depression. Short communication. *Journal of Neural Transmission*, 105, 537–42.

Tejkalova, H., Beneova, O., Kritofikova, Z., Klaschka, J., Panajotova, V. & Huek, P. (1998). Neurobehavioral effects of dehydroepiandrosterone in model experiments with old rats. *21st Collegium Internationale Neuro-Psychopharmacologicum Congress*. Glasgow, UK, Abstract No. PW11027.

Thomas, G., Frenoy, N., Legrain, S., Sebag-Lanoe, R., Baulieu, E. E. & Debuire, B. (1994). Serum dehydroepiandrosterone sulfate levels as an individual marker. *Journal of Clinical Endocrinology and Metabolism*, 79, 1273–6.

Tollefson, G. D., Haus, E., Garvey, M. J., Evans, M. & Tuason, V. B. (1990). 24 hour urinary dehydroepiandrosterone sulfate in unipolar depression treated with cognitive and/or pharmacotherapy. *Annals of Clinical Psychiatry*, 2, 39–45.

Uzunov, D. P., Cooper, T. B., Costa, E. & Guidotti, A. (1996). Fluoxetine-elicited changes in brain neurosteroid content measured by negative ion mass fragmentography. *Proceedings of the National Academy of Sciences*, USA, 93, 12599–604.

Uzunova, V., Sheline, Y., Davis, J. M., Rasmusson, A., Uzunovm D. F., Costa E. & Guidotti, A.A. (1998). Increase in the cerebrospinal fluid content of neurosteroids in patients with unipolar major depression who are receiving fluoxetine or fluvoxamine. *Proceedings of the National Academy of Sciences*, USA, 95, 3239–44.

van Vollenhoven, R. F. (1997). Dehydroepiandrosterone: uses and abuses. In *Textbook of Rheumatology*, volume update series No. 25, ed. W. N. Kelley, E. D. Harris Jr, S. Ruddy & C. B. Sledge, pp. 1–25. Philadelphia: W.B. Saunders Co.

van Vollenhoven, R. F., Engleman, E. G. & McGuire, J. L. (1994). An open study of dehydroepiandrosterone in systemic lupus erythematosus. *Arthritis and Rheumatism*, 37, 1305–10.

van Vollenhoven, R. F., Morabito, L. M., Engleman, E. G. & McGuire, J. L. (1998). Treatment of systemic lupus erythematosus with dehydroepiandrosterone: 50 patients treated up to 12 months. *Journal of Rheumatology*, 25, 285–9.

Wolf, O. T., Koster, B., Kirschbaum, C., Pietrowsky, R., Kern, W., Hellhammer, D. H., Born, J. & Fehm, H. L. (1997a). A single administration of dehydroepiandrosterone does not enhance memory performance in young healthy adults, but immediately reduces cortisol levels. *Biological Psychiatry*, 42, 845–8.

Wolf, O. T., Kudielka, B. M., Hellhammer, D. H., Hellhammer, J. & Kirschbaum, C. (1998a). Opposing effects of DHEA replacement in elderly subjects on declarative memory and attention after exposure to a laboratory stressor. *Psychoneuroendocrinology*, 23, 617–29.

Wolf, O. T., Naumann, E., Hellhammer, D. H. & Kirschbaum, C. (1998b). Effects of dehydroepiandrosterone replacement in elderly men on event- related potentials, memory, and well-being. *Journals of Gerontology. Series A, Biological Sciences and Medical Sciences*, 53, M385–90.

Wolf, O. T., Neumann, O., Hellhammer, D. H., Pietrowsky, R., Kern, W., Hellhammer, D. H., Born, J. & Fehm, H. L. (1997b). Effects of a two-week physiological dehydroepiandrosterone substitution on cognitive performance and well-being in healthy elderly women and men. *Journal of Clinical Endocrinology and Metabolism*, 82, 2363–7.

Wolkowitz, O. M., Kramer, J. H., Reus, V. I., Costa, M. E., Yaffe, K., Walton, P., Raskind, M., Peskind, E., Newhouse, P., Sack, D., Sadowsky, C., De Souza, E. & Roberts, E. (1999a). Dehydroepiandrosterone (NPI-34133) treatment of Alzheimer's disease: a randomized, double-blind, placebo-controlled, parallel group study. [Abstract] Annual Convention of the American Psychiatric Association, Washington, DC.

Wolkowitz, O. M., Reus, V. I., Keebler, A., Nelson, N., Friedland, M., Brizendin, L. & Roberts, E. (1999b). Double-blind treatment of major depression with dehydroepiandrosterone (DHEA). *American Journal of Psychiatry*, 156, 646–9.

Wolkowitz, O. M., Reus, V. I., Manfredi, F. & Roberts, E. (1992). Antiglucocorticoid effects of DHEA-S in Alzheimer's Disease (reply). *American Journal of Psychiatry*, 149, 1126.

Wolkowitz, O. M., Reus, V. I., Roberts, E., Manfredi, F., Chan, T., Raum, W. J., Ormiston, S., Johnson, R., Canick, J., Brizendine, L. & Weingartner, H. (1997). Dehydroepiandrosterone (DHEA) treatment of depression. *Biological Psychiatry*, 41, 311–8.

Yaffe, K., Ettinger, B., Pressman, A., Seeley, D., Whooley, M., Schaefer, C. & Cummings, S. (1998a). Neuropsychiatric function and dehydroepiandrosterone sulfate in elderly women: a prospective study. *Biological Psychiatry*, 43, 694–700.

Yaffe, K., Sawaya, G., Lieberburg, I. & Grady, D. (1998b). Estrogen therapy in post-menopausal women: effects on cognitive function and dementia. *JAMA*, 279, 688–95.

Yanase, T., Fukahori, M., Taniguchi, S., Nishi, Y., Sakai, Y., Takayanagi, R., Haji, M. & Nawata, H. (1996). Serum dehydroepiandrosterone (DHEA) and DHEA-sulfate (DHEA-S) in Alzheimer's disease and in cerebrovascular dementia. *Endocrine Journal*, 43, 119–23.

8

Sex hormones, cognition, and dementia in the elderly

Kristine Yaffe

Introduction

At least 10% of persons over 65 years old and 50% of persons over 85 years old have some form of cognitive impairment ranging from mild deficits to dementia (Evans, 1990). Alzheimer's disease (AD), the most common cause of dementia, is estimated to affect 4 million people in the United States and to cost $70 billion annually (Ernst & Hay, 1994). AD affects women disproportionately to men with women having a slightly higher increased risk of AD, even after adjusting for age (Payami et al., 1996a, b). Despite the severity and prevalence of dementia and mild cognitive impairment, there are few effective treatments or prevention strategies.

Recent studies have suggested that postmenopausal estrogen therapy might improve cognition in nondemented perimenopausal and postmenopausal women, that it might prevent the development of dementia, or that it might improve the severity of dementia. While less studied, interest is growing in the role of testosterone in cognition and dementia treatment. In this chapter, the basic science on sex hormones and cognition, the clinical studies of estrogen for the prevention and treatment of dementia, and the studies of testosterone and cognitive function are reviewed.

Possible biological mechanisms of estrogen's effect on cognition

Estrogen receptors are found in the hypothalamus, the preoptic area, the anterior pituitary, the CA1 region of the hippocampus, and several other brain regions (McEwen & Woolley, 1994). How estrogens may affect neuropsychologic function remains unknown, but several mechanisms have been suggested. One mechanism is the modulation of neurotransmitters, particularly acetylcholine. Estradiol administration to oophorectimized rats is associated with an increase in choline acetyltransferase and potassium-stimulated acetylcholine release in certain brain regions and an increase in the survival of cholinergic neurons (Honjo et al., 1992; Luine, 1985; Gibbs et al., 1997). Estrogen-treated rats have superior performance on behavioral memory tasks compared to estrogen-deprived animals, and performance is associated with increased choline uptake and higher levels of choline acetyltransferase in the hippocampus and frontal cortex (Simpkins et al., 1994). Estradiol has also been found to affect other neurotransmitter systems' activity. In rats, estradiol decreases monoamine oxidase activity in the amygdala and basomedial hypothalamus and induces serotonin receptors in forebrain regions involved in cognition and behavior, including the frontal lobe, cingulate, and nucleus accumbens (Luine et al., 1975; Summer & Fink, 1995). These neurotransmitter alterations induced by estradiol have significant implications for AD prevention and treatment because reductions in acetylcholine, serotonin, dopamine, and norepinephrine are a hallmark feature of patients with AD (Coyle et al., 1983; Palmer & DeKosky, 1993).

Another possible mechanism of estrogen's role in cognition is by promoting neuronal growth and synaptic reorganization. Estrogen regulates synaptic plasticity by stimulating axonal sprouting and dendritic spine formation in the adult rat hypothalamus and CA1 hippocampal pyramidal neurons (McEwen & Woolley, 1994; Gould et al., 1990). Early neuron loss in the CA1 region of the hippocampus, a region associated with memory and learning, is found in patients with AD and age-related cognitive dysfunction. In addition to promoting neuronal circuitry, estrogen may prevent cerebral ischemia. Estrogens may protect against cerebral ischemia by inducing vasodilatation, reducing platelet aggregation, or limiting oxidative stress related injury induced by excitotoxins and beta amyloid (Goodman et al., 1996; Gangar et al., 1991). Postmenopausal estrogen therapy reduces serum LDL-cholesterol and increases HDL-cholesterol (Applebaum-Bowden et al., 1989). These lipoprotein changes may slow progression of cerebral atherosclerosis and prevent dementia and other cognitive decline. Estrogen also modulates the expression of the apolipoprotein E gene in rodent tissues and theoretically could reduce risk of AD in humans via apolipoprotein E alterations (Srivastava et al., 1997). Thus, estrogens may reduce the risk of AD and other forms of cognitive decline through a variety of mechanisms.

Estrogen and cognition in non-demented women

Four cross-sectional observational studies have evaluated the association of estrogen therapy and cognitive performance. Three of the studies reported inconclusive results (Kampen & Sherwin, 1994; Robinson et al., 1994; Schmidt et al., 1996), and one found that estrogen use improved cognitive function (Kimura, 1995). Kampen and Sherwin administered 14 cognitive tests to 71 healthy, recently postmenopausal women and found that scores on only one of the tests (Paragraph Recall) were significantly higher in women taking estrogen compared to non-users (Kampen &

Sherwin, 1994). There were no other differences between the estrogen users and non-users, and there was no association of test scores with serum estrogen levels. The analyses were not adjusted for education or depression. If estrogen users are better educated or less depressed than non-users, these factors could account for differences in cognitive performance. Robinson et al. (1994) conducted a cross-sectional study of 72 postmenopausal estrogen users and 72 non-users matched for age and education to examine the association of estrogen use and performance on two recall tests. Women treated with estrogen performed significantly better on proper names recall but not on word recall compared to those not receiving estrogen. Another cross-sectional study found that of 222 postmenopausal women, those taking estrogen had better scores on 18 tests or subtests (Schmidt et al., 1996). When multivariate analyses were conducted including age, education, blood pressure, and self-reported activity, however, most of the differences became nonsignificant. Kimura assessed performance on ten cognitive tests and one mood scale in 21 postmenopausal women on estrogen replacement and 33 postmenopausal women not on estrogen. The author concluded that the estrogen group had better overall performance on the cognitive tests but no specific test scores or statistical analyses were reported (Kimura, 1995).

Four prospective studies of estrogen use and cognitive function have been conducted, allowing for a comparison of rates of cognitive decline between estrogen and non-estrogen users over time. Two studies found that estrogen users had less cognitive decline than non-users (Jacobs et al., 1998; Resnick et al., 1997), and two found no difference between the two groups (Paganini-Hill & Henderson, 1996; Barrett-Connor & Kritz-Silverstein, 1993). Paganini-Hill and Henderson (1996) conducted a nested case-control study of 214 elderly upper-middle-class women to assess the association of estrogen replacement therapy and performance on Clock-Drawing, a visual–spatial task. There was no statistically significant difference in percentage of normal and abnormal clock drawers in the estrogen users compared to the women not using estrogen. In one of the largest studies, Barrett-Connor and Kritz-Silverstein (1993) tested cognitive function with a battery of 12 cognitive function tests in 800 elderly women. Age- and education-adjusted comparisons showed no difference between estrogen users and non-users, and no effect of dose or duration of estrogen use. Another study administered four measures from three cognitive tests to 727 elderly women at baseline and again an average of 2.5 years later (Jacobs et al., 1998). At baseline, estrogen users (past and current) had better scores on all four measures; at follow-up the estrogen users had less decline on the Selective Reminding Test, Immediate and Delayed, but not on the other two tests. The baseline scores were adjusted for age, education, and race; however the longitudinal analyses were not adjusted for these potential confounders. As part of the Baltimore Longitudinal Study of Aging, 282 women received cognitive testing at baseline and biannually with the Benton Visual Retention Test, a test of visual memory (Resnick et al., 1997). Women currently taking estrogen had better baseline scores and had less decline over the average 6.5-year follow-up period, but these differences became non-significant after adjusting for education.

The results of these observational studies highlight some important issues in determining whether estrogen use improves cognitive performance and lessens cognitive decline. Observational studies such as these are susceptible to confounding, especially by such strong predictors of cognitive performance as age, education, and depression (Kittner et al., 1986). While all of the studies adjusted for age, many did not adjust for education, and in some cases the results became non-significant after adjustments (Schmidt et al., 1996; Resnick et al., 1997). Since women who take estrogen tend to be younger, better educated, less depressed, and more interested in health promotion, it is critical to take these differences into account when comparing cognitive testing among estrogen users and non-users (Barrett-Connor, 1991). Another methodological concern is that many of the studies compared estrogen users to non-users based on the results of multiple cognitive tests. Such multiple comparisons between users and non-users substantially increase the probability of obtaining at least one positive result by chance alone.

Randomized trials may avoid some of these methodological concerns. Eight randomized, controlled trials and one non-randomized, controlled trial of the effect of estrogen therapy on cognitive function have been published (Caldwell & Watson, 1952; Rauramo et al., 1975; Hackman & Galbraith, 1976; Campbell & Whitehead, 1977; Fedor-Freybergh, 1977; Sherwin, 1988; Ditkoff et al., 1991; Phillips & Sherwin, 1992; Polo-Kantola et al., 1998). Six of these nine trials concluded that estrogen therapy improved cognitive function (Caldwell & Watson, 1952; Hackman & Galbraith, 1976; Campbell & Whitehead, 1977; Fedor-Freybergh, 1977; Sherwin, 1988; Phillips & Sherwin, 1992). However, substantial methodologic problems make the results of these trials difficult to evaluate. The trials are small, including only 18 to 70 subjects. Two of the trials concluded that estrogen use improved cognitive function, despite the fact that there was improvement in only one or two of multiple cognitive tests (Caldwell & Watson, 1952; Phillips & Sherwin, 1992). Participants in most of the studies who reported benefit from estrogen therapy included many recently menopausal women who had menopausal symptoms. Relief of vasomotor symptoms and insomnia by estrogen therapy might have resulted in improved cognitive performance. A recent placebo-controlled trial in asymptomatic postmenopausal women found little or no effect of estrogen therapy on cognitive test scores (Ditkoff et al., 1991). Finally, several of these trials reported that scores on cognitive tests improved after treatment with estrogen but did not compare these changes in the estrogen-treated group to results in the placebo-treated group (Hackman & Galbraith, 1976; Ditkoff et al., 1991, Phillips & Sherwin, 1992).

Estrogen therapy and dementia risk

The possible beneficial effects of estrogen on cognition in non-demented postmenopausal women along with the observation that women may be at increased risk for AD led to the hypothesis that estrogen deficiency associated with menopause may contribute to the development of dementia. There have been eight case-control studies and two prospective cohort studies conducted to evaluate the association between AD and other dementias and postmenopausal estrogen therapy. The results of these studies are variable; some suggest a protective effect of estrogen on development of AD while others suggest an increased risk. One of the case-control studies (Henderson et al., 1994) and the two prospective studies (Tang et al., 1996; Kawas et al., 1997) found a statistically lower risk of developing dementia in postmenopausal women who had taken estrogen compared to those who had not. Of the seven other case-control studies, two showed a non-significant increased risk of dementia among estrogen users compared to non-users (Heyman et al., 1984; Amaducci et al., 1986); two showed no difference in the risk of dementia (Graves et al., 1990; Brenner et al., 1994); and three found a non-significant decreased risk of dementia among estrogen users compared to non-users (Paganini-Hill & Henderson, 1994; Mortel & Meyer, 1995). All of these observational studies either matched cases and controls for age or statistically adjusted for age, but most were not adjusted for education, and none of the studies was adjusted for depression. The one case-control study that found an association between estrogen use and reduced risk for dementia found this association only for current estrogen users compared to non-users (OR = 0.3; 95% confidence intervals 0.1–0.7) (Henderson et al., 1994). Current use of estrogen might appear to be protective if physicians stop hormone therapy in women who develop cognitive dysfunction or dementia. In addition, retrospective studies might find an association between estrogen use and reduced risk for dementia if women with dementia do not report using estrogen in the past because they cannot remember. Two case-control studies that addressed this problem by using pharmacy records or a verified medication history reported conflicting results (Henderson et al., 1994; Brenner et al., 1994). Prospective studies also avoid recall bias, and both prospective cohort studies found a decreased risk of AD in estrogen users. In one of the prospective studies, estrogen use was recorded among 1124 elderly community-dwelling women who were evaluated for dementia 1 to 5 years later. Women who had ever used estrogen had a 50% reduction (adjusted OR 0.5, 95% confidence interval 0.25–0.9) in risk of developing AD (Tang et al., 1996). The other prospective study found a similar reduction in risk of developing AD (adjusted OR 0.46, 95% confidence interval 0.21–1.0) among 472 postmenopausal women enrolled in the Baltimore Longitudinal Study of Aging who were followed for up to 16 years (Kawas et al., 1997). Both prospective studies and one case-control study examined whether increasing duration of estrogen use was associated with increasing protection from dementia and found conflicting results (Tang et al., 1996; Kawas et al., 1997; Paganini-Hill & Henderson, 1994).

A meta-analysis of these observational studies of estrogen and dementia was recently published (Yaffe et al., 1998). The summary odds ratio for all types of dementia was 0.71 (95% CI 0.53 – 0.96, p for heterogeneity = 0.10) and for AD only, the summary odds ratio was 0.71 (95% CI 0.52 – 0.98, p for heterogeneity = 0.11). This 29% decreased risk of developing dementia among estrogen users may be of major public health importance; summary finding from meta-analysis, however, are only as reliable as the findings of the individual studies. Unfortunately, the observational studies that were summarized are susceptible to confounding and compliance bias. For example, women who choose to take estrogen have been reported to be better educated and healthier than non-users (Cauley et al., 1990), differences that may result in a lower risk for developing AD (Mortimer & Graves, 1993). Nonetheless, the results from the meta-analysis support the hypothesis that postmenopausal estrogen use protects against the development of AD.

Estrogen for treatment of Alzheimer's disease

Epidemiologic evidence suggesting that estrogen use may prevent development of AD and improve cognitive function has sparked interest in estrogen as a treatment for AD. There have been four small trials of estrogen therapy in women with AD. In two uncontrolled trials that included 7 and 15 participants, severity of dementia was measured at baseline and after 6 weeks of estrogen therapy (Fillit et al., 1986; Honjo et al., 1989). Each of these studies found improvement on some, but not all measures of dementia severity after treatment. Because there was no control group for comparison, this improvement may represent a practice or a learning effect. In addition, these two trials were not blinded, which may have biased the outcome. In another trial, 15 women with AD were treated with estrogen and the change in their dementia severity was compared with 15 untreated controls matched for age and dementia severity at baseline (Ohkura et al., 1994). While the control group did not improve, the treatment group improved on one cognitive scale and on one dementia rating scale compared to scores prior to treatment, but changes in the severity of dementia in the estrogen treated group were not compared to changes in the untreated group. In the only placebo-controlled trial, Honjo et al. (1993) randomly assigned 14 women with AD to estrogen (1.25 mg conjugated oral estrogen per day) or placebo and found greater improvement on one dementia scale but not on two other scales in the estrogen-treated group compared to the placebo-treated group. All four of these studies are limited by very small sample size and short duration of therapy (3 to 6 weeks). Larger and longer duration randomized placebo-controlled trials of estrogen for AD treatment are under way.

Estrogen and Apolipoptrotein E

The apolipoprotein E (ApoE) isoform e4 has recently been identified as a major biological risk factor for AD and preclinical cognitive decline (Roses, 1995; Yaffe et al., 1997). Several lines of basic science evidence support the hypothesis that estrogen and ApoE may act synergistically. Estrogen modulates the expression of the ApoE gene in rodent tissues (Srivastava et al., 1997), and the estradiol enhancement of synaptic sprouting in response to injury in rats may operate through an ApoE-dependent mechanism (Stone et al., 1998). Another series of experiments using ApoE knockout mice has shown that transgenic e4 mice have marked behavioral and cognitive deficits and that these abnormalities are more pronounced in female rats (Raber et al., 1998). In humans, women who are heterozygous for ApoE e4 have a greater risk of developing AD than heterozygous men, especially those with the 2–4 genotype (Payami et al., 1996a, b; Farrer et al., 1997). The effect of cholinesterase treatment for AD has been reported to vary for women according to their ApoE e4 status but not in men (Farlow et al., 1998). Compared to subjects without an e4 allele, women with an e4 allele had less of a treatment effect. The mechanism for this gender-specific ApoE genotype interaction is not clear but could be related to estrogen.

Selective estrogen receptor modulators

Recently, several selective estrogen receptor modulators (SERMS) have been developed that have estrogen agonist and antagonist action in estrogen responsive tissues. The two most widely recognized SERMS are tamoxifen and raloxifene. Both have estrogen–agonist properties on bone and lipids and estrogen–agonist effects on breast; whereas raloxifene, unlike tamoxifen, has estrogen-agonist effects on the uterus (Bryant & Dere, 1998). Although several studies are under way, there have been no reported observational studies or trials of SERMS for prevention or treatment of dementia or other cognitive disorders.

Testosterone

The role of testosterone in modulating cognitive performance has been less well studied than estrogen, and much of the published results are conflicting and confusing. Androgen receptors tend to co-localize with estrogen receptors in the rat brain and are distributed in the hypothalamus, thalamus, hippocampus, and the deep layers of the cerebral cortex (Simerly et al., 1990). In men, testosterone levels decrease somewhat with age, declining from a mean of 23.5 nmol/liter in young adults to 5 nmol/liter in octogenarians (Vermeulen, 1991). Testosterone is converted by aromatase to estrogens that are present throughout the body including the central nervous system. In rodent models, aromatase enzymes are concentrated in the amygdala, hypothalamus, and stria terminalis (MacLusky et al., 1994). Because of the conversion from testosterone to estrogens, men, unlike women, maintain a fairly constant level of serum estrogens as they age (Gray et al., 1991). More recent studies suggest, however, that with aging, the bioavailable (non-sex hormone-binding globulin bound) testosterone and estrogen may decline by 50% (Khosla et al., 1998).

Men tend to perform better on tests of visuospatial skills whereas women tend to perform better on verbal fluency (Hampson & Kimura, 1992). This gender difference has led researchers to speculate that testosterone is related to visuospatial abilities. Shute and colleagues (1983) were among the first to indicate that there was a gender difference on testosterone levels and visuospatial abilities. They found that, in young men, low testosterone was associated with better visuospatial testing whereas the opposite was found for young women. Similarly, in young adults (mean age 22 years), Gouchie and Kimura found that lower salivary testosterone levels were associated with better visuospatial performance in men but worse performance in women (Gouchie & Kimura, 1991). Another study supported the findings that testosterone levels are negatively correlated with spatial performance in men and positively correlated with spatial abilities in women (Moffat & Hampson, 1996). These studies have led to the hypothesis that there is a curvilinear relationship of testosterone's effect on visuospatial performance, and that a mid-point is the optimal level. Others hypothesize that it is the conversion to estrogens that explains the negative visuospatial performance associated with high testosterone levels. While controversial, some studies have found that serum estradiol levels are negatively associated with visuospatial abilities and positively associated with verbal abilities (Hampson & Kimura, 1988; Hampson, 1990). However, other studies have not found an association between serum testosterone levels or estrogen levels and visuospatial performance (McKeever & Deyo, 1990; Gordon & Lee, 1986).

Only one randomized controlled trial of testosterone for cognitive function has been conducted in healthy men (Janowsky et al., 1994). Healthy older men (mean age 67 years) were administered testosterone or placebo for 3 months. In the treatment group, testosterone levels increased to 150% of baseline (approximately to the level of young, healthy men) and were associated with improved spatial cognition but not on any other measures of cognition. Interestingly, the exogenous testosterone administration suppressed estradiol levels in the treated group. The authors speculated that the lowered estradiol levels could have explained the improvements on visuospatial performance. They reanalyzed the data, assessing whether serum testosterone or serum estradiol was associated with visuospatial performance. They found that estradiol levels significantly correlated to performance, but not testosterone levels. The authors argue that, unlike previous studies of young men in which high testosterone is associated with worse visuospatial performance, the elderly men were relatively hypogonadal and that testosterone administration restored their levels to that of normal young men. They suggest that both high and low testosterone levels are negatively associated with visuospatial abilities and the midpoint ideal. When testosterone is very high, some testosterone could be aromatized to estrogens and negatively influence visuospatial performance; when testosterone is very low, and repleted, visuospatial abilities improve. Thus, evidence suggests that testosterone given to elderly men may improve visuospatial abilities, either due to testosterone itself or by a reduction in estrogen. Presumably, the ratio of estradiol to testosterone should be investigated, although few studies have attempted to do so. Furthermore, the association of serum testosterone and cognitive abilities in older women remains to be examined.

There has only been one trial of the effects of androgens on cognitive function in women. Sherwin (1988) administered estradiol, testosterone, both, or placebo to recently surgically menopausal women and found that all of the hormone-treated groups had stable scores on several memory tests, whereas the placebo group had declines on cognitive testing. The groups were compared to baseline scores but not to each other. No studies have explored the relationship between testosterone and dementia, including AD. However, based on the assumption that testosterone is converted to estrogens, a study is underway to explore whether testosterone treatment in men with AD improves severity of dementia.

Conclusions

There are plausible biological mechanisms that might account for a beneficial effect of estrogen therapy on cognition and dementia. Studies in women, however, have substantial methodologic problems and have produced conflicting results. Large, controlled, blinded trials are necessary to determine if estrogen therapy can reduce the risk of developing AD. The Women's Health Initiative Randomized Trial, which is currently enrolling participants, will include the Women's Health Initiative Memory Study. This ancillary trial will determine the effect of hormone replacement therapy on cognitive function and the risk for developing AD and other dementias among approximately 8000 postmenopausal women treated for 10 years. Based on the conflicting evidence and the potential side effects of estrogen therapy – including endometrial abnormalities (Grady et al., 1992), gallbladder disease

(Petitti et al., 1988), venous thromboembolic events (Daly et al., 1996), and breast cancer (Grady & Ernster, 1991; Colditz et al., 1995) – it is premature to recommend that estrogen be used to treat women with AD. However, given the lack of available treatment options for women with AD and the suggestive preliminary findings of benefit, large randomized trials of estrogen therapy should be completed as soon as possible. Whether or not estrogen therapy might improve other forms of dementia, such as vascular dementia, should also be explored. Since progestins are typically added to the estrogen regimen in women with a uterus, the role of this hormone must also be evaluated in future studies. Finally, testosterone may have an effect on cognition in both men and women and needs to be studied further. Its role as treatment for AD and other types of dementia is under investigation.

REFERENCES

Amaducci, L. A., Fratiglioni, L., Rocca, W. A., Fieschi, C., Livrea, P, Pedone, D., Bracco, L., Lippi, A., Grandolfo, C., Bino, G. et al. (1986). Risk factors for clinically diagnosed Alzheimer's disease: a case control study of an Italian population. *Neurology*, **36**(7), 922–31.

Applebaum-Bowden, D., McLean, P., Steinmetz, A., Fontana, D., Matthys, C., Warnick, G. R., Cheung, M., Albers, J. J., Hazzard, W. R. (1989). Lipoprotein, apolipoprotein, and lipolytic enzyme changes following estrogen administration in postmenopausal women. *Journal of Lipid Research*, **30**(12), 1895–906.

Barrett-Connor, E. (1991). Postmenopausal estrogen and prevention bias. *Annals of Internal Medicine*, **115**, 455–6.

Barrett-Connor, E. & Kritz-Silverstein, D. (1993). Estrogen replacement therapy and cognitive function in older women. *Journal of the American Medical Association* **269**, 2637–41.

Brenner, D. E., Kukull, W. A., Stergachis, A., van Belle, G., Bowen, J. O., McCormick, W. C., Terri, L. & Larson, E. B. (1994). Postmenopausal estrogen replacement therapy and the risk of Alzheimer's disease: a population-based case-control study. *American Journal of Epidemiology*, **14**(3), 262–7.

Bryant, H. U. & Dere, W. H. (1998). Selective estrogen receptor modulators: an alternative to hormone replacement therapy. *Proceedings of the Society for Experimental Biology and Medicine*, **217**(1), 45–52.

Caldwell, B. & Watson, R. (1952). An evaluation of psychologic effects of sex hormone administration in aged women: results after six months. *Journal of Gerontology*, **7**, 228–44.

Campbell, S. & Whitehead, M. (1977). Oestrogen therapy and the menopausal syndrome. *Clinical Obstetetrics and Gynaecology*, **4**(1), 31–47.

Cauley, J. A., Cummings, S. R., Black, D. M., Mascioli, S. R. & Seeley, D. G. (1990). Prevalence and determinants of estrogen replacement therapy in elderly women. *American Journal of Obstetrics and Gynecology*, **163**, 1438–44.

Colditz, G. A., Hankinson, S. E., Hunter, Willett, W. C., Manson, J. E., Stampfer, M. J., Hennekens, C., Rosner, B. & Speizer, F. E. (1995). The use of estrogen and progestins and the risk of breast cancer in postmenopausal women. *New England Journal of Medicine*, 332(24), 1589–93.

Coyle, J. T., Price, D. L. & DeLong, M. R. (1983). Alzheimer's disease: a disorder of cortical cholinergic innervation. *Science*, 219, 1184–90.

Daly, E., Vessey, M. P., Hawkins, M. M., Carson, J. L., Gough, P. & Marsh, S. (1996). Risk of venous thromboembolism in users of hormone replacement therapy. *Lancet*, 348(9033), 977–80.

Ditkoff, E. C., Crary, W. G., Cristo, M. & Lobo, R. A. (1991). Estrogen improves psychological function in asymptomatic postmenopausal women. *Obstetrics and Gynecology*, 78(6), 991–5.

Ernst, R. L. & Hay, J. W. (1994). The US economy and social costs of Alzheimer's disease revisited. *American Journal of Public Health*, 84(8), 1261–4.

Evans D. A. (1990). Estimated prevalence of Alzheimer's disease in the United States. *Milbank Quarterly*, 68, 267–89.

Farlow, M. R., Lahiri, D. K., Poirier, J., Davignon, J., Schnieder, L. & Hui, S. L. (1998). Treatment outcome of tacrine therapy depends on apolipoprotein genotype and gender of the subjects with Alzheimer's disease. *Neurology*, 50(3), 669–77.

Farrer, L. A., Cupples, L. A., Haines, J. L., Hyman, B., Kukull, W. A., Mayeuz, R., Myers, R.. H., Pericak-Vance, M. A., Risch, N. & van Duijn, C. M. (1997). Effects of age, sex, and ethnicity on the association between apolipoprotein E genotype and Alzheimer's disease. A meta-analysis. APOE and Alzheimer Disease Meta Analysis Consortium. *Journal of the American Medical Association* 278(16), 1349–56.

Fedor-Freybergh, P. (1977). The influence of oestrogens on the wellbeing and mental performance in climacteric and postmenopausal women. *Acta Obstetrics and Gynecology Scandin. Supplement*, 64, 1–91.

Fillit H., Weinreb, H., Cholst, I., Luine, V., McEwen, B., Amador, R. & Zabriskie, J. (1986). Observations in a preliminary open trial of estradiol therapy for senile dementia – Alzheimer's type. *Psychoneuroendocrinology*, 11(3), 337–45.

Gangar, K. F., Vyas, S., Whitehead, M., Crook, D., Meire, H. & Campbell, S. (1991). Pulsatility index in internal carotid artery in relation to transdermal oestradiol and time since menopause. *Lancet*, 338(8771), 839–42.

Gibbs, R. B., Hashash, A. & Johnson, D. A. (1997). Effects of estrogen on potassium-stimulated acetylcholine release in the hippocampus and overlying cortex of adult rats. *Brain Research*, 749(1), 143–6.

Goodman, Y., Bruce, A. J., Cheng, B. & Mattson, M. P. (1996). Estrogens attenuate and corticosterone exacerbates excitotoxicity, oxidative injury, and amyloid beta-peptide toxicity in hippocampal neurons. *Journal of Neurochemistry*, 66(5), 1836–44.

Gordon, H. & Lee, P. (1986). A relationship between gonadotropins and visuospatial function. *Neuropsychologia*, 24, 563–76.

Gouchie, C. & Kimura, D. (1991). The relationship between testosterone levels and cognitive ability patterns. *Psychoneuroendocrinology*, 16(4), 323–34.

Gould, E., Woolley, C. S., Frankfurt, M. & McEwen, B. S. (1990). Gonadal steroids regulate dendritic spine density in hippocampal pyramidal cells in adulthood. *Journal of Neuroscience*, 10(4), 1286–91.

Grady, D., Rubin, S. M., Petitti, D. B., Fox, C. S., Black, D., Ettinger, B., Ernster, V. L. & Cummings, W. R. (1992). Hormone therapy to prevent disease and prolong life in postmenopausal women. *Annals of Internal Medicine*, 117(12), 1016–37.

Grady, E. & Ernster, V. (1991). Does postmenopausal hormone replacement therapy cause breast cancer? *American Journal of Epidemiology*, 134, 1396–400.

Graves, A. B., White, E., Koepsell, T. D., Reifler, B. V., van Belle, G., Larson, E. B. & Raskind, M. (1990). A case-control study of Alzheimer's disease. *Annals of Neurology*, 28, 766–74.

Gray, A., Feldman, H., McKinlay, J. & Longcope, C., (1991). Age, disease, and changing sex hormone levels in middle-aged men: results of the Massachusetts Male Aging Study. *Journal of Clinical Endocrinology and Metabolism*, 73(5), 1016–25.

Hackman, B. W. & Galbraith, D. (1976). Replacement therapy and piperazine oestrone sulphate ('Harmogen') and its effect on memory. *Current Medical Research Opinion*, 4(4), 303–6.

Hampson, E. (1990). Estrogen-related variations in human spatial and articulatory–motor skills. *Psychoneuroendocrinology*, 15, 97–111.

Hampson, E. & Kimura, D. (1988). Reciprocal effects of hormonal fluctuations on human motor and perceptual skills. *Behavioral Neuroscience*, 102, 456–9.

Hampson, J. & Kimura, D. (1992). Sex differences and hormonal influences on cognitive function in humans. In *Behavioral Endocrinology*, ed. J. Becker, S. Breedlove & D. Crews, pp. 357–98. Cambridge, MA.: MIT Press.

Henderson, V. W., Paganini, H. A., Emanuel, C. K., Dunn, M. E. & Buckwalter, J. G. (1994). Estrogen replacement therapy in older women. Comparisons between Alzheimer's disease cases and nondemented control subjects. *Archives of Neurology*, 51, 896–900.

Heyman, A., Wilkinson, W. E., Stafford, J. A., Helms, M. J., Sigmon, A. H. & Weinberg, T. (1984). Alzheimer's disease: a study of epidemiological aspects. *Annals of Neurology*, 15, 353–41.

Honjo, H., Ogino, Y., Tanaka, K., Urabe, M., Kashiwagi, T., Ishihara, S., Okada, H., Araki, K., Fushiki, S., Nakajima, K., Hayashi, K., Hayashi, M. & Sasaki, T. (1993). An effect of conjugated estrogen to cognitive impairment in women with senile dementia-Alzheimer's type: a placebo-controlled double blind study. *Journal of the Japanese Menopause Society*, 1, 167–71.

Honjo, H., Ogino, Y., Naitoh, K., Urabe, M., Kitawaki, J., Yasuda, J., Yamamoto, T., Ishihara, S., Okada, H., Yonezawa, T. et al. (1989). *In vivo* effects by estrone sulfate on the central nervous system–senile dementia (Alzheimer's type). *Journal of Steroid Biochemistry*, 34, 521–5.

Honjo, H., Tamura, T., Matsumoto, Y., Kawata, M., Ogino, Y., Tanaka, K., Yamamoto, T. Ueda, S. & Okada, H. (1992). Estrogen as a growth factor to central nervous cells. Estrogen treatment promotes development of acetylcholinesterase-positive basal forebrain neurons transplanted in the anterior eye chamber. *Journal of Steroid Biochemistry and Molecular Biology*, 41, 633–5.

Jacobs, D. M., Tang, M. X., Stern, Y., Sano, M., Marder, K., Bell, K. L., Schofield, P., Dooneief, G., Gurland, B. & Mayeux, R. (1998). Cognitive function in nondemented older women who took estrogen after menopause. *Neurology*, 50, 368–73.

Janowsky, J. S., Oviatt, S. K. & Orwoll, E. S. (1994). Testosterone influences spatial cognition in older men. *Behavioral Neuroscience*, 108, 325–32.

Kampen, D. L. & Sherwin, B. B. (1994). Estrogen use and verbal memory in health postmenopausal women. *Obstetrics and Gynecology*, 83, 979–83.

Kawas, C., Resnick, S., Morrison, A., Brookmeyer, R., Corrada, M., Zonderman, A., Bacal, C., Lingle, D. D. & Metter, E. (1997). A prospective study of estrogen replacement therapy and the risk of developing Alzheimer's disease: the Baltimore Longitudinal Study of Aging. *Neurology*, 48, 1517–21.

Khosla, S., Melton, L. J. 3rd, Atkinson, E. J., O'Fallon, W. M., Klee, G. G. & Riggs, B. L. (1998). Relationship of serum sex steroid levels and bone turnover markers with bone mineral density in men and women: a key role for bioavailable estrogen. *Journal of Clinical Encocrinology and Metabolism*, 83, 2266–74.

Kimura, D. (1995). Estrogen replacement therapy may protect against intellectual decline in postmenopausal women. *Hormones and Behavior*, 29, 312–21.

Kittner, S. J., White, L. R., Farmer, M. E., Wolz, M., Kaplan, E., Moes, E., Brody, J. A. & Feinleib, M. (1986). Methodological issues in screening for dementia: the problem of education adjustment. *Journal of Chronic Diseases*, 39, 163–70.

Luine, V. N. (1985). Estradiol increases choline acetyltransferase activity in specific basal forebrain nuclei and projection areas of female rats. *Experimental Neurology*, 89, 484–90.

Luine, V. N., Khylchevskaya, R. I. & McEwen, B. S. (1975). Effect of gonadal steroid on activities of monoamine oxidase and choline acetylase in rat brain. *Brain Research*, 86, 293–306.

MacLusky, N. J., Walters, M. J., Clark, A. S. & Toran-Allerand, C. D. (1994). Aromatase in the cerebral cortex, hippocampus, and mid-brain: Ontogeny and developmental implications. *Molecular and Cellular Neuroscience*, 5, 691–8.

McEwen, B. S. & Woolley, C. S. (1994). Estradiol and progesterone regulate neuronal structure and synaptic connectivity in adult as well as developing brain. *Experimental Gerontology*, 29, 431–6.

McKeever, W. & Deyo, R. (1990). Testosterone, dihydrotestosterone, and spatial task performances of males. *Bulletin of the Psychonomic Society*, 25, 438–40.

Moffatt, S. D. & Hampson, E. (1996). A curvilinear relationship between testosterone and spatial cognition in humans: possible influence of hand preference. *Psychoneuroendocrinology*, 21, 323–7.

Mortel, K. F. & Meyer, J. S. (1995). Lack of postmenopausal estrogen replacement therapy and the risk of dementia. *Journal of Neuropsychiatry and Clinical Neurosciences*, 7, 334–7.

Mortimer, J. A. & Graves, A. B. (1993). Education and other socioeconomic determinants of dementia and Alzheimer's disease. *Neurology*, 43(suppl 4), S39–44.

Ohkura, T., Isse, K., Akazawa, K. Hamamoto, M., Yanoi, Y. & Hagino, N. (1994). Evaluation of estrogen treatment in female patients with dementia of the Alzheimer type. *Endocrinology Journal*, 41, 361–71.

Paganini-Hill, A. & Henderson, V. W. (1994). Estrogen deficiency and risk of Alzheimer's disease in women. *American Journal of Epidemiology*, 140, 256–61.

Paganini-Hill, A. & Henderson, V. W. (1996). The effects of hormone replacement therapy, lipoprotein cholesterol levels, and other factors on a clock drawing task in older women. *Journal of the American Geriatric Society*, 44, 818–22.

Palmer, A. M. & DeKosky, S. T. (1993). Monoamine neurons in aging and Alzheimer's disease. *Journal of Neural Transmission. General Section*, 91, 135–59.

Payami, H., Montee, K, Grimslid, H., Shattuc, S. & Kaye, J. (1996a). Increased risk of familial late-onset Alzheimer's disease in women. *Neurology*, 46, 126–9

Payami, H., Zaraparsi, S., Montee, K. R., Sexton, G. J., Kaye, J. A., Bird, T. D., Yu, C. E., Wijsman, E. M., Heston, L. L. Litt, M. & Schellenberg, G. D. (1996b). Gender differences in apolipoprotein E-associated risk for familial Alzheimer's disease: a possible clue to the higher incidence of Alzheimer's disease in women. *American Journal of Human Genetics*, 58, 803–11.

Petitti, D. B., Sidney, S. & Perlman, J. A. (1988). Increased risk of cholecystectomy in users of supplemental estrogen. *Gastroenterology*, 94, 91–5.

Phillips, S. M. & Sherwin, B. B. (1992). Effects of estrogen on memory function in surgically menopausal women. *Psychoneuroendocrinology*, 17, 485–95.

Polo-Kantola, P., Portin, R., Polo, O., Helenius, H., Irjala, K. & Erkkola, R. (1998). The effect of short-term estrogen replacement therapy on cognition: a randomized double-blind, cross-over trial in postmenopausal women. *Obstetrics and Gynecology*, 91, 459–66.

Raber, J., Wong, D., Buttini, M., Orth, M., Bellosta, S., Atas, R. E., Mahley, R. W. & Mucke, L. (1998). Isoform-specific effects of human apolipoprotein E on brain function revealed in ApoE knockout mice: increased susceptibility of females. *Proceedings of the National Academy of the Sciences, USA*, 95(18), 10914–19.

Rauramo, L. Lagerspetz, K., Engblom, P. & Punnonen, R. (1975). The effect of castration and peroral estrogen therapy on some psychological functions. *Frontiers in Hormone Research*, 3, 94–104.

Resnick, S. M., Metter, E. J. & Zonderman, A. B. (1997). Estrogen replacement therapy and longitudinal decline in visual memory. A possible protective effect? *Neurology*, 49, 1491–7.

Robinson, D., Friedman, L., Marcus, R., Tinklenberg, J. & Yesavage, J. (1994). Estrogen replacement therapy and memory in older women. *Journal of the American Geriatric Society*, 42, 919–22.

Roses, A. D. (1995). Apolipoprotein E genotyping in the differential diagnosis, no prediction of Alzheimer's disease. *Annals of Neurology*, 38, 6–14.

Schmidt, R., Fazekas, F., Reinhart, B., kapeller, P., Fazekas, G., Offenbacher, H., Eber, B., Schumacher, M. & Freidl, W. (1996). Estrogen replacement therapy in older women: a neuropsychological and brain MRI study. *Journal of the American Geriatric Society*, 44, 1307–13.

Sherwin, B. B. (1988). Estrogen and/or androgen replacement therapy and cognitive functioning in surgically menopausal women. *Psychoneuroendocrinology*, 13, 345–57.

Shute, V., Pellegrino, J., Hubert, L. & Reynolds, R. (1983). The relationship between androgen levels and human spatial abilities. *Bulletin of the Psychonomic Society*, 21, 465–8.

Simerly, R., Chang, C., Muramatsu, M. & Swanson, L. (1990). Distribution of androgen and estrogen receptor mRNA-containing cells in the rat brain: an in situ hybridization study. *Journal of Comparative Neurology*, 294, 76–95.

Simpkins, J. W., Singh, M. & Bishop, J. (1994). The potential role for estrogen replacement therapy in the treatment of the cognitive decline and neurodegeneration associated with Alzheimer's disease. *Neurobiology of Aging*, S195–7.

Srivastava, R. A., Srivastava, N., Averna, M., Lin, R. C., Korach, K. S., Lubahn, D. B. & Schonfeld, G. (1997). Estrogen up-regulates apolipoprotein E (ApoE) gene expression by increasing ApoE mRNA in the translating pool via the estrogen receptor alpha-mediated pathway. *Journal of Biological Chemistry*, 27, 33360–6.

Stone, D. J., Rozovsky, I., Morgan, T. E., Anderson, C. P. & Finch, C. E. (1998). Increased synaptic sprouting in response to estrogen via the apolipoprotein E-dependent mechanism: implications for Alzheimer's disease. *Journal of Neuroscience*, 18, 3180–5.

Summer, B. E. & Fink, G. (1995). Estrogen increases the density of 5-hydroxytryptamine(2A) receptors in cerebral cortex and nucleus accumbens in the female rat. *Journal of Steroid Biochemistry and Molecular Biology*, 54, 15–20.

Tang, M. X., Jacobs, D., Stern, Y., Marder, K., Schodield, P., Gurland, B., andrews, H. & Mayeux, R. (1996). Effect of oestrogen during menopause on risk and age at onset of Alzheimer's disease. *Lancet*, 348, 429–32.

Vermeulen, A. (1991). Clinical review 24: androgens in the aging male. *Journal of Clinical Endocrinology and Metabolism*, 73, 221–4.

Yaffe, K., Cauley, J., Sands, L. & Browner, W. (1997). Apolipoprotein E phenotype and cognitive decline in a prospective study of elderly community women. *Archives of Neurology*, 54, 1110–4.

Yaffe, K., Sawaya, G., Lieterburg, I. & Grady, D. (1998). Estrogen therapy in postmenopausal women: effects on cognitive function and dementia. *Journal of the American Medical Association* 279, 688–95.

9

Effects of estrogen on basal forebrain cholinergic neurons and cognition: implications for brain aging and dementia in women

Robert B. Gibbs

Introduction

Research over the past 30 years has demonstrated that the brain is an important target organ for estrogen effects. Studies using sensitive autoradiographic and immunohistochemical techniques have documented the presence of estrogen receptors throughout the brain (Brown et al., 1995; Österlund et al., 1998; Pfaff, 1968; Rainbow et al., 1982). The highest levels of receptors are often detected in brain areas involved in gonadal regulation, physiologic homeostasis, and reproductive behavior. Receptors have also been detected throughout the neocortex, hippocampus, and amygdala – regions of the brain long known to be associated with higher cognitive functions such as learning, memory, and attention. Some of the effects of estrogen recently described include changes in neurotransmitter production and release, changes in the number and frequency of synaptic contacts, and changes in the expression and regulation of second messengers and transcription factors, as well as effects on cell survival and growth.

Given the variety of estrogen effects throughout the brain, it is not surprising that estrogen should affect cognitive processes or that the loss of estrogen would play a role in the biology of brain aging in women. Consider that women in the United States reach menopause at approximately 51 years of age, and that the average lifespan for women in the United States is 79 years. This means that approximately 28 years of a woman's life are postmenopausal and reflect a hypoestrogenic state.

Given these facts, it is surprising how little we know about the effects of prolonged estrogen deprivation on the aging brain. Of particular concern is the possibility that the long-term loss of estrogen has adverse effects on the brain, contributing to neuronal loss with age and exacerbating the risk and severity of cognitive decline.

Such concerns have been brought to the forefront by recent studies suggesting that estrogen replacement therapy may help to reduce the risk and severity of Alzheimer's disease (AD)-related dementia in women (Baldereschi et al., 1998; Henderson et al., 1996; Honjo et al., 1995; Kawas et al., 1997; Ohkura et al., 1994, 1995a; Paganini-Hill & Henderson, 1996; Tang et al., 1996), and by studies in animals showing beneficial effects of estrogen replacement on both physiology and behavior (see below). Though the results of these studies are still highly controversial, the issues are forcing both clinicians and policy makers to consider how best to evaluate the risks and benefits of estrogen replacement in postmenopausal women.

This brief review summarizes recent animal research pertaining to potential mechanisms by which estrogen may help to reduce the risk and severity of AD-related dementia in women. The bulk of the review focuses on work demonstrating significant estrogen effects on cholinergic neurons projecting to the hippocampus and cortex, and places this work in context with recent studies demonstrating beneficial effects of estrogen replacement on the performance of certain learning and memory tasks. Also discussed are other potential mechanisms by which estrogen may help to reduce the risk and severity of AD-related dementia.

Cholinergic neurons and cognition

Cholinergic neurons in the medial septum (MS), the diagonal band of Broca (DBB), and the nucleus basalis magnocellularis (NBM) are the major source of cholinergic innervation to the hippocampus and cortex (Woolf, 1991). Numerous studies have demonstrated that these cholinergic projections play an important role in cognitive processes. More than 20 years ago, studies by Drachman and co-workers demonstrated that systemic administration of the muscarinic receptor antagonist scopolamine produced learning and memory deficits in humans consistent with the suspected role of central cholinergic projections in learning and memory (Drachman & Leavitt, 1974; Drachman, 1977; Drachman et al., 1980). Subsequent studies on lower primates demonstrated similar delay-dependent memory impairments following systemic administration of either scopolamine or atropine, comparable to memory deficits seen in normal-aged monkeys (Aigner & Mishkin, 1986; Aigner et al., 1991; Bartus, 1978; Bartus & Johnson, 1976; Penetar & McDonough, 1983). Notably, deficits were not observed following injections of methylscopolamine (Bartus & Johnson, 1976), a muscarinic antagonist which does not cross the blood–brain barrier, suggesting that the impairments observed were due specifically to the disruption of central, not peripheral, cholinergic processes. In addition, significant and consistent deficits in cholinergic parameters including decreases in the number and size of basal forebrain cholinergic neurons (Altavista et al., 1990; Fischer et al., 1989, 1991; Mesulam et al., 1987; Stroessner-Johnson et al., 1992), decreases in high affinity choline uptake (Kristofiková et al., 1992; Sherman & Friedman, 1990), acetylcholine synthesis (Gibson et al., 1981; Sherman et al., 1981; Sims et al., 1983), acetylcholine release (Araujo et al., 1990; Takei et al., 1989; Wu et al., 1988), and cholinergic synaptic transmission (Taylor & Griffith, 1993), have been detected in the brains of aged mammals, all of which suggest a role for central cholinergic neurons in the development of age-related cognitive decline.

Evidence for the specific involvement of basal forebrain cholinergic projections in the etiology of memory dysfunction has grown significantly since the discovery that AD is associated with a significant loss of cholinergic neurons in the MS and NBM (Davies & Maloney, 1976; Perry et al., 1977; Whitehouse et al., 1982). AD is an age-dependent neurodegenerative disease characterized by a progressive neuropathology with a corresponding loss of learning and memory and other cognitive processes. AD is also the most common cause of dementia in the elderly accounting for approximately 50% to 60% of all cases of dementia (Häfner, 1990). Animal studies have demonstrated that neurochemical lesions of basal forebrain cholinergic nuclei produce consistent, robust learning and memory deficits in rats (Dekker et al., 1991), many of which can be attenuated by muscarinic receptor agonists or acetylcholinesterase inhibitors (Matsuoka et al., 1991; McGurk et al., 1991; Murray & Fibiger, 1985, 1986). The extent to which these effects reflect specific cholinergic effects on learning and memory processes is still uncertain. Increasing evidence suggests that the cholinergic neurons may be more intimately involved in attentional processes, and that some of the deficits observed following basal forebrain cholinergic lesions are due to attentional deficits as opposed to learning and memory deficits per se (Holland, 1997; Jones et al., 1995; Lawrence & Sahakian, 1995; Voytko, 1996; Wenk, 1997). Hence the precise nature of the cognitive impairment associated with the loss of basal forebrain cholinergic neurons remains unclear. Nevertheless, both basic and clinical data continue to support the idea that sufficient loss of basal forebrain cholinergic projections has a negative impact either directly or indirectly on cognition, and that agents that enhance cholinergic function, such as tacrine and donepezil, can help to reduce cognitive impairments in some AD patients (Barner & Gray, 1998; Conway, 1998; Farlow et al., 1992; Rogers et al., 1998; Schneider, 1994).

Estrogen and basal forebrain cholinergic neurons

We and others have hypothesized that one mechanism by which estrogen may help to reduce the risk and severity of AD-related dementia in women is by enhancing and maintaining the functional status of basal forebrain cholinergic projections

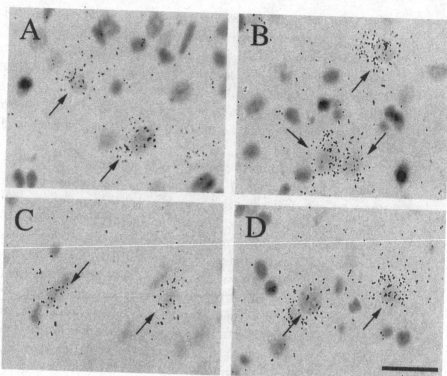

Figure 9.1.   Photomicrographs showing ChAT mRNA-containing cells in the medial septum (MS) (a) and the nucleus basilis magnocellularis (b) and NBM (c and d) of ovariectomized non-E-treated animals (a and c) and ovariectomized animals which received 10 μg 17-ß-E$_2$ either 24 hours (b) or 72 hours (d) prior to sacrifice. Hybridization signal consists of dark silver grains overlying lightly stained nuclei. Note the increased numbers of grains overlying cells (arrows) in the E-treated animals compared with the non-estrogen-treated controls, indicating increased levels of ChAT mRNA. Scale bar = 40 μm.

emanating from the MS and NBM. Work has shown that, in adult ovariectomized rats, continuous treatment with 17–ß-estradiol produces increases in choline acetyltransferase (ChAT) mRNA and protein in the MS and NBM (Gibbs, 1997; Gibbs & Pfaff, 1992; Gibbs et al., 1994; Luine, 1985; see Figs. 9.1–9.3), as well as increases in high affinity choline uptake (HACU) in the hippocampus and overly-ing cortex (O'Malley et al., 1987; Singh et al., 1994). Increases in ChAT mRNA typ-ically range between 20% to 30%, whereas increases in HACU have been reported to range from 46% in the hippocampus to 82% in the frontal cortex (Singh et al., 1994). In addition, some of these effects are dependent on the dose and duration of estrogen treatment. For example, increased numbers of ChAT-like immunoreactive (IR) cells were detected in the MS and NBM after short-term treatment with low levels of estradiol, but not after longer-term treatment or treatment with higher doses (Gibbs, 1997; Gibbs & Pfaff, 1992; see Fig. 9.3). These findings suggest that

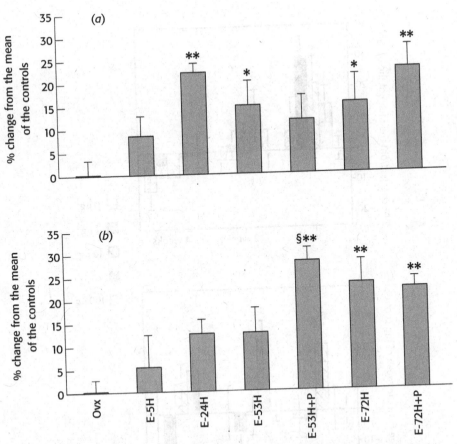

Figure 9.2. Effects of estrogen and estrogen + progesterone on relative levels of ChAT mRNA in the medial septum (MS) (a) and the nucleus basilis magnocellularis (NBM) (b). Animals received a single injection of 17-ß-E$_2$ (10 µg s.c.) and were sacrificed at different times postinjection. Some animals received an additional injection of progesterone (500 µg s.c.) 48 hours after receiving estrogen and were sacrificed 5 hours or 24 hours later. Bars represent percent change from the mean of the ovariectomized controls. Note the increase in ChAT mRNA detected in the MS 24 hours after receiving E$_2$ and in the NBM 72h after receiving E$_2$. Note also the ability of progesterone to enhance the effects of E$_2$ in both the MS and NBM. *$P < 0.05$ relative to ovariectomized controls. **$P < 0.01$ relative to ovariectomized controls. §$P < 0.05$ relative to E-53H. (Adapted from Gibbs, 1996b).

estrogen replacement can produce an increase in the functional status of basal fore-brain cholinergic neurons projecting to the hippocampus and cortex, but they also suggest that the efficacy may depend on the dose and regimen of estrogen treatment.

Evidence has also shown that estrogen plays a role in the normal physiological regulation of basal forebrain cholinergic neurons. Recently, we demonstrated that relative levels of ChAT mRNA in the rat MS fluctuate significantly across the estrous cycle (Gibbs, 1996b). Notably, peak levels of ChAT mRNA were detected on

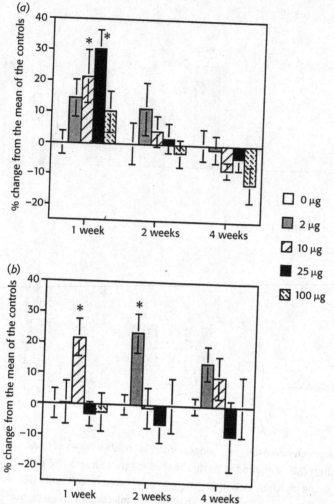

Figure 9.3.   Changes in the number of ChAT-like immunoreactive (IR) cells detected in the medial septum (MS) (*a*) and the nucleus basilis magnocellularis (NBM) (*b*) after receiving different doses and durations of estrogen treatment. Estrogen was administered every other day for a period of 1, 2, or 4 weeks. Bars represent percent change from the mean of the ovariectomized controls. Note the increased numbers of ChAT-IR cells detected in the MS and NBM after treating for 1 or 2 weeks with low physiological doses of E_2. In contrast, increased numbers of ChAT-IR cells were not detected after treating with higher doses of E_2, or after treating with lower doses of E_2 for a longer period of time. *$P<0.05$ relative to non-estrogen-treated controls. (Adapted from Gibbs, 1997.)

the morning of diestrus 1, approximately 36 hours following peak levels of circulating estradiol. In a companion study, peak levels of ChAT mRNA were detected in the MS of ovariectomized rats sacrificed 24 hours following a single injection of 17–ß-E_2 (see Fig. 9.2a). These data suggest that changes in circulating estrogens are responsible for normal physiological fluctuations in ChAT mRNA in the MS, and that there is a delay of approximately 24 hours between peak levels of circulating estradiol and peak levels of ChAT mRNA. Similar effects were observed in the NBM where peak levels of ChAT mRNA were detected 72 hours following the administration of 17–ß- E_2 (see Fig. 9.2b). Notably, progesterone was found to enhance the effects of estrogen by decreasing the time to achieve peak levels of ChAT mRNA in the NBM, and by prolonging the effects of estrogen on ChAT mRNA in the MS (see Fig. 9.2b). Collectively, these data suggest that both estrogen and progesterone play a role in the normal physiological regulation of basal forebrain cholinergic neurons. The data are consistent with the idea that estrogen replacement can enhance the functional status of cholinergic projections to the hippocampus and cortex.

Estrogen replacement and acetylcholine release

To determine whether the effects of estrogen replacement on ChAT and HACU reflect changes in cholinergic activity, we examined whether short-term treatment with 17–ß-E_2 produces changes in basal or evoked acetylcholine release in the hippocampus and overlying cortex. Ovariectomized animals received continuous estrogen replacement for 10 to 11 days to correspond with conditions producing elevated levels of ChAT mRNA and protein in the MS and NBM. Basal and potassium-evoked acetylcholine release in the hippocampus and overlying cortex were then measured using in vivo microdialysis and HPLC and compared with corresponding values from ovariectomized, non-estrogen-treated controls. No significant effects of 17–ß-E_2 on basal acetylcholine release were detected. Significantly greater potassium-evoked release, however, was detected in the estrogen-treated animals (see Table 9.1). It was detected particularly after a longer period of potassium-stimulated release (see Fig. 9.4).

These results suggest that estrogen replacement may enable the neurons to maintain elevated levels of acetylcholine release during periods of increased activation while, at the same time, having relatively little impact on basal cholinergic tone. This interpretation is consistent with the increases in ChAT and HACU, detected following short-term estrogen replacement, since increases in ChAT and HACU would help to maintain elevated levels of acetylcholine available for release. Ordinarily, the effects of estrogen on ChAT and HACU may have little impact on cholinergic function and cognitive processes in a young healthy brain. These effects may be of greater significance, however, in AD where the number of cholinergic

Table 9.1. Effects of estrogen replacement on baseline and potassium-stimulated acetylcholine release in the hippocampus and overlying cortex

	Ovx + NoE	Ovx + E
Average basal	6.2 ± 0.6	5.0 ± 0.7
Average stimulated	12.2 ± 1.3	11.9 ± 1.7
Average % change	97.5 ± 12.6	137.8 ± 12.6 *

Ovariectomized animals received capsules containing 17-ß-E$_2$ or sham surgery 10 days prior to in vivo microdialysis. Values indicate average acetylcholine release (pmol/sample) during a stable 60 min baseline period and during a 90 min period of potassium-stimulated release. Average percent change reflects the mean of the percent change in release calculated for each animal. $N=7$ animals/group. *$P=0.04$ relative to the non-estrogen-treated controls.

cells are substantially reduced and physiological demands on remaining cells are correspondingly increased.

Estrogen replacement and learning and memory

Other ways of assessing the biological significance of estrogen-mediated effects on basal forebrain cholinergic neurons are by correlating estrogen effects on behavior with changes in cholinergic parameters, and by examining the effects of estrogen replacement on behaviors known to be sensitive to cholinergic manipulations. Singh et al. (1994) recently examined the effects of ovariectomy and estrogen replacement on active avoidance behavior along with effects on ChAT activity and HACU. In this study, animals were ovariectomized and then 3 weeks later began receiving continuous 17–ß-E$_2$ replacement for either 2 weeks or 28 weeks. These animals were then compared with intact as well as ovariectomized non-E-treated controls. Results of this study demonstrated a significant estrogen-mediated enhancement of active avoidance behavior after both 2 weeks and 28 weeks of treatment. The results also demonstrated significant decreases in HACU in the frontal cortex and hippocampus at 5 weeks following ovariectomy. These decreases were reversed by 2 weeks of estrogen treatment. There was also a significant increase in ChAT activity in the frontal cortex following 28 weeks (but not 2 weeks) of estrogen treatment. These results demonstrate significant increases in cholinergic parameters, as well as a significant enhancement of active avoidance learning associated with estrogen treatment.

In other studies, Luine and co-workers have demonstrated that low levels of estrogen replacement significantly improve radial arm maze performance in female rats, particularly when delays are introduced to increase the difficulty of the task. Radial arm maze performance is a sensitive measure of spatial working memory in

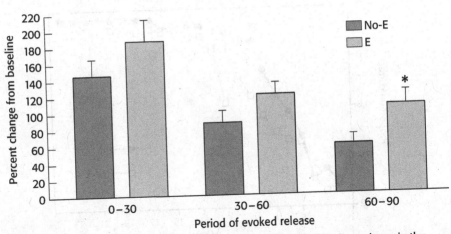

Figure 9.4.   Effects of estrogen replacement on potassium-stimulated acetylcholine release in the hippocampus and overlying cortex. Ovariectomized animals received either estrogen (subcutaneous capsules containing 17-ß-E$_2$) or empty capsules 10 days prior to measuring ACh release by in vivo microdialysis. Bars represent the average percent change from baseline during three successive 30 minute periods of potassium-stimulated release. Note that the increase in release produced by elevated potassium is greater for the estrogen-treated animals compared with the non-estrogen-treated controls, particularly during the last 30 minutes of stimulated release. *$P < 0.05$ relative to non-estrogen-treated animals. (Adapted from Gibbs et al., 1997.)

rats and has been shown in numerous studies to be sensitive to manipulations of basal forebrain cholinergic projections. Interestingly, higher levels of estrogen replacement produced an enhancement of radial arm maze performance in males, but not in females (Luine & Rodriguez, 1994), suggesting that the effects of estrogen on this task are both dose and sex specific. Daniel et al. (1998) likewise demonstrated that low levels of estrogen replacement significantly enhance acquisition of an 8-arm radial maze by ovariectomized female rats. Notably, in this study estrogen replacement was just as effective when administered for 30 days prior to training as when administered throughout training, suggesting that estrogen can induce neural changes and behavioral effects beyond the period of treatment. Estradiol replacement has also been shown to increase the number of correct reinforced alternations in a T-maze, which is another task used to test spatial working memory in rats (Fader et al., 1998).

Since rats have a natural tendency to alternate, it is possible that the enhancement of radial arm maze acquisition and alternation in a T-maze reflect an increase in the tendency to alternate as opposed to an increase in spatial memory per se. Recently, we examined the effects of estrogen replacement on acquisition of a

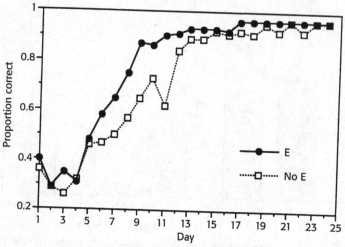

Figure 9.5. Learning curves showing the rate of acquisition of a delayed matching-to-position T-maze task for estrogen-treated and non-estrogen-treated animals. Animals received eight trial pairs/day. Data points indicate the proportion of correct responses on each day of testing. Note that, after the first 5 days of training, the estrogen-treated animals acquired the task at a faster rate than the non-estrogen-treated controls.

delayed matching-to-position task using a T-maze. The DMP task consists of trial pairs. On the first trial, an animal is forced to enter a particular arm of the T-maze to receive a food reward. On the second trial, the animal must choose between the two arms of the T-maze and is rewarded for entering the arm visited on the immediately preceding trial. Note that acquisition of this task requires animals to overcome their natural tendency to alternate as well as to remember which arm of the maze was entered on the immediately preceding trial. Animals received eight trial pairs each day and were trained to a criterion of 15 out of 16 correct choices on two consecutive days. Results indicate that ovariectomized, estrogen-treated animals required significantly fewer days to reach criterion than the ovariectomized, non-estrogen-treated controls (11.0 ± 1.1 vs. 15.0 ± 1.0; $P = 0.01$). Furthermore, inspection of the learning curves shows that performance of the estrogen-treated and non-estrogen-treated animals were nearly identical during the first 5 days of training and then diverged (see Fig. 9.5). This indicates an estrogen-mediated effect on the rate of acquisition as opposed to merely an estrogen-mediated effect on performance. Like the studies by Daniel et al. (1998), these results suggest that estrogen replacement enhances the animals' ability to acquire the spatial memory task.

Studies like those described above are useful for assessing the effects of estrogen replacement on the performance of specific well-characterized behavioral paradigms. Several investigators have also examined the ability for estrogen replacement to reduce behavioral deficits produced by the muscarinic receptor antagonist scopolamine, in order to examine the functional implications of estrogen-mediated effects on cholinergic neurons. In one study, Dohanich et al. (1994) reported that estrogen replacement significantly reduced the effects of systemic scopolamine administration on reinforced alternation in a T-maze. In this study, ovariectomized animals were first trained to alternate for a food reward between the arms of a T-maze. After reaching criterion, some animals received estrogen for 3 days, or a combination of estrogen for 3 days plus progesterone 4 to 6 hours before testing. Results showed that ovariectomized, untreated animals administered scopolamine (0.2 mg/kg) 15 minutes prior to testing failed to alternate for food reward above chance levels. In contrast, hormone-treated animals administered scopolamine prior to testing alternated successfully.

In a subsequent study, Fader et al. (1998) demonstrated that estrogen replacement could also mitigate the effects of scopolamine administered directly into the hippocampus. In this study, intrahippocampal scopolamine was shown to reduce T-maze alternation to chance levels in ovariectomized, non-estrogen-treated animals, but did not affect alternation in the estrogen-treated animals. Intracortical administration of scopolamine had no effect on alternation in either estrogen-treated or non-estrogen-treated animals, suggesting that estrogen specifically attenuated the effects of cholinergic inhibition in the hippocampus.

Using similar techniques, we have recently examined the ability of estrogen replacement to attenuate deficits in the acquisition and retention of inhibitory avoidance behavior produced by systemic administration of scopolamine (Gibbs et al., 1998). In this study, ovariectomized animals received either continuous 17–ß-E_2 replacement or vehicle for 10 days and were then trained using a step-through multiple trial passive avoidance paradigm. Animals received either scopolamine (1 mg/kg) or vehicle 20 to 30 minutes prior to training. Animals were then trained to criterion and tested for retention one week later. Our studies indicate that estrogen replacement attenuated a small but significant scopolamine-induced impairment in passive avoidance acquisition, but did not attenuate a scopolamine-induced impairment of retention. Interestingly, estrogen replacement was not effective at attenuating the scopolamine-induced impairment in passive avoidance acquisition when circulating levels of estradiol were very high (>400 pg/ml) (Gibbs et al., 1998). This is reminiscent of the effects reported by Luine & Rodriguez (1994) in which low, but not high, levels of estradiol replacement enhanced the performance of female rats in a radial arm maze (Luine, 1997). Like the studies described above, this result is consistent with an ability of estrogen replacement to attenuate learning deficits associated with muscarinic cholinergic impairment.

Collectively, these studies demonstrate that estrogen replacement can significantly affect performance on a variety of spatial and non-spatial learning and memory tasks, and that estrogen can mitigate behavioral impairments associated with systemic, as well as intrahippocampal, cholinergic inhibition. These findings combined with the data showing estrogen-mediated effects on ChAT activity, HACU, and potassium-evoked acetylcholine release continue to support the idea that one mechanism by which estrogen can influence cognitive processes is by influencing the functional status of cholinergic projections emanating from the basal forebrain.

Mechanisms of estrogen effects on cholinergic neurons

How estrogen affects basal forebrain cholinergic neurons and whether the effects are direct or indirect are still largely unclear. Studies suggest that cholinergic neurons in the MS, DBB, and NBM contain high affinity estrogen binding sites (Toran-Allerand et al., 1992) and estrogen receptor-like immunoreactivity (Gibbs, 1996a), suggesting that estrogen may directly influence the cholinergic neurons via binding to intracellular receptors followed by direct, steroid-mediated effects on gene transcription. Honjo et al. (1992) reported evidence of a trophic effect of estrogen on embryonic cholinergic neurons transplanted to the anterior chamber of the eye, which would be consistent with a direct trophic effect of estrogen on the developing cholinergic neurons. The possibility, however, that estrogen influences basal forebrain cholinergic neurons indirectly must also be considered.

Effects on growth factors and growth factor receptors

Several studies have investigated the possibility that estrogen influences basal forebrain cholinergic neurons by affecting growth factors and growth factor receptors. Nerve growth factor (NGF) is a target-derived polypeptide growth factor which is produced in the hippocampus and cortex, and which has been shown to support the survival and function of basal forebrain cholinergic neurons (Varon & Conner, 1994). Intraventricular infusions of NGF have been shown to increase ChAT mRNA and protein in the MS and NBM (Cavicchioli, 1991; Dekker & Maloney, 1992; Fusco et al., 1989), to maintain ChAT and p75^{NTR} (neurotrophin receptor)-expressing cells in the MS following injury (Hefti, 1986; Kromer, 1987; Williams et al., 1986), and to increase ACh release and HACU in the hippocampus and cortex (Araujo et al., 1993; Rylett et al., 1993).

Effects of NGF are mediated by binding to two cell-surface receptors referred to as p75^{NTR} and TrkA. P75^{NTR} binds NGF and other related neurotrophins and is a member of a family of receptors, including fas and TNFR1, that mediate cellular differentiation and apoptosis (Chao, 1994). TrkA is a protein tyrosine kinase receptor that is an essential component of functional, high affinity NGF binding sites (Barbacid et al., 1991; Chao & Hempstead, 1995). Studies have shown that the binding of NGF to TrkA, the activation of the receptor tyrosine kinase, and the autophosphorylation of the receptor are essential for mediating biological effects of NGF (for review see Segal & Greenberg, 1996). The role of the $p75^{NTR}$ receptor in mediating biological effects of NGF is more controversial. Several studies have demonstrated significant effects of $p75^{NTR}$ receptor expression on the sensitivity and specificity of NGF effects in some cells (Benedetti et al., 1993; Chao & Hempstead, 1995; Davies et al., 1993; Hantzopoulos, 1994; Lee, K-F. et al., 1994; Verdi et al., 1994). The $p75^{NTR}$ receptor has also been implicated in the regulation of cell death, and it is reportedly involved in the brain-derived neurotrophic factor (BDNF)-induced cell death of developing sympathetic neurons (Bamji et al., 1998), as well as in the ischemia-induced death of hippocampal CA1 pyramidal cells (Lee et al., 1994).

Ross et al. (1998) recently reported evidence for a model in which, in the absence of ligand, the $p75^{NTR}$ and TrkA receptors exist as a heteroreceptor complex that binds NGF with high affinity and prevents the autophosphorylation of TrkA and other receptor mediated effects. According to their model, the binding of NGF to the heteroreceptor complex causes the complex to undergo a conformational change and/or dissociate. This enables the formation of $p75^{NTR}$ and TrkA homoreceptor complexes, which then produce receptor-mediated effects. This model can explain how NGF normally does not induce apoptosis via $p75^{NTR}$ unless cells are lacking TrkA, or unless $p75^{NTR}$ homodimers are favored (e.g. via an increased ratio of $p75^{NTR}$/TrkA). The model can also explain why, in the absence of NGF, cells expressing both $p75^{NTR}$ and TrkA do not exhibit high levels of TrkA autophosphorylation, a phenomenon that is known to occur in the absence of ligand with TrkA homodimers. According to this model, effects of NGF on a given cell would then be a function of the proportion of $p75^{NTR}$ and TrkA homoreceptor complexes that are formed in response to binding with NGF and other neurotrophins, which in turn would be related to the relative proportion of $p75^{NTR}$ and TrkA molecules and to the number of receptors bound to the different neurotrophins. Consequently, changes in the relative levels of $p75^{NTR}$ and TrkA, as well as changes in neurotrophin expression, may have a significant effect on NGF responsive cells.

Studies indicate that most (>90%) of the cholinergic cells detected in the MS and NBM contain both $p75^{NTR}$ and TrkA receptors, and that nearly all $p75^{NTR}$ and TrkA expressing cells in the MS and NBM are cholinergic (Dawbarn et al., 1988; Gibbs & Pfaff, 1994; Sobreviela et al., 1994). Several studies have demonstrated that continuous treatment with relatively high levels of estradiol for 2 or more weeks results in significant decreases in $p75^{NTR}$ mRNA and protein in the MS (Gibbs, 1997; Gibbs & Pfaff, 1992). Like the effect on ChAT-like immunoreactive (IR) cells, changes in the number of $p75^{NTR}$-IR cells appear to be dose and time dependent with greater decreases observed with higher doses and longer periods of treatment (Gibbs, 1997) (see Fig. 9.6). Notably, estrogen has also been reported to produce a decrease in $p75^{NTR}$ expression in dorsal root ganglion (DRG) neurons (Sohrabji et

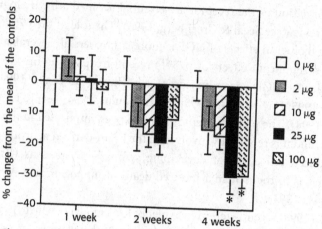

Figure 9.6. Changes in the number of p75^{NTR}-like immunoreactive (IR) cells detected in the medial septum (MS) after receiving different doses and durations of estrogen treatment. Estrogen was administered every other day for a period of 1, 2, or 4 weeks. Bars represent percent change from the mean of the ovariectomized controls. Note the decreased numbers of p75^{NTR}-IR cells detected in the MS after treating for 4 weeks with the higher doses of E$_2$. *$P < 0.05$ relative to non-estrogen-treated controls. (Adapted from Gibbs, 1997.)

al., 1994), suggesting that estrogen effects on p75^{NTR} expression are not limited to the basal forebrain.

Evidence for estrogen regulation of trkA mRNA expression has also been reported. McMillan et al. (1996) recently reported an increase in relative levels of trkA mRNA in the horizontal limb of the diagonal band and the NBM following short-term estrogen replacement. Sohrabji et al. (1994) have likewise reported an increase in trkA mRNA in DRG neurons following estrogen replacement. More recently we have examined changes in the levels of trkA mRNA in the MS and NBM across the estrous cycle, and in response to acute as well as continuous hormone replacement (Gibbs, 1998b; Gibbs et al., 1994). Significant fluctuations in trkA mRNA were detected in the MS across the estrous cycle (see Fig. 9.7a). The fluctuations corresponded with increases in trkA mRNA detected in the MS following acute treatment with estrogen or estrogen plus progesterone (see Fig. 9.8b). As with the changes in ChAT mRNA described above, a significant increase in trkA mRNA was detected in the MS 24 hours after estrogen administration and persisted in response to treatment with estrogen followed by progesterone (see Fig. 9.7b). In contrast, a separate study showed that longer-term continuous treatment with estradiol resulted in significant decreases in trkA mRNA in the MS (see Fig. 9.7c). This was comparable to the decreases in p75^{NTR} previously described (Gibbs et al., 1994).

Collectively, these studies demonstrate that estrogen replacement can have a

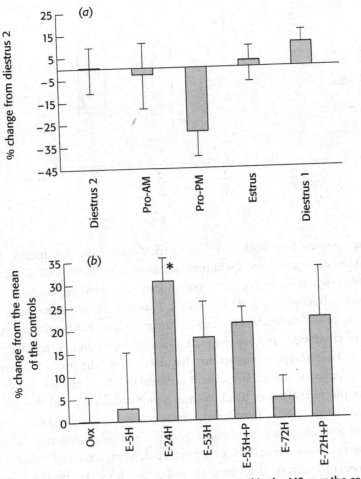

Figure 9.7.   Changes in relative levels of trkA mRNA detected in the MS over the course of the estrus cycle (a) and in response to treatment with estrogen or estrogen plus progesterone (b and c). Bars in (a) represent percent change relative to diestrus 2. Bars in (b) and (c) represent percent change relative to ovariectomized, non-E-treated controls. Panel (a) shows significant fluctuation in the levels of trkA mRNA detected in the medial septum (MS) over the course of the estrous cycle, with peak levels detected on the morning of diestrus 1, approximately 36 hours after peak levels of circulating estrogen. Panel (b) shows that, in ovariectomized animals, a significant increase in trkA mRNA was detected in the MS 24 h (but not 5 h) after a single injection of 17-ß-E$_2$, demonstrating a delay between peak levels of circulating estrogen and the subsequent increase in trkA mRNA consistent with the fluctuation observed during the estrous cycle. Note also that the increase in trkA mRNA was partially maintained for up to 72 h following a subsequent injection of progesterone. Panel (c) (overleaf) shows that, in contrast to the increase in trkA mRNA observed following acute estrogen administration, continuous estrogen replacement for 1 or 2 weeks resulted in significant decreases in trkA mRNA in the MS. *$P < 0.05$ relative to ovariectomized controls. (Adapted from Gibbs, 1998b; Gibbs et al., 1994.)

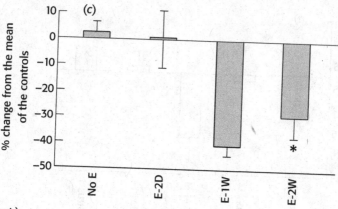

Figure 9.7 (cont.)

significant impact on both p75^{NTR} and trkA expression. Specifically, acute and short-term estrogen replacement produce an increase in trkA mRNA in the basal forebrain, whereas longer-term continuous estrogen replacement produces decreases in both p75^{NTR} and trkA mRNA. This suggests that estrogen has multiple effects on basal forebrain cholinergic neurons that may influence the functional status of cholinergic projections to the hippocampus and cortex. Based on the model of NGF receptor interactions discussed above, the initial increase in trkA mRNA expression and the subsequent decrease in p75^{NTR} expression may serve to increase the formation of TrkA homoreceptor complexes and thereby increase TrkA-mediated effects. Conversely, the decrease in trkA mRNA expression observed following more prolonged estrogen administration may subsequently decrease the formation of TrkA homoreceptor complexes and thereby decrease TrkA-mediated effects. This may be mitigated, however, by the concomitant decrease in p75^{NTR}. It is interesting to note that the increase in trkA mRNA following acute hormone replacement corresponds with the increases in ChAT mRNA and protein detected in the MS and NBM, and that the decreases in trkA mRNA and p75^{NTR} correspond with the return of ChAT-IR to control levels following prolonged estrogen administration (Gibbs, 1997; Gibbs & Pfaff, 1992).

Evidence for estrogen-mediated effects on neurotrophin expression have also been described, but are somewhat less consistent. Singh and co-workers (1993) recently reported a decrease in NGF mRNA in the rat frontal cortex and hippocampus. In contrast, Gibbs et al. (1994) reported a significant decrease in hippocampal levels of NGF mRNA following 1 to 2 weeks of continuous 17–ß-E$_2$ administration, comparable to the effects on p75^{NTR} and trkA mRNA. Singh et al. (1995) have also reported a decrease in BDNF mRNA in the frontal and temporal cortex and hippocampus following ovariectomy, and an increase in BDNF mRNA in the dentate gyrus, CA3, and CA4 regions of the hippocampus following long-term (25 weeks) estrogen replacement.

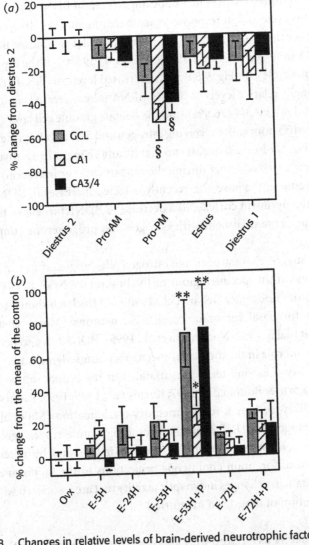

Figure 9.8. Changes in relative levels of brain-derived neurotrophic factor (BDNF) mRNA detected in three regions of the hippocampus over the course of the estrus cycle (*a*) and in response to treatment with estrogen or estrogen plus progesterone (*b*). Bars in (*a*) represent percent change relative to diestrus 2. Bars in (*b*) and (*c*) represent percent change relative to ovariectomized, non-estrogen-treated controls. (*a*) Note the significant fluctuation in the levels of BDNF mRNA detected in regions CA1 and CA3/4 over the course of the estrus cycle with peak levels detected on diestrus 2, approximately 60 hours after peak levels of circulating estrogen. (*b*) Note the significant increase in BDNF mRNA detected in all three regions of the hippocampus in animals sacrificed 53 hours after receiving E_2 and 5 hours after receiving progesterone. §$P<0.05$ relative to the mean at diestrus 2. *$P<0.05$ relative to ovariectomized controls. **$P<0.01$ relative to ovariectomized controls. GCL = granule cell layer of the dentate gyrus. CA1 – CA1 pyramidal cell layer of the hippocampus. CA3/4 – CA3/4 pyramidal cell layer of the hippocampus. (Adapted from Gibbs, 1998b.)

Recently, we examined changes in hippocampal levels of BDNF and NGF mRNA across the estrous cycle and in response to acute treatment with estrogen or estrogen plus progesterone (Gibbs, 1998). The results revealed significant fluctuations in BDNF mRNA in regions CA1 (51.7%) and CA3/4 (39.7%) of the hippocampus across the estrous cycle (see Fig. 9.8a) with decreased levels on the afternoon proestrus. Surprisingly, relative levels of BDNF mRNA were increased significantly in regions CA1 (28.1%), CA3/4 (76.9%), and the dentate granule cell layer (73.4%) of animals sacrificed 53 hours after receiving estrogen and 5 hours after receiving progesterone (see Fig. 9.8b). In contrast, no significant changes in relative levels of NGF mRNA were detected either during the estrous cycle or in response to acute hormone replacement. We have also recently detected increases in BDNF mRNA and protein in the pyriform cortex and a decrease in BDNF protein in the hippocampus following acute treatment with estrogen and progesterone (unpublished observations).

These studies suggest that estrogen and estrogen plus progesterone can influence BDNF expression within specific regions of the brain. Like NGF, BDNF binds to the $p75^{NTR}$ receptor (Rodriguez-Tebar et al., 1990) and has been shown to provide trophic support for basal forebrain cholinergic neurons (Morse et al., 1993; Nonomura & Hatanaka, 1992; Nonomura et al., 1995). BDNF has also been shown to play an important role in the molecular mechanisms underlying activity-dependent neuroplasticity (i.e. long-term potentiation) in the hippocampus (Kang & Schuman, 1995; Korte & Bonhoeffer, 1997; Korte et al., 1995, 1996; Patterson et al., 1996), and may likewise have a role in memory consolidation (Ma et al., 1998). Consequently, changes in BDNF expression resulting from estrogen replacement may help to enhance learning and memory processes in two ways: by increasing the functionality of basal forebrain cholinergic projections to the hippocampus and cortex, and by enhancing changes in synaptic activity that are associated with learning and the formation of long-term memories.

Changes in cholinergic parameters associated with long-term loss of ovarian function

The studies described above demonstrate that estrogen influences basal forebrain cholinergic neurons under normal physiological conditions, and that short-term estrogen replacement can produce increases in cholinergic parameters, enhance spatial memory ability, and mitigate behavioral impairments associated with cholinergic inhibition. Fewer studies have examined the effects that the long-term loss of ovarian function has on brain aging and the ability for estrogen replacement to enhance cholinergic function and cognition in aged animals.

Singer et al. (1998) recently reported that short-term estrogen replacement (100 μg E_2 every other day for 1 week) produced a modest but significant increase in both ChAT and trkA mRNA in the NBM of aged (24 month old) ovariectomized

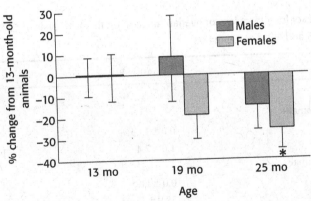

Figure 9.9.   Effect of aging on relative levels of trkA mRNA detected in the medial septum (MS) of gonadally intact males and females. Bars represent percent change from the corresponding 13-month-old animals. Note the significant decrease in trkA mRNA in the MS of females, but not males, between 13 and 25 months of age. *$P<0.05$ relative to 13-month-old animals of the same sex. (Adapted from Gibbs, 1998a.)

rats and corresponding young adult rats. In this study, animals were ovariecto-mized one week prior to treatment. A similar increase in ChAT (but not trkA) mRNA was also detected in the horizontal limb of the diagonal band. This suggests that estrogen can up-regulate both ChAT and trkA mRNA in aged animals when administered shortly following ovariectomy.

Recently we completed a study in which the effects of aging on cholinergic neurons were compared between male and female rats, and between ovariecto-mized animals and age-matched, gonadally intact controls (Gibbs et al., 1998). The goal was to determine whether the loss of ovarian function contributes to a loss and/or impairment of basal forebrain cholinergic neurons beyond the effects of normal aging. In the first part of the study, male and female rats were sacrificed at 13, 19, and 25 months of age and compared. Parameters which were measured included the number and size of ChAT-IR profiles and relative levels of ChAT and trkA mRNA in the MS and NBM. In the second part of the study, 16- and 19-month-old animals were sacrificed 3 and 6 months following ovariectomy and compared with age-matched, gonadally intact controls.

The results revealed no significant change in the number or size of ChAT-IR profiles in the MS or NBM between 13 to 25 months of age or in response to ova-riectomy. This suggests that neither sex nor ovarian status directly affect the number or size of cholinergic neurons in the MS and NBM as a function of age. A significant decrease in relative levels of trkA mRNA was detected, however, in the MS of gonadally intact females between 13 to 25 months of age, but not in males (see Fig. 9.9). In addition, significant decreases in the levels of ChAT and trkA

Table 9.2. Effects of long-term loss of ovarian function on Relative levels of ChAT and trkA mRNA in the MS and NBM of aging rats

	ChAT mRNA	trkA mRNA
Medial septum		
16-month-old animals:		
Controls	0.0 ± 13.3	0.0 ± 12.8
Ovx – 3 Mo	-1.0 ± 7.4	-11.3 ± 12.0
19-month-old animals:		
Controls	0.0 ± 11.5	0.0 ± 14.3
Ovx – 6 Mo	$-38.9 \pm 12.9†$	$-34.0 \pm 9.4†$
Ovx – 6 Mo + E	-15.1 ± 7.9	$-37.6 \pm 14.3†$
Nucleus basalis		
16-month-old animals:		
Controls	0.0 ± 4.1	0.0 ± 8.8
Ovx – 3 Mo	-11.9 ± 7.2	-4.1 ± 14.5
19-month-old animals:		
Controls	0.0 ± 11.1	0.0 ± 6.3
Ovx – 6 Mo	$-33.5 \pm 3.5†$	$-32.3 \pm 7.9†$
Ovx – 6 Mo + E	$-37.5 \pm 6.1†$	-24.2 ± 15.3

Animals received either ovariectomy or sham surgery at 13 months of age. E-treated animals were estrogen-free for 6 months and then received 17-ß-E_2 for 3 days prior to sacrifice. Values represent percent change from the mean of the age-matched, gonadally intact controls. †$P<0.05$ relative to age-matched, gonadally intact controls.

mRNA were detected in the MS and NBM of animals sacrificed 6 months, but not 3 months, following ovariectomy (see Table 9.2). This suggests that females may be more apt to experience a decline in TrkA receptors in the MS with age than males, and that the long-term loss of ovarian function results in decreased levels of both ChAT and trkA mRNA in the MS and NBM beyond the effects of normal aging. Short-term (3 days) treatment with 17–ß-E_2 partially restored levels of ChAT mRNA in the MS and trkA mRNA in the NBM, but not to the extent predicted by the effects of estrogen replacement in young adults. One possibility is that the effectiveness of acute estrogen replacement is diminished following the long-term loss of ovarian function. These findings suggest that ovarian hormones play a role in maintaining normal levels of ChAT and trkA expression in the MS and NBM, and that long-term hormone deprivation combined with aging produces significant decreases in both ChAT and trkA expression which, in turn, may adversely affect basal forebrain cholinergic projections.

Summary of effects of estrogen on basal forebrain cholinergic neurons

Studies to date have demonstrated that estrogen significantly affects basal forebrain cholinergic neurons projecting to the hippocampus and cortex. Collectively, these studies have demonstrated that physiological levels of estrogen influence the expression of growth factors and growth factor receptors, produce changes in cholinergic parameters, and influence behavior in ways that are consistent with the ability of estrogen to enhance the functional status of basal forebrain cholinergic projections. In addition, there is evidence that the long-term loss of ovarian function has negative effects on basal forebrain cholinergic neurons that go beyond the effects of normal aging. Whether these effects occur in humans still needs to be determined. Notably, many of the processes affected by estrogen are processes adversely affected by AD. For example, AD is associated with decreases in ChAT (Perry et al., 1977, 1978; Whitehouse et al., 1982) and trkA (Mufson et al., 1996, 1997), decreases in HACU (Rylett et al., 1983; Sims et al., 1983), and decreases in BDNF mRNA (Phillips et al., 1991). One possibility is that decreases in TrkA receptors lead to a reduction in trophic support for the cholinergic neurons, making them more susceptible to the effects of injury and disease. This would suggest that the decreases in cholinergic function, as well as the cholinergic cell loss, that are associated with AD may be exacerbated by decreases in TrkA. In rats, estrogen replacement increases trkA mRNA, ChAT, HACU, and BDNF mRNA. We hypothesize that similar effects in humans would help to maintain cholinergic projections to the hippocampus and cortex and thereby help to reduce the risk and severity of AD-related dementia in women.

Other effects of estrogen

While the focus of this review has been to summarize the effects of estrogen on basal forebrain cholinergic neurons and related learning and memory function, it must be emphasized that the effects of estrogen on cholinergic neurons are but one mechanism by which estrogen can affect the aging brain, and that other effects of estrogen have been reported that may contribute significantly to effects on aging and AD-related cognitive decline.

Other effects of estrogen recently reported include effects on other neurotransmitter systems (Fink et al., 1996; Luine et al., 1997; McDermott et al., 1994b; Shimizu & Bray, 1993; Wilson, 1996), neuroprotective effects of estrogen and estrogen-related compounds (Alkayed et al., 1998; Behl et al., 1997; Green et al., 1997a, 1997b; Shi et al., 1997; Simpkins et al., 1997), alterations in ß-amyloid and lipoprotein metabolism (Applebaum-Bowden et al., 1989; Jaffe et al., 1994; Kushwaha et al., 1991; Muesing et al., 1992; Xu et al., 1998), increased cerebral blood flow

(Belfort et al., 1995; Ohkura et al., 1995b), anti-inflammatory effects (Bauer et al., 1992), antioxidant effects (Mooradian, 1993; Niki & Nakano, 1990), and effects on hippocampal connectivity (Gould et al., 1990; McEwen, 1996; Woolley & McEwen, 1992) and lesion-induced plasticity (Morse et al., 1986; Stone et al., 1998). Some of these effects are discussed below.

Effects on other neurotransmitter systems

In addition to affecting basal forebrain cholinergic neurons, estrogen affects a variety of other neurotransmitter systems including dopamine (Dluzen et al., 1996; Lindamer et al., 1997; McDermott et al., 1997, McDermott et al., 1994a, 1994b; Shimizu & Bray, 1993), serotonin (Fink et al., 1996; Maswood et al., 1995; Pecins-Thompson et al., 1996; Shimizu & Bray, 1993), norepinephrine (Shimizu & Bray, 1993), glutamate (Carbone et al., 1995; Luine et al., 1997; Thind & Goldsmith, 1997), and gamma aminobutyric acid (GABA; Herbison, 1997; Wilson, 1996), any of which may influence the effects of estrogen on brain aging and cognitive decline. Serotonin in particular plays an important role in the etiology of depression and mood disorders. Given that the incidence of depression and mood disorders in aging women is much higher than in aging men, there is considerable interest in the possibility that estrogen replacement may help to reduce the risk of depression in late life by increasing the functionality of serotoninergic systems (see Chapter 5). Such an effect could in turn improve cognition secondarily to improvements in mood.

Evidence for estrogen effects on GABAergic neurons, GABA turnover, glutamic acid decarboxylase (GAD) mRNA, and GABA receptors has also been reported (Canonaco et al., 1989; Grattan et al., 1996; Hamon et al., 1983; Luine et al., 1997; McCarthy et al., 1995; Perez et al., 1988). Recently we reported that estrogen replacement significantly reduced the amnestic effects of lorazepam, a benzodiazepine, on passive avoidance retention (Gibbs et al., 1998). Lorazepam, like other benzodiazepines, facilitates GABAergic effects by binding to the GABA–A receptor and enhancing GABA-mediated effects on chloride conductance. In our initial studies, ovariectomized animals received either estrogen replacement or vehicle for 10 days and were then trained using a multiple trial passive avoidance paradigm. Lorazepam (0.375 mg/kg, i.p.) or vehicle was administered 30 minutes prior to training, and animals were tested for retention one week later. Results from this study indicated that while lorazepam produced a significant deficit in passive avoidance retention in the ovariectomized non-estrogen-treated animals, lorazepam failed to significantly affect passive avoidance retention in the estrogen-treated animals (see Fig. 9.10). Subsequent studies confirmed this result and demonstrated that the effect was associated with estrogen treatment prior to and during training,

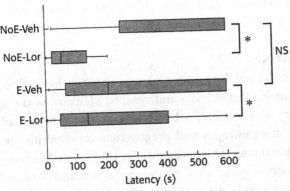

Figure 9.10. Box plots showing the effects of lorazepam on passive avoidance retention in ovariectomized estrogen-treated and non-estrogen-treated animals. Decreased latency reflects poorer retention. Note that lorazepam significantly impaired passive avoidance retention in the non-estrogen-treated animals, but did not significantly impair retention in the estrogen-treated animals, suggesting that the estrogen treatment counteracted the memory impairing effects of the benzodiazepine. (Adapted from Gibbs et al., 1998.)

but not during retention testing, and the effect was not due to an effect of estrogen on lorazepam kinetics.

One possible explanation is that estrogen may reduce the effects of the benzodiazepine on the GABA–A receptor. Bitran and Dowd (1996) have reported that treatment with estradiol prevented a stress-induced potentiation of flunitrazepam binding in cortical and cerebellar membranes, suggesting that estrogen replacement may reduce benzodiazepine effects following stress. This is consistent with a report by Nomikos and Spyraki (1988) that short-term estradiol replacement abolished the anxiolytic effect of diazepam as measured with an elevated plus maze. Hence estrogen may attenuate the effects of lorazepam on passive avoidance retention by preventing a stress-induced increase in lorazepam binding to the GABA–A receptor complex.

Another possibility is that estrogen may reduce GABAergic transmission via effects on GAD mRNA and GABA release. Murphy et al. (1998) have demonstrated a significant decrease in the expression of GAD by aspiny inhibitory interneurons in the hippocampus following acute estrogen replacement in vitro. The estrogen-mediated decrease in GAD was correlated with a reduction in the size and frequency of GABAergic miniature inhibitory post synaptic currents (IPSCs) and an increase in the frequency of miniature excitatory post synaptic currents (EPSCs). Furthermore, these effects were correlated with an increase in dendritic spine density on hippocampal neurons, an effect that was also observed after pharmacologically blocking GABA synthesis. These findings suggest that an estrogen-mediated decrease in GABAergic activity results in an increase in excitatory potentials followed by an increase in dendritic spine density on hippocampal neurons.

Effects on hippocampal connectivity

Another mechanism by which estrogen replacement may help to prevent cognitive decline is by enhancing connectivity and synaptic plasticity in the aging brain. Studies by Woolley and co-workers have demonstrated a remarkable dynamic influence of circulating estrogen and progesterone on dendritic structure and synapse formation in the adult hippocampus. Specifically, studies have shown that the density of dendritic spines on CA1 pyramidal cells increases and decreases throughout the estrous cycle in accordance with fluctuating levels of estrogen and progesterone (Woolley et al., 1990), and that ovariectomy produces a decrease in dendritic spine density which can be prevented (Gould et al., 1990) or reversed (Woolley & McEwen, 1993) by treatment with estradiol. Studies have likewise demonstrated a significant estrogen-mediated increase in the number of axospinous synapses on hippocampal CA1 pyramidal cells (Woolley & McEwen, 1992) which is due primarily to an increase in the number of synaptic contacts formed by pre-existing synaptic boutons (Woolley et al., 1996).

More recent reports have demonstrated estrogen-mediated increases in N-methyl-D-aspartate (NMDA), but not AMPA, binding in stratum radiatum and oriens (Woolley & McEwen, 1993). Increases in NMDAR1 (glutamate receptor) expression (Gazzaley et al., 1996), and an increase in the sensitivity of CA1 pyramidal cells to NMDA receptor-mediated synaptic input (Woolley & McEwen, 1993) have also been reported, suggesting that the new synapses that are formed in response to estrogen treatment are functional and support an increase in excitatory NMDA responses. This is consistent with one recent report showing an enhancement of long term potentiation during the proestrus phase of the estrous cycle (Warren et al., 1995). As mentioned above, studies by Murphy et al. (1998) suggest that increased spine density in CA1 results from an estrogen-mediated decrease in GABA transmission by hippocampal interneurons and a corresponding decrease in GABA-mediated inhibition of CA1 pyramidal neurons. One possibility is that a decrease in GABA-mediated inhibition of CA1 pyramidal cells results in increased pyramidal cell activity and increased trophic activity (Isackson et al., 1991; Nibuya et al., 1995), which in turn facilitates the formation of additional dendritic spines and synapses.

Collectively, these studies suggest a model in which estrogen produces a decrease in GABA-mediated inhibition of CA1 pyramidal neurons in the hippocampus along with an increased number of dendritic spines, synapses, and NMDA receptors in region CA1, resulting in increased effects of glutamate at NMDA receptors and an increase in activity dependent synaptic plasticity. It is hypothesized that similar effects in humans could help to reduce synapse loss and enhance synaptic plasticity in the hippocampus and thereby help to reduce cognitive decline associated with aging and AD.

Effects on ß-amyloid processing

One of the pathological hallmarks of AD is the deposition in the brain of numerous ß-amyloid (Aß)-containing senile plaques (Selkoe, 1993). Aß is a 40–42 amino acid polypeptide produced by enzymatic cleavage of a ~700 amino acid precursor protein (ßAPP) (Haass & Selkoe, 1993). This precursor protein can undergo cleavage by a variety of proteolytic enzymes. Production of the Aß (amyloidogenic) peptide results from N-terminal cleavage of the ßAPP precursor protein by ß-secretase, followed by further cleavages by γ-secretases. Alternatively, ßAPP can be metabolized by an enzyme 'α-secretase' which cleaves ßAPP within its Aß region releasing a soluble (non-amyloidogenic) sßAPP and precluding the formation of Aß peptides. In vitro studies have demonstrated toxic effects of Aß on neurons in some (Gao et al., 1998; Lorenzo & Yankner, 1994; Malouf, 1992; Ueda et al., 1994; Zhang et al., 1994), but not all (Wujek et al., 1996), culture systems. Central administration of the synthetic amyloid peptides has also been shown to have neurotoxic effects (Giordano et al., 1994; Smyth et al., 1994), and to produce learning and memory deficits in mice. Some of these deficits are reversible by systemic administration of either the acetylcholinesterase inhibitor tacrine or the cholinergic agonist nicotine (Maurice et al., 1996), suggesting that cholinergic enhancement can ameliorate effects associated with Aß toxicity. These findings are consistent with the idea that Aß deposition contributes to the neurodegeneration and cognitive impairment characteristic of AD.

Recent evidence suggests that estrogen can influence ßAPP processing in vitro. Jaffe et al. (1994) initially reported that the treatment of cells containing high levels of estrogen receptor with estrogen resulted in the accumulation of soluble ßAPP in the medium. More recently, Xu et al. (1998) reported that estradiol (2–3 nM) increased the production of soluble ßAPP peptides and reduced the production of insoluble Aß peptides in neuroblastoma cells, as well as in rat, mouse, and human embryonic neocortical cultures. Effects were both dose- and time-dependent with maximal effects observed at a concentration of 200 nM administered for 7 to 10 days (but not 30 days). Conversely, estradiol had no effect on the levels of ßAPP mRNA or protein. These studies suggest that estrogen can decrease Aß production by altering metabolism of the ßAPP precursor protein to favor production of the non-amyloidogenic secreted form. Hence another mechanism by which estrogen may help to delay or prevent AD is by decreasing the production and accumulation of non-soluble Aß peptides in the brain.

Neuroprotective effects

Many studies have shown that estrogen can have neurotrophic or neuroprotective effects both in vivo and in vitro. Recent in vivo studies suggest that estrogen can help reduce mortality and protect against ischemic injury following middle cerebral artery (MCA) occlusion. In one study (Simpkins et al., 1997), ovariectomized rats received 17–ß-E_2 replacement or vehicle in conjunction with MCA occlusion. Estrogen replacement either prior to or shortly after occlusion significantly reduced mortality and significantly decreased the ischemic area of the brain as determined by H&E staining. Notably, similar effects were produced by 17-α-E_2 which is much less potent at the estrogen receptor, suggesting that classical estrogen receptors are not involved. Another recent study reported that gonadally intact female rats had a smaller infarct size and increased cerebral blood flow following MCA occlusion than either gonadally intact males or ovariectomized females (Alkayed et al., 1998).

Different mechanisms for the neuroprotective effects of estrogen have been proposed based on the effects of estrogen on cells in culture. Several recent studies suggest that estrogen can help to protect neurons by guarding them from the effects of lipid peroxidation. In one recent study, pretreatment of cultured hippocampal neurons with 0.1–10 μM 17–ß-E_2, estriol, or progesterone, significantly attenuated neurotoxic effects of glutamate, glucose deprivation, $FeSO_4$, and Aß peptides (Goodman et al., 1996). Treatment with estrogen and progesterone also significantly reduced lipid peroxidation produced by Aß and $FeSO_4$ in both neurons and isolated membranes, suggesting that some of the neuroprotective effects of estrogen were due to its ability to protect against oxidative damage. In another recent study, 17–ß-E_2 was shown to significantly attenuate the death of SK-N-SH cells produced by the Aß fragment Aß[25–35] (Gridley et al., 1997). As in the previous study, effects of Aß were correlated with an increase in lipid peroxidation which was significantly attenuated by treatment with 17–ß-E_2. Mattson et al. (1997) also recently demonstrated the ability of 17–ß-E_2 and estriol to protect PC12 cells expressing mutant presenilin-1 from apoptosis induced by Aß[25–35] and trophic factor withdrawal. These effects were correlated with the ability of 17–ß-E_2 to preserve mitochondrial function and reduce the formation of reactive oxygen species (i.e. oxidative stress).

As with the neuroprotective effects of estrogen observed in vivo, the effects observed in vitro are probably not mediated via binding to classical estrogen receptors. Studies by Behl et al. (1997) recently demonstrated that 17-ß-E_2, 17-α-E_2, and other structurally related compounds significantly enhanced survival and reduced intracellular peroxide accumulation in primary hippocampal and cortical cultures treated with H_2O_2, Aß[25–35], glutamate, and buthionine sulfoxide. Similar effects were observed in HT22 cells, a murine neuronal cell line which lacks functional estrogen receptors. The effects of estrogen and related compounds did not correlate with estrogenic potency at the estrogen receptor, but did correlate with the presence of an OH group at the C3 position on the A ring of the steroid molecule. These studies suggest that the ability of estrogen and related compounds to protect against oxidative damage is not mediated by a classical estrogen receptor-mediated mechanism.

Similar studies by Green and co-workers (1997a, b) have shown that 17–ß-E$_2$ protects SK-N-SH cells from the toxic effects of serum deprivation and that similar effects are produced by the less estrogenic compound, 17-α-E$_2$, as well as by non-estrogenic compounds with similar structures. These effects were only partially attenuated by the estrogen receptor antagonist tamoxifen, suggesting that classical estrogen receptors are not involved. In this case, the authors conclude that the neuroprotective effect of estrogen is related to the presence of a phenolic A ring along with at least three rings of the steroid nucleus and is not related to the estrogenic potency of the molecule. Green et al. (1998) subsequently showed that treatment of HT-22 cells with 17-ß-E$_2$, 17-α-E$_2$, or estratrien-3-ol resulted in a significant dose-dependent protection against the toxic effects of Aß peptide. Whether all of these effects are related to the antioxidant effects of estradiol and other phenolic A ring steroid compounds is still unclear. In the studies by Green and co-workers (1997a, b), the concentrations of estrogen and related compounds needed to produce neuroprotective effects were considerably lower than the concentrations needed to produce antioxidant effects, suggesting that another mechanism must also be involved. It is notable that several studies have demonstrated the ability of estrogen to protect neurons from the toxic effects of Aß in culture, and one study has reported the ability of estrogen to reduce toxic effects associated with the expression of mutant presenilin-1. Similar effects in vivo could help to reduce neuronal loss associated with Aß deposition and presenilin-1 expression in the aging brain, and may therefore be another mechanism by which estrogen can help to delay or prevent AD-related cognitive decline in postmenopausal women.

Summary and conclusions

Animal studies have demonstrated that estrogen influences CNS neurons in a multitude of ways that can affect brain function and cognition. Specifically, studies have demonstrated physiological effects of ovariectomy and estrogen replacement on cholinergic neurons in the MS and NBM, as well as estrogen-mediated increases in cholinergic parameters in the hippocampus and cortex. Estrogen has also been shown to attenuate behavioral impairments produced by cholinergic inhibition, and to enhance performance on spatial memory tasks and other tasks known to be sensitive to cholinergic manipulations. Based on these findings, we hypothesize that estrogen plays a role in the normal regulation and maintenance of basal forebrain cholinergic function, and that estrogen-mediated enhancement of basal forebrain cholinergic neurons can enhance certain cognitive processes that are adversely affected by cholinergic cell loss or cholinergic inhibition. Likewise, we suspect that similar effects in humans can help to reduce the risk and severity of AD-related dementia in postmenopausal women.

Estrogen may also influence brain function and cognition, including having an effect on other neurotransmitter systems such as serotonin and GABA, on growth factors and synapses in the hippocampus, and on ßAPP and lipoprotein metabolism. Estrogen may also have neuroprotective effects. Note that none of these effects is mutually exclusive, and the extent to which each of these contribute to the maintenance of normal brain function and cognition has yet to be determined. Even so, it is tempting to speculate that estrogen may have similar effects in the human brain, effects that collectively can help to maintain normal brain function and reduce the risk of cognitive decline.

In spite of the many recent studies that have examined the effects of ovariectomy and estrogen replacement on the brain, there is still little known about the long-term effects of estrogen deprivation on brain function and cognition, and about how best to prevent or ameliorate the negative effects of estrogen deprivation through the use of hormone replacement therapy. One of the emerging themes from the basic research is that the effects of estrogen on neurons and brain function are often very much dependent on the dose and duration of treatment, and that giving more estrogen for longer periods of time is not always more effective. This has been demonstrated in a variety of systems and for a variety of endpoints ranging from estrogen effects on ChAT and trkA expression (Gibbs, 1997; Gibbs, 1998b; Gibbs & Pfaff, 1992; Gibbs et al., 1994) and effects on spatial memory ability (Luine & Rodriguez, 1994; Luine, 1997) and inhibitory avoidance (Gibbs et al., 1998), as well as neuroprotective and neurotrophic effects in culture (Brinton et al., 1997; Xu et al., 1998) and neuroprotective effects in vivo (Sudo et al., 1997). In many of these studies, treatment with low levels of estrogen for short periods of time was more effective than treatment with higher doses for longer periods of time. Although it is not known whether similar effects occur in humans, the issue has relevance to the use of estrogen replacement in postmenopausal women and to the design of future clinical studies looking to assess the effectiveness of estrogen replacement therapy for the prevention and treatment of aging- and AD-related cognitive decline.

In conclusion, animal research continues to support the idea that estrogen replacement has beneficial effects on the brain that can help to maintain normal brain function and reduce the risk of aging- and AD-related cognitive decline. Many questions still need to be addressed, however, before the role of estrogen replacement in the prevention and treatment of cognitive decline in women becomes apparent. Does long-term estrogen deprivation cause neurons to be more vulnerable to the effects of aging and AD? Can long-term or short-term hormone replacement prevent adverse effects associated with long-term hormone deprivation and reduce the risk of aging- and AD-related cognitive decline? What dose and regimen of estrogen replacement is likely to be most beneficial for the aging brain and consequently, most effective for the prevention and treatment of AD-related cognitive decline? These are some of the questions that will help to shape future research focused on understanding the effects of hormone replacement on the aging brain.

ACKNOWLEDGMENT

This work was supported by NIH Grant RO1-NS28896, NIH Grant P50-AG05133, and NSF Grant IBN-9630851. Special thanks to Douglas Nelson, Denise Gillen-Caralli, Judith Balcita, and Jessica Check for their excellent technical assistance.

REFERENCES

Aigner, T. G. & Mishkin, M. (1986). The effects of physostigmine and scopolamine on recognition memory in monkeys. *Behavioral and Neural Biology*, 45, 81–7.

Aigner, T. G., Walker, D. L. & Mishkin, M. (1991). Comparison of the effects of scopolamine administered before and after acquisition in a test of visual recognition memory in monkeys. *Behavioral and Neural Biology*, 55(1), 61–7.

Alkayed, N. J., Harukuni, I., Kimes, A. S., London, E. D., Traystman, R. J. & Hurn, P. D. (1998). Gender-linked brain injury in experimental stroke. *Stroke*, 29, 159–66.

Altavista, M. C., Rossi, P., Bentivoglio, A. R., Crociani, P. & Albanese, A. (1990). Aging is associated with a diffuse impairment of forebrain cholinergic neurons. *Brain Research*, 508, 51–9.

Applebaum-Bowden, D., McLean, P. & Steinmetz, A. (1989) Lipoprotein, apolipoprotein, and lipolytic enzyme changes following estrogen administration in postmenopausal women. *Journal of Lipid Research*, 30, 1895–906.

Araujo, D. M., Lapchak, P. A. & Hefti, F. (1993). Effects of chronic basic fibroblast growth factor administration to rats with partial fimbrial transections on presynaptic cholinergic parameters and muscarinic receptors in the hippocampus: comparison with nerve growth factor. *Journal of Neurochemistry*, 61(3), 899–910.

Araujo, D. M., Lapchak, P. A., Meaney, M. J., Collier, B. & Quirion, R. (1990). Effects of aging on nicotinic and muscarinic autoreceptor function in the rat brain: relationship to presynaptic cholinergic markers and binding sites. *Journal of Neuroscience*, 10, 3069–78.

Baldereschi, M., DiCarlo, A., Lepore, V., Bracco, L. Maggi, S., Grigoletto, F., Scarlato, G. & Amaducci, L. (1998). Estrogen replacement therapy and Alzheimer's disease in the Italian longitudinal study on aging. *Neurology*, 50(4), 996–1002.

Bamji, S. X., Majdan, M., Pozniak, C. D., Belliveau, D. J., Aloyz, R., Kohn, J., Causing, C. G. & Miller, F. D. (1998). The P75 Neurotrophin receptor mediates neuronal apoptosis and is essential for naturally occurring sympathetic neuron death. *Journal of Cell Biology*, 140(4), 911–23.

Barbacid, M., Lamballe, F., Pulido, D. & Klein, R. (1991). The *trk* family of tyrosine kinase receptors. *Biochemica et Biophysiologica Acta*, **1072**, 115–27.

Barner, E. L. & Gray, S. L. (1998). Donepezil use in Alzheimer disease. *Annals of Pharmacotherapy*, **32**(1), 70–7.

Bartus, R. T. (1978). Short-term memory in the rhesus monkey: effects of dopamine blockade vs acute haloperidol administration. *Pharmacology, Biochemistry and Behavior*, **9**(3), 353–7.

Bartus, R. T. & Johnson, H. R. (1976). Short-term memory in the rhesus monkey: disruption from the anti-cholinergic scopolamine. *Pharmacology, Biochemistry and Behavior*, **5**(1), 39–46.

Bauer, J., Ganter, U., Strauss, S., Stadmuller, G., Frommberger, U., Bauer, H., Volk, B. & Berger, M. (1992). The participation of interleukin-6 in the pathogenesis of Alzheimer's disease. *Research in Immunology*, **143**, 650–7.

Behl, C., Skutella, T., Lezoualch, F., Post, A., Widmann, M., Newton, C. J. & Holsboer, F. (1997). Neuroprotection against oxidative stress by estrogens – structure–activity relationship. *Molecular Pharmacology*, **51**(4), 535–41.

Belfort, M. A., Saade, G. R., Snabes, M., Dunn, R., Moise, K. J. Jr., Cruz, A. & Young, R. (1995). Hormonal status affects the reactivity of the cerebral vasculature. *American Journal of Obstetrics and Gynecology*, **172**, 1273–8.

Benedetti, M., Levi, A. & Chao, M. V. (1993). Differential expression of nerve growth factor receptors leads to altered binding affinity and neurotrophin responsiveness. *Proceedings of the National Academy of Sciences*, USA, **90**, 7859–63.

Bitran, D. & Dowd, J. A. (1996). Ovarian steroids modify the behavioral and neurochemical responses of the central benzodiazepine receptor. *Psychopharmacology*, **125**(1), 65–73.

Brinton, R. D., Tran, J., Proffitt, P. & Montoya, M. (1997). 17 beta-estradiol enhances the outgrowth and survival of neocortical neurons in culture. *Neurochemical Research*, **22**(11), 1339–51.

Brown, T. J., Sharma, M., Heisler, L. E., Karsan, N., Walters, M. J. & MacLusky, N. J. (1995). *In vitro* labeling of gonadal steroid hormone receptors in brain tissue sections. *Steroids*, **60**, 726–37.

Canonaco, M., O'Connor, L. H., Pfaff, D. W. & McEwen, B. S. (1989). GABA$_A$ receptor level changes in female hamster forebrain following in vivo estrogen progesterone and benzodiazepine treatment: a quantitative autoradiography analysis. *Experimental Brain Research*, **75**(3), 644–52.

Carbone, S., Szwarcfarb, B., Losada, M. & Moguilevsky, J. A. (1995). Effect of ovarian hormones on the hypothalamic excitatory amino acids system during sexual maturation in female rats. *Neuroendocrinology*, **61**(3), 235–42.

Cavicchioli, L., Flanigan, T. P., Dickson, J. G., Vantini, G., Toso, R. D., Fusco, M., Walsh, F. S. & Leon, A. (1991). Choline acetyltransferase messenger RNA expression in developing and adult rat brain: regulation by nerve growth factor. *Molecular Brain Research*, **9**, 319–25.

Chao, M. V. (1994). The p75 neurotrophin receptor. *Journal of Neurobiology*, **25**, 1373–85.

Chao, M. V. & Hempstead, B. L. (1995). p75 and Trk: a two-receptor system. *Trends in Neurological Sciences*, **18**(7), 321–26.

Conway, E. L. (1998). A review of the randomized controlled trials of tacrine in the treatment of Alzheimer's disease: methodologic considerations. *Clinical Neuropharmacology*, **21**(1), 8–17.

Daniel, J. M., Fader, A. J., Spencer, A. L. & Dohanich, G. P. (1998). Estrogen enhances performance of female rats during acquisition of a radial arm maze. *Hormones and Behavior*, 32, 217–25.

Davies, A. M., Lee, K-F. & Jaenisch, R. (1993). p75-deficient trigeminal sensory neurons have an altered response to NGF but not to other neurotrophins. *Neuron*, 11, 565–74.

Davies, P. & Maloney, A. J. F. (1976). Selective loss of central cholinergic neurons in Alzheimer's disease. *Lancet*, ii, 1403.

Dawbarn, D., Allen, S. J. & Semenenko, F. M. (1988). Coexistence of choline acetyltransferase and nerve growth factor receptors in the rat basal forebrain. *Neuroscience Letters*, 94, 138–44.

Dekker, A. J. & Thal, L. J. (1992). Effect of delayed treatment with nerve growth factor on choline acetyltransferase activity in the cortex of rats with lesions of the nucleus basalis magnocellularis: dose requirements. *Brain Research*, 584, 55–63.

Dekker, J. A. M., Connor, D. J. & Thal, L. J. (1991). The role of cholinergic projections from the nucleus basalis in memory. *Neuroscience Biobehavior Review*, 15, 299–317.

Dluzen, D. E., McDermott, J. L. & Liu, B. (1996). Estrogen alters MPTP-induced neurotoxicity in female mice: effects on striatal dopamine concentrations and release. *Journal of Neurochemistry*, 66, 658–66.

Dohanich, G. P., Fader, A. J. & Javorsky, D. J. (1994). Estrogen and estrogen-progesterone treatments counteract the effect of scopolamine on reinforced T-maze alternation in female rats. *Behavioral Neuroscience*, 108(5), 988–92.

Drachman, D. & Leavitt, J. (1974). Human memory and the cholinergic system: a relationship to aging? *Archives of Neurology*, 30(2), 113–21.

Drachman, D. A. (1977). Memory and cognitive function in man: does the cholinergic system have a specific role? *Neurology*, 27(8), 783–90.

Drachman, D. A., Noffsinger, D., Sahakian, B. J., Kurdziel, S. & Fleming, P. (1980). Aging, memory and the cholinergic system: a study of dichotic listening. *Neurobiology of Aging*, 1(1), 39–43.

Fader, A. J., Hendricson, A. W. & Dohanich, G. P. (1998). Estrogen improves performance of reinforced T-maze alternation and prevents the amnestic effects of scopolamine administered systemically or intrahippocampally. *Neurobiology, Learning and Memory*, 69(3), 225–40.

Farlow, M., Gracon, S. I., Hershey, L. A., Lewis, K. W., Sadowsky, C. H. & Dolan-Ureno, J. (1992). A controlled trial of tacrine in Alzheimer's disease. *Journal of the American Medical Association* 268(18), 2523–29.

Fink, G., Sumner, B. E., Rosie, R., Grace, O. & Quinn, J. P. (1996). Estrogen control of central neurotransmission: effect on mood, mental state, and memory. *Cellular and Molecular Neurobiology*, 16(3), 325–44.

Fischer, W., Chen, K. S., Gage, F. H. & Björklund, A. (1991). Progressive decline in spatial learning and integrity of forebrain cholinergic neurons in rats during aging. *Neurobiology of Aging*, 13, 9–23.

Fischer, W., Gage, F. H. & Björklund, A. (1989). Degenerative changes in forebrain cholinergic nuclei correlate with cognitive impairments in aged rats. *European Journal of Neuroscience*, 1(1), 34–45.

Fusco, M., Oderfeld-Nowak, B., Vantini, G., Schiavo, N., Gradkowska, M., Zaremba, M. & Leon, A. (1989). Nerve growth factor affects uninjured, adult rat septohippocampal cholinergic neurons. *Neuroscience*, 33, 45–52.

Gao, Z-Y., Collins, H. W., Matschinsky, F. M., Lee, V. M-Y. & Wolf, B. A. (1998). Cytotoxic effect of ß-amyloid on a human differentiated neuron is not mediated by cytoplasmic Ca^{2+} accumulation. *Journal of Neurochemistry*, **70**, 1394–400.

Gazzaley, A. H., Weiland, N. G., McEwen, B. S. & Morrison, J. H. (1996). Differential regulation of NMDAR1 mRNA and protein by estradiol in the rat hippocampus. *Journal of Neuroscience*, **16**, 6830–8.

Gibbs, R. B. (1996a). Expression of estrogen receptor-like immunoreactivity by different subgroups of basal forebrain cholinergic neurons in gonadectomized male and female rats. *Brain Research*, **720**, 61–8.

Gibbs, R. B. (1996b). Fluctuations in relative levels of choline acetyltransferase mRNA in different regions of the rat basal forebrain across the estrous cycle: effects of estrogen and progesterone. *Journal of Neuroscience*, **16**(3), 1049–55.

Gibbs, R. B. (1997). Effects of estrogen on basal forebrain cholinergic neurons vary as a function of dose and duration of treatment. *Brain Research*, **757**, 10–16.

Gibbs, R. B. (1998a). Impairment of basal forebrain cholinergic neurons associated with aging and long-term loss of ovarian function. *Experimental Neurology*, **151**, 289–302.

Gibbs, R. B. (1998b). Levels of trkA and BDNF mRNA, but not NGF mRNA, fluctuate across the estrous cycle and increase in response to acute hormone replacement. *Brain Research*, **787**, 259–68.

Gibbs, R. B. & Pfaff, D. W. (1992). Effects of estrogen and fimbria/fornix transection on p75^{NGFR} and ChAT expression in the medial septum and diagonal band of Broca. *Experimental Neurology*, **116**, 23–39.

Gibbs, R. B. & Pfaff, D. W. (1994). In situ hybridization detection of trkA mRNA in brain: distribution, co-localization with p75^{NGFR} and up-regulation by nerve growth factor. *Journal of Comparative Neurology*, **341**, 324–39.

Gibbs, R. B., Burke, A. M. & Johnson, D. A. (1998). Estrogen replacement attenuates effects of scopolamine and lorazepam on memory acquisition and retention. *Hormones and Behavior*, **34**, 112–25.

Gibbs, R. B., Hashash, A. & Johnson, D. A. (1997). Effects of estrogen on potassium-evoked acetylcholine release in the hippocampus and overlying cortex of adult rats. *Brain Research*, **749**(1), 143–6.

Gibbs, R. B., Wu, D-H., Hersh, L. & Pfaff, D. W. (1994). Effects of estrogen replacement on relative levels of ChAT, TrkA and nerve growth factor messenger RNAs in the basal forebrain and hippocampal formation of adult rats. *Experimental Neurology*, **129**(1), 70–80.

Gibson, G. E., Peterson, C. & Jenden, D. J. (1981). Brain acetylcholine declines with senescence. *Science*, **213**, 674–6.

Giordano, T., Pan, J. B., Monteggia, L. M., Holzman, T. F., Snyder, S. W., Krafft, G., Ghanbari, H. & Kowall, N. W. (1994). Similarities between ß amyloid peptides 1–40 and 40–1: effects on aggregation, toxicity *in vitro*, and injection in young and aged rats. *Experimental Neurology*, **125**, 175–82.

Goodman, Y., Bruce, A. J., Cheng, B. & Mattson, M. P. (1996). Estrogens attenuate and corticosterone exacerbates excitotoxicity, oxidative injury, and amyloid beta-peptide toxicity in hippocampal neurons. *Journal of Neurochemistry*, **66**(5), 1836–44.

Gould, E., Woolley, C.S., Frankfurt, M. & McEwen, B. S. (1990). Gonadal steroids regulate dendritic spine density in hippocampal pyramidal cells in adulthood. *Neuroscience*, 10, 1286–91.

Grattan, D. R., Rocca, M. S., Strauss, K. I., Sagrillo, C. A., Selmanoff, M. & McCarthy, M. M. (1996). GABAergic neuronal activity and mRNA levels for both forms of glutamic acid decarboxylase (GAD65 and GAD67) are reduced in the diagonal band of Broca during the afternoon of proestrus. *Brain Research*, 733(1), 46–55.

Green, P. S., Bishop, J. & Simpkins, J. W. (1997a). 17-alpha-estradiol exerts neuroprotective effects on SK-N-SH cells. *Journal of Neuroscience*, 17(2), 511–15.

Green, P. S., Gordon, K. & Simpkins, J. W. (1997b). Phenolic A ring requirement for the neuroprotective effects of steroids. *Journal of Steroid Biochemistry and Molecular Biology*, 63(4–6), 229–35.

Green, P. S., Gridley, K. E. & Simpkins, J. W. (1998). Nuclear estrogen receptor-independent neuroprotection by estratrienes: a novel interaction with glutathione. *Neuroscience*, 1998; 84(1), 7–10.

Gridley, K. E., Green, P. S. & Simpkins, J. W. (1997). Low concentrations of estradiol reduce beta-amyloid (25–35)-induced toxicity, lipid peroxidation and glucose utilization in human SK-N-SH neuroblastoma cells. *Brain Research*, 778(1), 158–65.

Haass, C. & Selkoe, D. J. (1993). Cellular processing of ß-amyloid precursor protein and genesis of the amyloid-ß-peptide. *Cell*, 75, 1039–42.

Häfner, H. (1990). Epidemiology of Alzheimer's Disease. In *Alzheimer's Disease, Epidemiology, Neuropathology, Neurochemistry, and Clinics*, ed. K. Maurer, R. Riederer & H. Beckmann, pp. 23–39. Federal Republic of Germany: Springer-Verlag.

Hamon, M., Goetz, C., Euvard, C., Pasqualini, C., Le Dafniet, M., Kerdelhue, B., Cesselin, F. & Peillon, F. (1983). Biochemical and functional alterations of central GABA receptors during chronic estradiol treatment. *Brain Research*, 279(1–2), 141–52.

Hantzopoulos, P. A., Suri, C., Glass, D. J., Goldfarb, M. P. & Yancopoulos, G. D. (1994). The low affinity NGF receptor, p75, can collaborate with each of the Trks to potentiate functional responses to the neurotrophins. *Neuron*, 13, 187–201.

Hefti, F. (1986). Nerve growth factor promotes survival of septal cholinergic neurons after fimbrial transections. *Journal of Neuroscience*, 6, 2155–62.

Henderson, V. W., Watt, L. & Buckwalter, J. G. (1996). Cognitive skills associated with estrogen replacement in women with Alzheimer's disease. *Psychoneuroendocrinology*, 21(4), 421–30.

Herbison, A. E. (1997). Estrogen regulation of GABA transmission in rat preoptic area. *Brain Research Bulletin*, 44(4), 321–6.

Holland, P. (1997). Brain mechanisms for changes in processing of conditioned stimuli in Pavlovian conditioning: implications for behavior theory. *Animal Learning and Behavior*, 25(4), 373–99.

Honjo, J., Tamura, T., Matsumoto, Y., Kawata, M., Ogino, Y., Tanaka, K., Yamamoto, T., Ueda, S. & Okado, H. (1992). Estrogen as a growth factor to central nervous cells. *Journal of Steroid Biochemistry*, 41, 633–5.

Honjo, H., Tanaka, K., Kashiwagi, T., Urabe, M., Hayashi, O. M. & Hayashi, K. (1995). Senile dementia – Alzheimer's type and estrogen. *Hormone and Metabolism Research*, 27, 204–7.

Isackson, P. J., Huntsman, M. M., Murray, K. D. & Gall, C. M. (1991). BDNF mRNA expression is increased in adult rat forebrain after limbic seizures: temporal patterns of induction distinct from NGF. *Neuron*, 6, 937–48.

Jaffe, A. B., Toran-Allerand, C. D., Greengard, P. & Gandy, S. E. (1994). Estrogen regulates metabolism of Alzheimer amyloid beta precursor protein. *Journal of Biological Chemistry*, 269(18), 13065–8.

Jones, D. N., Barnes, J. C., Kirkby, D. L. & Higgins, G. A. (1995). Age-associated impairments in a test of attention: evidence for involvement of cholinergic systems. *Journal of Neuroscience*, 15(11), 7282–92.

Kang, H. & Schuman, E. M. (1995). Long-lasting neurotrophin-induced enhancement of synaptic transmission in the adult hippocampus. *Science*, 267, 1658–62.

Kawas, C., Resnick, S., Morrison, A., Brookmeyer, R., Corrada, M., Zonderman, A., Bacal, C., Lingle, D. L. & Metter, E. (1997). A prospective study of estrogen replacement therapy and the risk of developing Alzheimer's disease: the Baltimore Longitudinal Study of Aging. *Neurology*, 48, 1517–21.

Korte, M. & Bonhoeffer, T. (1997). Activity-dependent synaptic plasticity: a new face of action for neurotrophins. *Molecular Psychiatry*, 2, 197–9.

Korte, M., Carroll, P., Wolf, E., Brem, G., Thoenen, H. & Bonhoeffer, T. (1995). Hippocampal long-term potentiation is impaired in mice lacking brain-derived neurotrophic factor. *Proceedings of the National Academy of Sciences*, 92, USA, 8856–60.

Korte, M., Griesbeck, O., Gravel, C., Carroll, P., Staigner, V., Thoenen, H. & Bonhoeffer, R. (1996). Virus-mediated gene-transfer into hippocampal CA1 region restores LTP in BDNF-mutant mice. *Proceedings of the National Academy of Sciences*, USA, 93, 12547–52.

Kristofiková, Z., Klaschka, J., Tejkalová, H. & Benesová, O. (1992). High-affinity choline uptake and muscarinic receptors in rat brain during aging. *Archives of Gerontology and Geriatrics*, 15, 87–97.

Kromer, L. F. (1987). Nerve growth factor treatment after brain injury prevents neuronal death. *Science*, 235, 214–6.

Kushwaha, R. S., Foster, D. M., Barrett, P. H. R., Carey, K. D. & Bernard, M. G. (1991). Metabolic regulation of plasma apolipoprotein E by estrogen and progesterone in the baboon. *Metabolism*, 40, 93–100.

Lawrence, A. D. & Sahakian, B. J. (1995). Alzheimer disease, attention, and the cholinergic system. *Alzheimer's Disease and Associated Disorders*, 9(Suppl 2), 43–9.

Lee, K-F., Davies, A. M. & Jaenisch, R. (1994). p75-deficient embryonic dorsal root sensory and neonatal sympathetic neurons display a decreased sensitivity to NGF. *Development*, 120, 1027–33.

Lee, T. H., Abe, K., Nakamura, M., Kogure, K. & Itoyama, Y. (1994). Reduction of nerve growth factor receptor immunoreactivity in ischaemic gerbil hippocampal CA1 neurons after treatment with L-threo-3,4-dihydroxyphenylserine (DOPS). *Neurological Research*, 16, 201–4.

Lindamer, L. A., Lohr, J. B., Harris, M. J. & Jeste, D. V. (1997). Gender, estrogen, and schizophrenia. *Psychopharmacology Bulletin*, 33(2), 221–8.

Lorenzo, A. & Yankner, B. A. (1994). ß-Amyloid neurotoxicity requires fibril formation and is inhibited by Congo red. *Proceedings of the National Academy of Sciences*, USA, 91, 12243–7.

Luine, V. & Rodriguez, M. (1994). Effects of estradiol on radial arm maze performance of young and aged rats. *Behavioral and Neural Biology*, 62, 230–6.

Luine, V. N. (1985). Estradiol increases choline acetyltransferase activity in specific basal fore-brain nuclei and projection areas of female rats. *Experimental Neurology*, 89, 484–90.

Luine, V. N. (1997). Steroid hormone modulation of hippocampal dependent spatial memory. *Stress*, 2(1), 21–36.

Luine, V. N., Grattan, D. R. & Selmanoff, M. (1997). Gonadal hormones alter hypothalamic GABA and glutamate levels. *Brain Research*, 747, 165–8.

Ma, Y. L., Wang, H. L., Wu, H. C., Wei, C. L. & Lee, E. H. (1998). Brain-derived neurotrophic factor antisense oligonucleotide impairs memory retention and inhibits long-term potentiation in rats. *Neuroscience*, 82(4), 957–67.

Malouf, A. T. (1992). Effect of beta amyloid peptides on neurons in hippocampal slice cultures. *Neurobiology of Aging*, 13, 543–51.

Maswood, S., Stewart, G. & Uphouse, L. (1995). Gender and estrous cycle effects of the 5–HT1A agonist, 8–OH-DPAT, on hypothalamic serotonin. *Pharmacology, Biochemistry and Behavior*, 51(4), 807–13.

Matsuoka, N., Maeda, N., Ohkubo, Y. & Yamaguchi, I. (1991). Differential effects of physostigmine and pilocarpine on the spatial memory deficits produced by two septo-hippocampal deafferentations in rats. *Brain Research*, 559, 233–40.

Mattson, M. P., Robinson, N. & Guo, Q. (1997). Estrogens stabilize mitochondrial function and protect neural cells against the pro-apoptotic action of mutant presenilin-1. *NeuroReport*, 8, 3817–21.

Maurice, T., Lockhart, B. P. & Privat, A. (1996). Amnesia induced in mice by centrally administered ß-amyloid peptides involves cholinergic dysfunction. *Brain Research*, 706, 181–93.

McCarthy, M. M., Kaufman, L. C., Brooks, P. J., Pfaff, D. W. & Schwartz-Giblin, S. (1995). Estrogen modulation of mRNA levels for the two forms of glutamic acid decarboxylase (GAD) in female rat brain. *Journal of Comparative Neurology*, 360, 685–97.

McDermott, J. L., Anderson, L. I. & Dluzen, A. E. (1997). Interactive effects of tamoxifen and estrogen upon the nigrostriatal dopamine system. *Neuroendocrinology*, 105, 1–7.

McDermott, J. L., Kreutzberg, J. D., Liu, B. & Dluzen, D. E. (1994a). Effects of estrogen treatment on sensorimotor task performance and brain dopamine concentrations in gonadectomized male and female CD-1 mice. *Hormones and Behavior*, 28, 16–28.

McDermott, J. L., Liu, B. & Dluzen, D. E. (1994b). Sex differences and effects of estrogen on dopamine and DOPAC release from the striatum of male and female CD-1 mice. *Experimental Neurology*, 125, 306–11.

McEwen, B. S. (1996). Gonadal and adrenal steroids regulate neurochemical and structural plasticity of the hippocampus via cellular mechanisms involving NMDA receptors. *Cellular and Molecular Neurobiology*, 16(2), 103–16.

McGurk, S. R., Levin, E. D. & Butcher, L. L. (1991). Impairment of radial-arm maze performance in rats following lesions involving the cholinergic medial pathway: reversal by arecoline and differential effects of muscarinic and nicotinic antagonists. *Neuroscience*, 44(1), 137–47.

McMillan, P. J., Singer, C. A. & Dorsa, D. M. (1996). The effects of ovariectomy and estrogen replacement on trkA and choline acetyltransferase mRNA expression in the basal forebrain of adult female Sprague-Dawley rat. *Journal of Neuroscience*, 16(5), 1860–5.

Mesulam, M. M., Mufson, E. J. & Rogers, J. (1987). Age-related shrinkage of cortically projecting cholinergic neurons: a selective effect. *Annals of Neurology*, 22, 31–6.

Mooradian, A. D. (1993). Antioxidant properties of steroids. *Journal of Steroid Biochemistry and Molecular Biology*, 45, 509–11.

Morse, J. K., Scheff, S. W. & DeKosky, S. T. (1986). Gonadal steroids influence axon sprouting in the hippocampal dentate gyrus: a sexually dimorphic response. *Experimental Neurology*, 94, 649–58.

Morse, J. K., Wiegand, S. J., Anderson, K., You, Y., Cai, N., Carnahan, J., Miller, J., DiStefano, P. S., Altar, C. A., Lindsay, R. M. & Alderson, R. F. (1993). Brain-derived neurotrophic factor (BDNF) prevents the degeneration of medial septal cholinergic neurons following fimbria/fornix transection. *Journal of Neuroscience*, 13(10), 4146–56.

Muesing, R. A., Miller, V. T., LaRosa, J. C., Stoy, D. B. & Phillips, E. A. (1992). Effects of unopposed conjugated equine estrogen on lipoprotein composition and apolipoprotein-E distribution. *Journal of Clinical Endocrinology and Metabolism*, 75, 1250–4.

Mufson, E. J., Lavine, N., Jaffar, S., Kordower, J. H., Quirion, R. & Saragovi, H. U. (1997). Reduction in p140–TrkA receptor protein within the nucleus basalis and cortex in Alzheimer's disease. *Experimental Neurology*, 146(1), 91–103.

Mufson, E. J., Li, J-M., Sobreviela, T. & Kordower, J. H. (1996). Decreased trkA gene expression within basal forebrain neurons in Alzheimer's disease. *NeuroReport*, 8, 25–9.

Murphy, D. D., Cole, N. B., Greenberger, V. & Segal. M. (1998). Estradiol increases dendritic spine density by reducing GABA neurotransmission in hippocampal neurons. *Journal of Neuroscience*, 18(7), 2550–9.

Murray, C. L. & Fibiger, H. C. (1985). Learning and memory deficits after lesions of the nucleus basalis magnocellularis: reversal by physostigmine. *Neuroscience*, 14(4), 1025–32.

Murray, C. L. & Fibiger, H. C. (1986). Pilocarpine and physostigmine attenuate spatial memory impairments produced by lesions of the nucleus basalis magnocellularis. *Behavioral Neuroscience*, 100(1), 23–32.

Nibuya, M., Morinobu, S. & Duman, R. S. (1995). Regulation of BDNF and trkB mRNA in rat brain by chronic electroconvulsive seizure and antidepressant drug treatments. *Journal of Neuroscience*, 15(11), 7539–47.

Niki, E. & Nakano, M. (1990). Estrogens as antioxidants. *Methods in Enzymology*, 186, 330–3.

Nomikos, G. G. & Spyraki, C. (1988). Influence of oestrogen on spontaneous and diazepam-induced exploration of rats in an elevated plus maze. *Neuropharmacology*, 27(7), 691–6.

Nonomura, T. & Hatanaka, H. (1992). Neurotrophic effect of brain-derived neurotrophic factor on basal forebrain cholinergic neurons in culture from postnatal rats. *Neuroscience Research*, 14, 226–33.

Nonomura, T., Nishio, C., Lindsay, R. M. & Hatanaka, H. (1995). Cultured basal forebrain cholinergic neurons from postnatal rats show both overlapping and non-overlapping responses to the neurotrophins. *Brain Research*, 683, 129–39.

O'Malley, C. A., Hautamaki, R. D., Kelley, M. & Meyer, E. M. (1987). Effects of ovariectomy and estradiol benzoate on high affinity choline uptake, ACh synthesis, and release from rat cerebral cortical synaptosomes. *Brain Research*, 403, 389–92.

Ohkura, T., Isse, K., Akazawa, K., Hamamoto, M., Yaoi, Y. & Hagino, N. (1994). Evaluation of estrogen treatment in female patients with dementia of the Alzheimer type. *Endocrine Journal*, 41(4), 361–71.

Ohkura, T., Isse, K., Akazawa, K., Hamamoto, M., Yaoi, Y. & Hagino, N. (1995a). Long-term estrogen replacement therapy in female patients with dementia of the Alzheimer type: 7 case reports. *Dementia*, 6, 99–107.

Ohkura, T., Teshima, Y., Isse, K., Matsuda, H., Inoue, T., Sakai, Y., Iwasaki, N. & Yaoi, Y. (1995b). Estrogen increases cerebral and cerebellar blood flows in postmenopausal women. *Menopause*, 2(1), 13–18.

Österlund, M., Kuiper, G. G. J. M., Gustafsson, J-Å. & Hurd, Y. L. (1998). Differential distribution and regulation of estrogen receptor-α and -ß mRNA within the female rat brain. *Molecular Brain Research*, 54, 175–80.

Paganini-Hill, A. & Henderson, V. W. (1996). Estrogen replacement therapy and risk of Alzheimer's disease. *Archives of Internal Medicine*, 156, 2213–7.

Patterson, S. L., Abel, T., Deuel, T. A. S., Martin, K. C., Rose, J. C. & Kandel, E.R. (1996). Recombinant BDNF rescues deficits in basal synaptic transmission and hippocampal LTP in BDNF knockout mice. *Neuron*, 16, 1137–45.

Pecins-Thompson, M., Brown, N. A. & Bethea, C. L. (1996). Regulation of serotonin reuptake transporter (SERT) mRNA expression by estrogen (E) and progesterone (P) in rhesus macaques. *Society for Neuroscience*, Abstr. 22, 1441.

Penetar, D. M. & McDonough, J. H. J. (1983). Effects of cholinergic drugs on delayed matching-to-sample performance of Rhesus monkeys. *Pharmacology, Biochemistry and Behavior*, 19, 963–7.

Perez, J. , Zucci, I. & Maggi, A. (1988). Estrogen modulation of the γ-aminobutyric acid receptor complex in the central nervous system. *Journal of Pharmacology and Experimental Therapeutics*, 244(3), 1005–10.

Perry, E. K., Perry, R. H., Blessed, G. & Tomlinson, B. E. (1977). Necropsy evidence of cholinergic deficits in senile dementia. *Lancet*, i, 189.

Perry, E. K., Tomlinson, B. E., Blessed, G., Bergmann, K., Gibson, P. H. & Perry, R. H. (1978). Correlation of cholinergic abnormalities with senile plaques and mental test scores in senile dementia. *British Medicine Journal*, 2, 1457.

Pfaff, D. W. (1968). Autoradiographic localization of radioactivity in rat brain after injection of tritiated sex hormones. *Science*, 161, 1355–6.

Phillips, H. S., Hains, J. M., Armanini, M., Laramee, G. R., Johnson, S. A. & Winslow, J. W. (1991). BDNF mRNA is decreased in the hippocampus of individuals with Alzheimer's disease. *Neuron*, 7, 695–702.

Rainbow, T. C., Parsons, B., MacLusky, N. J. & McEwen, B. S. (1982). Estradiol receptor levels in rat hypothalamic and limbic nuclei. *Journal of Neuroscience*, 2(10), 1439–45.

Rodriguez-Tebar, A., Dechant, G. & Barde, Y-A. (1990). Binding of brain-derived neurotrophic factor to the nerve growth factor receptor. *Neuron*, 4, 487–92.

Rogers, S. L., Doody, R. S., Mohs, R. C. & Friedhoff, L. T. (1998). Donepezil improves cognition and global function in Alzheimer disease: a 15-week, double-blind, placebo-controlled study. Donepezil Study Group (see comments). *Archives of Internal Medicine*, 158(9), 1021–31.

Ross, G. M., Shamovsky, I. L., Lawrance, G., Solc, M., Dostaler, S. M., Weaver, D. F. & Riopelle, R. J. (1998). Reciprocal modulation of TrkA and P75(NTR) affinity states is mediated by direct receptor interactions. *European Journal of Neuroscience*, 10(3), 890–8.

Rylett, R. J., Ball, M. J. & Colhoun, E. H. (1983). Evidence for high affinity choline transport in synaptosomes prepared from hippocampus and neocortex of patients with Alzheimer's disease. *Brain Research*, 289(1–2), 169–75.

Rylett, R. J., Goddard, S., Schmidt, B. M. & Williams, L. R. (1993). Acetylcholine synthesis and release following continuous intracerebral administration of NGF in adult and aged Fischer-344 rats. *Journal of Neuroscience*, 13(9), 3956–63.

Schneider, L. S. (1994). Tacrine development experience: early clinical trials and enrichment and parallel designs. *Alzheimer's Disease and Associated Disorders*, 8(Suppl. 2), S12–S21.

Segal, R. A. & Greenberg, M. E. (1996). Intracellular signaling pathways activated by neurotrophic factors. *Annual Review of Neuroscience*, 19, 463–89.

Selkoe, D. J. (1993). Physiological production of the ß-amyloid protein and the mechanism of Alzheimer's disease. *Trends in Neurological Sciences*, 16(10), 403–9.

Sherman, K. A. & Friedman, E. (1990). Pre- and post-synaptic cholinergic dysfunction in aged rodent brain regions: new findings and an interpretative review. *International Journal of Developmental Neuroscience*, 8, 689–708.

Sherman, K. A., Kuster, J. E., Dean, R. L., Bartus, R. T. & Friedman, E. (1981). Presynaptic cholinergic mechanisms in brain of aged rats with memory impairments. *Neurobiology of Aging*, 2, 99–104.

Shi, J., Zhang, Y. Q. & Simpkins, J. W. (1997). Effects of 17-beta-estradiol on glucose transporter 1 expression and endothelial cell survival following focal ischemia in the rats. *Experimental Brain Research*, 117(2), 200–6.

Shimizu, H. & Bray, G. A. (1993). Effects of castration, estrogen replacement and estrus cycle on monoamine metabolism in the nucleus accumbens, measured by microdialysis. *Brain Research*, 621(2), 200–6.

Simpkins, J. W., Rajakamar, G., Zhang, Y. Q., Simpkins, C. E., Greenwald, D., Yu, C. J., Bodor, N. & Day, A. L. (1997). Estrogens may reduce mortality and ischemic damage caused by middle cerebral artery occlusion in the female rat. *Journal of Neurosurgery*, 87(5), 724–30.

Sims, N. R., Bowen, D. M., Allen, S. J., Smith, C. C., Neary, D., Thomas, D. J. & Davison, A. N. (1983). Presynaptic cholinergic dysfunction in patients with dementia. *Journal of Neurochemistry*, 40(2), 503–9.

Sims, N. R., Marek, K. L., Bowen, D. M. & Davison, A. N. (1982). Production of (^{14}C)acetylcholine and (^{14}C)carbon dioxide from (U-^{14}C)glucose in tissue prisms from aging rat brain. *Journal of Neurochemistry*, 26, 127–39.

Singer, C. A., McMillan, P. J., Dobie, D. J. & Dorsa, D. M. (1998). Effects of estrogen replacement on choline acetyltransferase and trkA mRNA expression in the basal forebrain of aged rats. *Brain Research*, 789, 343–6.

Singh, M., Meyer, E. M., Huang, F. S., Millard, W. J. & Simpkins. J. W. (1993). Ovariectomy reduces ChAT activity and NGF mRNA levels in the frontal cortex and hippocampus of the female Sprague Dawley rat. In *Program of the 23rd Annual Meeting of the Society for Neuroscience*, pp. 1254. Washington, DC.

Singh, M., Meyer, E. M., Millard, W. J. & Simpkins, J. W. (1994). Ovarian steroid deprivation results in a reversible learning impairment and compromised cholinergic function in female Sprague–Dawley rats. *Brain Research*, 644, 305–12.

Singh, M., Meyer, E. M. & Simpkins, J. W. (1995). The effects of ovariectomy and estradiol replacement on brain-derived neurotrophic factor messenger ribonucleic acid expression in cortical and hippocampal brain regions of female Sprague–Dawley rats. *Endocrinology*, 136(5), 2320–4.

Smyth, M. D., Kesslak, P., Cummings, B. J. & Cotman, C. W. (1994). Analysis of brain injury following intrahippocampal administration of ß-amyloid in streptotocin-treated rats. *Neurobiology of Aging*, 15(2), 153–59.

Sobreviela, T., Clary, D. O., Reichardt, L. F., Brandabur, M. M., Kordower, J. H. & Mufson, E. J. (1994). TrkA-immunoreactive profiles in the central nervous system: colocalization with neurons containing p75 nerve growth factor receptor, choline acetyltransferase, and serotonin. *Journal of Comparative Neurology*, 350(4), 587–611.

Sohrabji, F., Miranda, R. C. & Toran-Allerand, C. D. (1994). Estrogen differentially regulates estrogen and nerve growth factor receptor mRNAs in adult sensory neurons. *Journal of Neuroscience*, 14(2), 459–71.

Stone, D. J., Rozovsky, I., Morgan, T. E., Anderson, C. P. & Finch, C. E. (1998). Increased synaptic sprouting in response to estrogen via an apolipoprotein E-dependent mechanism: implications for Alzheimer's disease. *Journal of Neuroscience*, 18(9), 3180–5.

Stroessner-Johnson, H. M., Rapp, P. R. & Amaral, D. G. (1992). Cholinergic cell loss and hypertrophy in the medial septal nucleus of the behaviorally characterized aged Rhesus monkey. *Journal of Neuroscience*, 12(5), 1936–44.

Sudo, S., Wen, T. C., Desaki, J., Matsuda, S., Tanaka, J., Arai, T., Maeda, N. & Sakanaka, M. (1997). Beta-estradiol protects hippocampal CA1 neurons against transient forebrain ischemia in gerbil. *Neuroscience Research*, 29(4), 345–54.

Takei, N., Nihonmatsu, I. & Kawamura, H. (1989). Age-related decline of acetylcholinesterase release evoked by depolarizing stimulation. *Neuroscience Lett.* 101, 182–6.

Tang, M-X., Jacobs, D., Stern, Y., Marder, K., Schofield, P., Gurland, B., Andrews, H. & Mayeux, R. (1996). Effect of oestrogen during menopause on risk and age at onset of Alzheimer's disease. *Lancet*, 348, 429–32.

Taylor, L. & Griffith, W. H. (1993). Age-related decline in cholinergic synaptic transmission in hippocampus. *Neurobiology of Aging*, 14, 509–15.

Thind, K. K. & Goldsmith, P. C. (1997). Expression of estrogen and progesterone receptors in glutamate and GABA neurons of the pubertal female monkey hypothalamus. *Neuroendocrinology*, 65(5), 314–24.

Toran-Allerand, D., Miranda, R. C., Bentham, W. D. L., Sohrabji, F., Brown, T. J., Hochberg, R. B. & MacLusky, N. J. (1992). Estrogen receptors colocalize with low-affinity nerve growth factor receptors in cholinergic neurons of the basal forebrain. *Proceedings of the National Academy of Sciences USA*, 89, 4668–72.

Ueda, K., Fukui, Y. & Kageyama, H. (1994). Amyloid ß protein-induced neuronal cell death: neurotoxic properties of aggregated amyloid ß protein. *Brain Research*, 639, 240–4.

Varon, S. & Conner, J. M. (1994). Nerve growth factor in CNS repair. *Journal of Neurotrauma*, 11(5), 473–86.

Verdi, J. M., Birren, S. J., Ibáñez, C. F., Persson, H., Kaplan, D. R., Benedetti, M., Chao, M. V. & Anderson, D. J. (1994). p75[LNGFR] regulates Trk signal transduction and NGF-induced neuronal differentiation in MAH cells. *Neuron*, 12, 733–45.

Voytko, M. L. (1996). Cognitive functions of the basal forebrain cholinergic system in monkeys: memory or attention? *Behavioural Brain Research*, 75(1–2), 13–25.

Warren, S. G., Humphreys, A. G., Juraska, J. M. & Greenough, W. T. (1995). LTP varies across the estrous cycle: enhanced synaptic plasticity in proestrus. *Brain Research*, 703, 26–40.

Wenk, G. L. (1997). The nucleus basalis magnocellularis cholinergic system: one hundred years of progress. *Neurobiology of Learning and Memory*, 67(2), 85–95.

Whitehouse, P. J., Price, D. L., Struble, R. G., Clark, A. W., Coyle, J. T. & DeLong, M. R. (1982). Alzheimer's disease and senile dementia: loss of neurons in the basal forebrain. *Science*, 215, 1237–9.

Williams, L. R., Varon, S., Peterson, G. M., Wictorin, K., Fischer, W., Björklund, A. & Gage, F. H. (1986). Continuous infusion of nerve growth factor prevents basal forebrain neuronal death after fimbria fornix transection. *Proceedings of the National Academy of Sciences*, USA, 83, 9231–5.

Wilson, M. A. (1996). GABA physiology: modulation by benzodiazepines and hormones. Critical Reviews in *Neurobiology*, 10(1), 1–37.

Woolf, N. J. (1991). Cholinergic systems in mammalian brain and spinal cord. *Progress in Neurobiology*, 37, 475–524.

Woolley, C. S., Gould, E., Frankfurt, M. & McEwen, B. S. (1990). Naturally occuring fluctuation in dendritic spine density on adult hippocampal pyramidal neurons. *Journal of Neuroscience*, 10, 4035–9.

Woolley, C. S. & McEwen, B. S. (1992). Estradiol mediates fluctuation in hippocampal synapse density during estrus in the adult rat. *Journal of Neuroscience*, 12(7), 2549–54.

Woolley, C. S. & McEwen, B. S. (1993). Role of estradiol and progesterone in regulation of hippocampal dendritic spine density during the estrous cycle in the rat. *Journal of Comparative Neurology*, 336, 293–306.

Woolley, C. S., Weiland, N. G., McEwen, B. S. & Schwartzkroin, P. A. (1997). Estradiol increases the sensitivity of hippocampal CA1 pyramidal cells to NMDA receptor-mediated synaptic input: correlation with dendritic spine density. *Journal of Neuroscience*, 17(5), 1848–59.

Woolley, C. S., Wenzel, H. J. & Schwartzkroin, P. A. (1996). Estradiol increases the frequency of multiple synaptic boutons in the hippocampal CA1 region of the adult female rat. *Journal of Comparative Neurology*, 373, 108–17.

Wu, C. F., Bertorelli, R., Sacconi, M., Pepeu, G. & Consolo, S. (1988). Decrease of brain acetylcholine release in aging freely-moving rats detected by microdialysis. *Neurobiology of Aging*, 9, 357–61.

Wujek, J. R., Dority, M. D., Fredrickson, R. C. A. & Brunden, K. R. (1996). Deposits of Aß fibrils are not toxic to cortical and hippocampal neurons *in vitro*. *Neurobiology of Aging*, 17, 107–13.

Xu, H., Gouras, G. K., Greenfield, J. P., Vincent, B., Naslund, J., Mazzarelli, L., Fried, G., Jovanovic, J. N., Seeger, M., Relkin, N. R., Liao, F., Checler, F., Buxbaum, J. D., Chait, B. T., Thinakaran, G., Sisodia, S. S., Wang, R., Greengard, P. & Gandy, S. (1998). Estrogen reduces neuronal generation of Alzheimer beta-amyloid peptides. *Nature Medicine*, 4(4), 447–51.

Zhang, Z., Drzewiecki, G. J., Hom, J. T., May, P. C. & Hyslop, P. A. (1994). Human cortical neurnal (HCN) cell lines: a model for amyloid ß neurotoxicity. *Neuroscience Letters*, 177, 162–4.

10

Gender and schizophrenia

Laurie A. Lindamer, M. Jackuelyn Harris, Julie Akiko Gladsjo, Robert Heaton, Jane S. Paulsen, Shelley C. Heaton and Dilip V. Jeste

Introduction

The heterogeneity of schizophrenia has greatly challenged efforts to understand the etiology and pathophysiology of this disorder. Gender has been recognized for a long time as one of a number of factors that may contribute to the heterogeneity of schizophrenia, but only recently have researchers systematically examined the role of gender in the development of schizophrenia and in the modification of its expression. Recent literature reviews of gender differences in schizophrenia found gender differences in various aspects of the schizophrenic syndrome, including age of onset of illness, symptom presentation, course of illness, cognitive performance, neuroradiological abnormalities, and response to antipsychotic medication (Andia & Zisook, 1991; Yassa & Jeste, 1992; Yassa et al., 1991; Tamminga, 1997). A number of other published studies, as well, found gender differences in aspects of the schizophrenic syndrome (Szymanski et al., 1995; Gur et al., 1996; Hafner et al., 1998).

Our own findings suggest that gender accounts for some of the heterogeneity in the varying clinical presentations of schizophrenia; however, the lack of differences on neuropsychological measures suggests that the cognitive deficits seen in schizophrenia are similar in male and female patients (Andia et al., 1995).

Age of onset of schizophrenia

Age of onset of schizophrenia has usually been found to be later in women than in men, regardless of study design, culture, definition of schizophrenia, or definition of age of onset (Loranger, 1984; Castle & Murray, 1993; Hafner et al. 1989, 1998; Angermeyer & Kuhn, 1988; Hambrecht et al., 1992). A 4- to 5-year delay in age of onset of schizophrenia for women has been observed both in epidemiological studies, as well as in samples of convenience and in studies of inpatients, outpatients, first-episode patients, and more chronic patients (Castle & Murray, 1993; Hafner et al., 1998; Angermeyer & Kuhn, 1988; Lindamer et al., 1999). The gender difference in age of onset is seen regardless of the definition of schizophrenia (broad or narrow), classification system (ICD, DSM, or other), or age of onset (prodomal or positive symptoms or age of hospitalization) (Loranger, 1984). Furthermore, the gender difference in age of onset appears to be specific to schizophrenia relative to other psychotic disorders (Loranger, 1984; Bland et al., 1977). In addition to the delayed age of onset of schizophrenia in women, some researchers (Hafner et al., 1989; 1992; Lindamer et al., 1997) have reported a second smaller incidence peak for women but not for men after the age of 40 to 45. Moreover, the studies that included both male and female patients with late-onset schizophrenia reported a preponderance of women (Harris & Jeste, 1988).

It is unlikely that the small difference in the mean longevity between men and women provides an adequate explanation for the female predominance in late-onset schizophrenia. Seeman (1983) hypothesized that there might be specific biological protective factors in female patients with schizophrenia, such as less lateralization of cognitive functions or relative dopaminergic inhibition by estrogens. Riecher-Rossler and colleagues (1994) also proposed an antidopaminergic role for estrogen. These authors hypothesized that schizophrenic symptoms emerged when stress increased and/or protective factors decreased in an individual with a genetic predisposition for schizophrenia. High levels of estrogen in women between puberty and menopause would offer intrinsic protection against the development of schizophrenic symptoms, delaying the onset of the disorder. Adequate research examining the direct effects of estrogen on schizophrenic symptoms in postmenopausal women is, however, lacking.

Symptom presentation

While some studies have reported no gender differences in symptom presentation (Gift et al., 1985; Haas et al., 1989), most found that men had more severe symptoms of schizophrenia than women but that women had more severe positive or depressive symptoms than men (Goldstein et al., 1990). In one study, as the criteria for diagnosis became more stringent, more men were diagnosed with the disorder (Westermeyer & Harrow, 1984). Furthermore, it was noted that more women were classified as having 'reactive' schizophrenia; whereas more men were diagnosed as having 'process' schizophrenia (Harrow et al., 1986). Some investigators reported that men presented with 'amotivational syndrome' with more negative symptoms, more passivity, and greater loss of organization (Lewine, 1981, 1985; Runyon et al., 1985) than women. More recent studies of both younger and older patients with schizophrenia have found that women have fewer or less severe negative symptoms (Gur et al., 1996; Arnold et al., 1995; Shtasel et al., 1992). Several studies demonstrated more depression in women than in men with schizophrenia

(Lewine, 1981; Westermeyer & Harrow, 1984; Bland, 1977; Goldstein & Link, 1988; McGlashan & Bardenstein, 1990; Flor-Henry, 1990). More recent studies, however, have failed to find gender differences in depressive symptoms using the Hamilton Rating Scale for Depression (Shtasel et al., 1992). Some studies found that female patients with schizophrenia demonstrated more of Schneider's first-rank positive symptoms (Marneros, 1984), more paranoid symptoms (Goldstein & Link, 1988), or more positive symptoms than men with schizophrenia (Goldstein et al., 1990; McGlashan & Bardenstein, 1990). Some studies, however, have found no gender differences in positive symptoms (Gur et al., 1996; Arnold et al., 1995; Shtasel et al., 1992). In general, men with schizophrenia have more negative symptoms and women more positive symptoms. These gender differences in symptom presentation roughly parallel the positive/negative distinction hypothesized by Crow (1985), whereby positive symptoms are associated with increased dopaminergic activity in the brain and negative symptoms are associated with structural brain abnormalities. Longitudinal studies of positive and negative symptoms have indicated that negative symptoms increase with duration of illness (Cadet et al., 1987). The delayed onset of schizophrenia and shorter duration of illness might partially explain the predominance of positive symptoms in women. In short, despite these intriguing observations, the precise relationship among the positive/negative symptomatology, chronicity, and gender has yet to be determined.

Course of illness

The course of schizophrenia has been considered milder in women than in men (Goldstein, 1988). Several European research groups (Salokangas, 1983; Nyman & Jonsson, 1983; Prudo & Blum, 1987) and one Canadian group (Walter & Keward, 1985) reported female schizophrenic patients to have better social, as well as occupational, functioning than male schizophrenic patients. Several studies have found that women have better premorbid adjustment than men (Westermeyer & Harrow, 1984; Goldstein et al., 1989; Angermeyer et al., 1990; Fenton & McGlashan, 1991). More recent studies reported that women had better premorbid and current functioning, as well as better quality of life than men (Shtasel et al.,1992). Another study found no gender differences in age, duration of illness, symptom severity, neurocognitive functioning, or clinical MRI results in 85 outpatients between the ages of 18 and 45; these investigators did, however, note better psychosocial adjustment in female patients (Andia et al., 1995). Two large studies looking at gender differences in outcome in patients in the pre-neuroleptic treatment era, reported no relationship between gender and outcome (Loyd et al., 1985; Ciompi, 1980). Short-term outcome studies appear to show greater gender differences – such as better outcome in women – than do long-term ones (Yassa et al., 1991).

Cognitive performance

Gender differences in cognitive functioning have yielded inconsistent results with some studies finding that women with schizophrenia performed worse than men, others reporting that men were more impaired, and still others observing no gender differences. An early study of gender differences in cognitive performance in schizophrenia found that women performed worse on two tests of general intellectual ability (Progressive Matrices and the Mill-Hill vocabulary tests) than did men (Foulds & Dixon, 1962). This study included both inpatients and outpatients, but more detailed information regarding sample characteristics, such as age, duration of illness and severity of symptoms, was not provided.

More recent studies also have found that women with schizophrenia have more cognitive impairment than men. A sample of inpatient and outpatient women had worse performance on the Dementia Rating Scale, specifically on the Conceptualization and Attention subscales relative to men (Perlick et al., 1992). There were, however, no gender differences on the Construction, Memory, or Initiation/Perseveration subscales. The genders were equivalent with respect to ethnicity, socioeconomic status, and duration of illness. Similar results were obtained when the effects of age, overall psychopathology, and age of onset were taken into account in the statistical analysis. A significant gender by group interaction was observed with inpatient women performing worse than inpatient men, and with outpatient women performing better than outpatient men. The authors reasoned that since women with schizophrenia usually have later age of onset than men, the women with earlier onset who participated in this study may have been atypical in that they had more cognitive impairment relative to general sample of women with schizophrenia.

Using a comprehensive neuropsychological test battery, Lewine and colleagues (1996, 1997) also found that women inpatients and outpatients with schizophrenia or schizoaffective disorder had more cognitive impairment than men. The neuropsychological test battery included the following domains: language, executive function, verbal memory, spatial memory, visual processing, concentration, and motor function. While men had significantly earlier onset, there were no differences in positive or negative symptoms, amount of antipsychotic or anticholinergic medication. Overall, men had higher IQ scores than women and performed better than women on verbal memory, spatial memory, visual processing, and motor functioning when controlling for the level of education and duration of illness.

In contrast to studies that have found that women with schizophrenia are more cognitively impaired relative to men, many studies have found that men with schizophrenia have worse cognitive impairment. A meta-analysis of gender differences in cognitive performance in adults and children with schizophrenia

(Aylward et al., 1984) noted that males appeared to have lower average IQ than females on standardized intelligence tests. A comparison of patients with first-episode and chronic schizophrenia on selected subtests of WAIS-R found that men with chronic schizophrenia had more impairment than women with chronic schizophrenia but that there was no gender difference in the patients with first episode schizophrenia (Bilder et al., 1992). Thus, the authors concluded that men deteriorated cognitively at a faster rate than women did.

Several studies have failed to find gender differences in cognitive performance between men and women with schizophrenia. No gender difference was observed in a study of 46 first-episode schizophrenic patients on numerous measures of cognitive performance, including Progressive Matrices and Mill Hill Vocabulary (The Scottish Schizophrenia Research Group, 1987). Furthermore, no gender differences were noted on a wide range of neuropsychological tests in four cohorts of patients with schizophrenia: two groups of relatively treatment refractory inpatients, a group of inpatients privately hospitalized for an acute exacerbation, and a group of twins discordant for schizophrenia (Goldberg et al., 1995).

In a sample of outpatients with schizophrenia between the ages of 18 and 45 years, no gender differences were observed on any of the tests of the Halstead–Reitan battery or WAIS-R, using T-scores correcting for normal effects of age, education, and gender, although both men and women with schizophrenia had below average IQ scores (Andia et al., 1995). In a study of first episode patients and healthy controls, there were no gender by group differences on a battery of neuropsychological tests that measured verbal intelligence and other language skills; spatial organization, verbal memory, and learning; visual memory; visual–motor–processing speed and attention; and abstraction/flexibility (Albus et al., 1997). The authors concluded that gender did not appear to modify the cognitive impairment characteristic of schizophrenia.

The inconsistencies in gender differences in neuropsychological performance in schizophrenia may be due to several factors, including differences in test batteries, sample characteristics, and study design.

Neuroradiological abnormalities

Some studies directly compared neuroradiological abnormalities in women and men with schizophrenia. Larger ventricle brain ratios (VBR) in male schizophrenia patients were observed in some studies (Flaum et al., 1990; Nopoulous et al., 1997); whereas, other studies found larger VBRs in women (Gur et al., 1994; Nasrallah et al., 1990), and still other studies have found no gender differences in brain volume (Flaum et al., 1995). Gender differences in specific brain regions have been noted, yet these results are inconsistent. For example, one study (Lewine et al., 1990) reported that men with schizophrenia had a smaller corpus callosum than women patients; however another study (Hoff et al., 1994) reported that in women with schizophrenia, the corpus callosum size was decreased relative to men. Men with schizophrenia showed a trend toward smaller temporal lobe volume (Cowell et al., 1996) while women with schizophrenia showed reduced frontal volumes (Nasrallah et al., 1990). Numerous methodological differences in these studies, including the variation in male to female ratio (Nopoulos et al., 1997) and the dissimilarity in sample characteristics, most likely contribute to these inconsistencies.

Response to antipyschotic medication

The available literature concerning gender differences in response to antipyschotic medication is complex with different studies reporting variable results. In a number of investigations, women were reported to require higher dosages but to respond better to long-term neuroleptic treatment (Salokangas, 1983; Nyman & Jonsson, 1983; Affleck et al., 1976; Marriott & Hiep, 1978). Several other studies noted that women responded better to neuroleptics and also seemed to maintain their adjustment outside the hospital longer in the community than men (Hogarty et al., 1974; Seeman, 1986; Young & Meltzer, 1980). And some evidence suggests that premenopausal women need lower neuroleptic doses than men while the reverse is true with postmenopausal women (Marriott & Hiep, 1978). This may be related to protective antidopaminergic effects of estrogen in premenopausal women.

Tardive dyskinesia

A number of studies found the prevalence of tardive dyskinesia (TD) to be higher in neuroleptic-treated women than in men, while some studies found no gender difference (Yassa & Jeste, 1992). Yassa and Jeste (1992), in their literature review of 76 studies, noted that the reported average prevalence of TD was 26.6% in women and 21.6% in men. Women also had more severe forms of TD than men. The prevalence of TD seemed to increase with age in women while it appeared to decrease after age 70 in men. Interaction of age and gender may be related to estrogens such that premenstrual women may be less susceptible while postmenopausal women may be more susceptible to TD. Two recent investigations of TD in older patients, however, reported no significant gender differences in the incidence of TD (Saltz et al., 1991; Jeste et al., 1995).

Report of ongoing studies assessing gender differences in clinical and neuropsychological variables of schizophrenia

Below we report some of the findings from our ongoing studies assessing gender differences in clinical and neuropsychological variables in a large outpatient sample of schizophrenic patients. The methodology and the data have, in part, been published previously (Andia et al., 1995; Jeste et al., 1995; 1997; Heaton et al., 1994).

As would be expected in light of other studies on the topic, our findings suggest gender accounts for some of the heterogeneity in the varying clinical presentations of schizophrenia. Our data thus far showed women with schizophrenia had a significantly later age of onset and less severe negative symptoms than their male counterparts. There was a trend for women to have more severe positive symptoms while the findings regarding more depressive symptoms in women were equivocal. The female patients were treated with a significantly lower daily antipsychotic dose and tended to have fewer abnormal involuntary movements. There were no significant gender differences on any neuropsychological measures. The lack of differences on neuropsychological measures suggests that cognitive deficits seen in schizophrenia are similar in male and female patients.

Materials and methods

Subjects consisted of those patients recruited for participation in several studies from our Geriatric Psychiatry or Outpatient Clinical Research Centers (Andia et al., 1995; Jeste et al., 1995; Heaton et al., 1994). All the patients met DSM-III-R (American Psychiatric Association, 1987) or DSM-IV (American Psychiatric Association, 1994) criteria for schizophrenia or schizoaffective disorder and were recruited from the San Diego Veterans Affairs (VA) Medical Center; University of California, San Diego Medical Center and Psychiatry Outpatient Services; San Diego County Mental Health Services; and private physicians. A majority of the male patients came from the VA Medical Center, and most of the women were recruited from the non-VA sources. A clinical evaluation including the Structured Clinical Interview for DSM III-R (SCID) (Spitzer et al., 1990) was performed by a Psychiatry Fellow who was trained in this procedure. Subjects were included only if a consensus on diagnosis was reached by two Board Certified psychiatrists at a staffing meeting. Exclusion criteria were diagnosable dementia, seizure disorder, history of head injury with unconsciousness for greater than 30 minutes, and current substance abuse or dependence meeting DSM-III-R criteria (American Psychiatric Association, 1987). All the patients gave written informed consent for research participation.

The total sample of subjects ($n = 255$) was predominantly white (75.3%) and included 12.5% African American, 2.7% Asian American, and 7.1% Hispanic patients. The group consisted of 72 (28.2%) female and 183 (71.8%) male subjects. Within the total sample, 14.5% of the subjects had the diagnosis of schizoaffective disorder. Of the patients diagnosed with schizophrenia, 47.5% had paranoid subtype, 18.4% had undifferentiated, 14.1% had residual, and 5.5% other subtypes.

Clinical evaluation

Relevant demographic and socioeconomic data, as well as extensive medical, neurological, and pharmacological history, were obtained. A physical examination was performed on all the subjects, and appropriate laboratory evaluations were ordered if indicated.

The following rating scales were used: Brief Psychiatric Rating Scale (BPRS) for overall psychopathology (Overall & Gorham, 1988); Scales for the Assessment of Positive and Negative Symptoms (SAPS and SANS, respectively) (Andreasen & Olsen, 1982), Abnormal Involuntary Movement Scale (AIMS) for TD (National Institute of Mental Health, 1975), and Gittelman–Klein Scale for Premorbid Asocial Adjustment (1969) (Gittelman-Klein & Klein, 1969). The inter-rater reliability (intraclass correlation coefficient) ranged from 0.77 to 0.89 for these scales. The daily doses of different neuroleptics at the time of assessment were converted to mg chlorpromazine equivalents or (CPZE) (Jeste & Wyatt, 1982). All the assessments were performed by members of the research team who were not treating those patients and who were blind to the other data.

Neuropsychological assessment

All subjects underwent a comprehensive neuropsychological evaluation (Heaton et al., 1994) that included: Vocabulary, Arithmetic, Comprehension, Digit Symbol, Block Design, Digit Span, Picture Completion, and Picture Arrangement subtests from the Wechsler Adult Intelligence Scale-Revised (WAIS-R; Wechsler, 1981); as well as Trails A, Trails B, Grooved Pegboard, Digit Vigilance, and the Booklet Category Test from the Halstead-Reitan Battery (Reitan & Wolfson, 1985); and Learning and Memory components of the Story and Figure Memory Tests (Heaton et al., 1991). Testing was conducted after patients were psychiatrically, medically, and pharmacologically stable for several weeks. All the neuropsychological tests were administered by experienced psychometrists in a standardized fashion.

To correct for demographic differences among subjects, raw scores on each test in the battery were converted to age-, gender-, and education-corrected T-scores (Heaton et al., 1991). In neurologically normal subjects, the T-Scores are normally distributed with a mean of 50 and a standard deviation (SD) of 10. Lower T-scores reflect greater degrees of neuropsychological impairment.

Statistical methods

To examine gender differences, we performed Mann–Whitney U Tests for each continuous variable using SPSS/PC Software Package. Chi-square tests of independence were performed to examine the gender differences in categorical variables. All the statistical tests were two-tailed. We selected for analysis only those clinical variables that had a minimum total sample size of 195, with the exception of the Gittelman–Klein Premorbid Asocial Adjustment Scale ($n = 126$). All analyses on neuropsychological variables were conducted on a sample of 123 patients. We did not examine the interactions of age, gender, and age of onset of schizophrenia in this analysis; the interactions have been reported elsewhere (Lindamer et al., 1999).

Results

Table 10.1 presents results of the Mann–Whitney U Tests for women and men with schizophrenia on demographic and clinical variables.

The female schizophrenic patients had a significantly later age of onset, had higher scores on the BPRS-Depression subscale, lower scores on the BPRS Negative Symptom subscale, lower scores on the SANS-Total, and received lower doses of antipsychotic medication, compared to their male counterparts. There was a trend for women with schizophrenia to have higher scores on the SAPS total and lower scores on the AIMS total than men with schizophrenia. The two genders did not differ in reported premorbid adjustment.

No significant gender differences were observed for any of the neuropsychological measures (see Table 10.2).

Discussion and summary

Consistent with the literature, our data showed that women were diagnosed with the symptoms of schizophrenia at a later age than men (Lewine, 1981; Loranger, 1984; Castle & Murray, 1993; Hafner et al., 1989; 1998; Angermeyer & Kuhn, 1988; Hambrecht et al., 1992). In addition, consistent with results of previous studies, we found male schizophrenics had more negative symptoms (Lewine, 1981; 1985; Runyon et al., 1985; Gur et al., 1996; Arnold et al., 1995; Shtasel et al., 1992). The findings of higher positive symptom (SAPS) scores in this group of female schizophrenics, although significant at a trend level only, are consistent with previous reports (Lewine, 1981; 1985; Goldstein et al., 1990; Bland, 1977; McGlashan & Bardenstein, 1990; Marneros, 1984). Some researchers have suggested that positive symptoms are more prominent in the earlier stages of schizophrenia, while negative symptoms are more typical of a more chronic course. The differing presentations of schizophrenia in men and women may be related to differences in the age at the onset of symptoms and duration of illness.

While women with schizophrenia had higher scores on the depression subscale of the BPRS, there were no gender differences on the Ham-D. The BPRS depression subscale consisted of three items: emotional withdrawal, motor retardation, and blunted affect, which represented a limited characterization of depression. As women with schizophrenia demonstrated slower performance on the Grooved Pegboard Test, which measures motor speed, the gender difference seen on the BPRS depression subscale might be due mostly to motor slowing.

Women with schizophrenia in our studies received lower daily doses of antipsychotics than men with schizophrenia, which is consistent with several ports in the

Table 10.1. Comparison of women and men with schizophrenia on demographic variables, clinical rating scales and premorbid adjustment. Means with (standard deviations) or percentages

	Women (n = 72)	Men (n = 183)	M-W U or X² P-value
Age (years)	60.4 (11.3)	57.6 (9.4)	NS
Education (years)	12.5 (2.5)	12.5 (2.7)	NS
Age of onset of illness (years)	38.0 (17.5)	29. (12.8)	0.001
Subtype (% paranoid)	55.6%	44.3%	NS
Daily neuroleptic dose (mg CPZE)	335 (722)	674 (1368)	0.010*
% On neuroleptic medication	72.9%	77.1%	NS
BPRS (total)	33.7 (8.6)	33.1 (9.0)	NS
BPRS (disorganization subscale)	5.9 (3.0)	5.7 (3.0)	NS
BPRS (depression subscale)	7.0 (3.1)	6.1 (2.8)	0.050*
BPRS (negative symptoms subscale)	5.0 (2.5)	5.0 (2.8)	0.004*
BPRS (hostility subscale)	5.6 (2.4)	5.6 (2.4)	NS
SAPS (total)	6.8 (4.1)	5.8 (3.9)	0.083**
SANS (total)	6.7 (4.0)	8.4 (4.4)	0.013*
Ham-D	10.6 (5.5)	9.7 (6.7)	NS
AIMS (total)	3.9 (3.8)	4.7 (3.7)	0.080**
GK-preadolescent*	1.6 (1.1)	1.6 (1.3)	NS
GK-adolescent*	1.8 (1.4)	2.0 (1.4)	NS
GK-total*	1.7 (1.2)	1.9 (2.0)	NS

Notes:

NS = non-significant.

* = significant.

** = trend.

literature (Hogarty et al., 1974; Seeman, 1985; Young & Meltzer, 1980). One study (Zito et al., 1987) reported higher mean doses (CPZE equivalents) in schizophrenic women than men, but this finding only approached significance. The authors, however, also noted that a disproportionate number of women in their study were treated with high potency neuroleptics.

The lack of gender differences on neuropsychological measures is similar to the results of several studies that found no differences in cognitive performance with schizophrenia shortly after the first episode between men and women (The Scottish Schizophrenia Research Group, 1987; Goldberg et al., 1995; Andia et al., 1995; Albus et al., 1997). Heaton and colleagues (1994) have previously reported that neuropsychological performance is unrelated to current age, age of onset, or duration of illness. On average, both men and women with schizophrenia in our sample performed in the mildly impaired range for both visual and verbal learning, as well

Table 10.2. Comparison of women and men with schizophrenia on neuropsychological variables

Neuropsychological test results (T-scores)	Women ($n=49$)	Men ($n=74$)	M-W U P-value
Verbal IQ	40.9 (10.1)	42.2 (10.4)	NS
Performance IQ	41.5 (10.0)	42.0 (9.5)	NS
Full scale IQ	40.2 (10.2)	40.9 (10.0)	NS
Information	44.7 (9.4)	47.2 (10.7)	NS
Digit span	41.9 (9.1)	42.1 (10.0)	NS
Vocabulary	45.0 (8.9)	45.9 (10.6)	NS
Arithmetic	40.5 (11.3)	40.2 (10.5)	NS
Comprehension	41.4 (9.9)	42.6 (10.2)	NS
Digit symbol	40.3 (6.5)	41.3 (7.6)	NS
Picture arrangement	44.6 (7.8)	44.9 (11.0)	NS
Picture completion	43.2 (11.7)	42.2 (9.8)	NS
Block design	45.3 (8.4)	43.9 (9.9)	NS
Category	40.8 (12.0)	42.9 (12.6)	NS
Trails A	39.5 (11.1)	39.0 (9.2)	NS
Trails B	37.9 (12.2)	38.4 (10.1)	NS
Pegs (dominant)	31.0 (11.2)	35.7 (12.3)	0.030*
Pegs (non-dominant)	32.0 (10.7)	34.7 (10.5)	NS
Visual learning	39.4 (9.6)	36.2 (9.7)	0.060**
Visual memory	50.2 (8.7)	51.7 (7.0)	NS
Story learning	38.4 (11.8)	38.5 (11.7)	NS
Story meaning	48.6 (16.3)	49.2 (13.4)	NS

Notes:

NS = non-significant.

* = significant.

** = trend.

as in the mildly impaired range on Trails A and B; borderline normal mean scores were recorded on most other neuropsychological measures.

One limitation of our studies was the differential recruitment of male and female subjects. A majority of our male subjects were recruited from the VA Medical Center while a majority of the females were recruited from the UCSD Psychiatric Outpatient Clinic. Because of these recruitment constraints, our male and female subject groups may not be representative of the same population. In addition, our sample was limited to outpatient schizophrenics. More severely impaired patients with schizophrenia may yield different patterns or degree of gender differences. Furthermore, we did not examine the possible confounding effects of other factors (e.g. subtype of schizophrenia) on gender differences in clinical presentation.

Finally, there is a possibility of a Type I error because of multiple comparisons between men and women with schizophrenia.

One possible explanation for the later onset of schizophrenic symptoms, the predominance of positive symptoms, and lower neuroleptic dose in women may lie in the interaction of dopamine and estrogen. Gender differences in dopamine metabolism have been demonstrated in the basal ganglia in rats (Becker, 1990). Bazzett and Becker (1994) demonstrated that 17–β-estradiol down-regulated rat D-2 receptors. Another study reported gender differences in basal extracellular striatal dopamine levels, with castrated male rats having 20% higher levels than ovariectomized females (Castner et al., 1993). Estrogens may be anti-dopaminergic in humans, thus performing a protective role in the development of schizophrenia in women. Riecher-Rossler et al. (1994) have proposed that estrogen may exert a neuroleptic-like effect. These investigators noted a significant relationship between general psychopathologic measures, as well as specific measures of psychosis, and serum estrogen levels. The study also found no correlation between estrogen levels and depression measures.

A number of researchers (Feinberg, 1983; Weinberger, 1987; Murray et al., 1988) have proposed neurodevelopmental hypotheses to explain the development and course of schizophrenia. A modified version of such an hypothesis may explain, in part, the observed gender differences in the clinical picture of schizophrenia (see Table 10.3). The available data from the literature do not suggest any large or consistent gender differences in genetic (family history) or perinatal (obstetric complications) predisposition to schizophrenia. The overall risk of schizophrenia is believed to be similar for the two genders, and our estimate of the earliest manifestation of such a risk, preadolescent adjustment, was comparable in men and women with schizophrenia. The age of onset of illness (especially that of positive symptoms) is however, later in women than in men. Improper or inadequate pruning of dopaminergic neurons during late adolescence causing hyperdopaminergic activity has been proposed to be responsible for the clinical onset of schizophrenia in predisposed individuals (Mednick & Cannon, 1991). Such pruning is reported to occur later in women (Wong et al., 1984) and may explain the later onset of the illness in females.

Finally, hypodopaminergia due to aging-related loss of dopamine neurons could result in the development and chronicity of negative symptoms. Again, there is a suggestion that the loss of dopamine neurons with aging is delayed in women, thereby conceivably leading to later and milder development of a deficit-type schizophrenia with predominantly negative symptoms. This may explain the association of schizophrenia in women with paranoid subtype, better prognosis, and a need for lower dosages of neuroleptics.

One may suggest that estrogen exerts a protective effect in female schizophrenic patients in term of delayed onset, less severe negative symptoms, and better prog-

Table 10.3. *Possible neurobiologic explanations for the gender differences in schizophrenia*

Clinical manifestations in women with schizophrenia	Presumed neurobiology
Early childhood maladjustment similar to that in men	Genetic and perinatal predisposition in the form of fixed brain lesions
Onset of positive symptoms later than in men	(Delayed) increase in DA activity due to improper pruning of DA neurons in selected brain regions
Development and chronicity of negative symptoms later and less severe than in men	(Delayed and less severe) decrease in DA activity due to loss of DA neurons

Note:
DA = dopamine.

nosis. However, the fact that the two genders do not seen to differ in genetic and perinatal predisposition argues against the possibility that the 'female schizophrenia' is different from the 'male schizophrenia.' Rather, estrogen and other modifying factors may influence the clinical manifestations of the same illness in women. The above hypothesis is speculative at this stage, and is somewhat simplistic. For example, the contributions of other neurotransmitter abnormalities have not been considered.

Studies are needed to examine the direct effects of estrogen on positive and negative symptoms in patients with schizophrenia. Such investigations may help in furthering our understanding of the heterogeneity of the disorder.

ACKNOWLEDGMENT

This work was supported, in part, by NIMH Grants MH43693, MH51459, MH45131, MH49671, and by the Department of Veterans Affairs, MH01580 and National Alliance for Research on Schizophrenia and Depression (NARSAD) Young Investigator Award.

REFERENCES

Affleck, J. W., Burns, J., & Forrest, A. D. (1976). Long-term follow-up of schizophrenia patients in Edinburgh. *Acta Psychiatrica Scandinavica*, 53, 227–37.

Albus, M., Hubmann, W., Mohr, F., Scherer, J., Sobizack, N., Franz, U., Hecht, S., Borrmann, M. & Wahlheim, C. (1997). Are there gender differences in neuropsychological performance in patients with first-episode schizophrenia? *Schizophrenia Research*, 28, 39–50.

American Psychiatric Association. *Diagnostic and Statistical Manual of Mental Disorders*, third edition – revised. (1987). Washington, DC: American Psychiatric Press.

American Psychiatric Association. *Diagnostic Criteria from DSM-IV.* (1994). Washington, DC: American Psychiatric Press.

Andia, A. M. & Zisook, S. (1991). Gender differences in schizophrenia: A literature review. *Annals of Clinical Psychiatry*, **3**, 333–40.

Andia, A. M., Zisook, S., Heaton, R. K., Hesselink, J., Jernigan, T., Kuck, J., Moranville, J. & Braff, D. L. (1995). Gender differences in schizophrenia. *Journal of Nervous and Mental Disease*, **183**, 522–8.

Andreasen, N. C. & Olsen, S. (1982). Negative vs. positive schizophrenia: definition and validation. *Archives of General Psychiatry*, **39**, 789–94.

Angermeyer, M. C. & Kuhn, L. (1988). Gender differences in age at onset of schizophrenia. *European Archives of Psychiatry and Clinical Neuroscience*, **237**, 351–64.

Angermeyer, M. C., Kuhn, L. & Goldstein, J. M. (1990). Gender and the course of schizophrenia: differences in treated outcomes. *Schizophrenia Bulletin*, **16**, 293–307.

Arnold, S. E., Gur, R. E., Shapiro, R. M, Fisher, K. R. Moberg P. J., Gibney, M. R., Gur, R. C., Blackwell P. & Trojanowski, J. Q. (1995). Prospective clinicopathologic studies of schizophrenia: accrual and assessment of patients. *American Journal of Psychiatry*, **152**, 731–7.

Aylward, E., Walker, E. & Bettes, B. (1984). Intelligence in schizophrenia: Meta-analysis of the research. *Schizophrenia Bulletin*, **10**(3), 430–59.

Bazzett, T. J. & Becker, J. B. (1994). Sex differences in the rapid and acute effects of estrogen on striatal D2 dopamine receptor binding. *Brain Research*, **637**, 163–72.

Becker, J. B. (1990). Direct effect of 17 beta-estradiol on striatum: sex differences in dopamine release. *Synapse*, **5**, 157–64.

Bilder, R. M., Turkel, E., Lipschutz-Broch, L. & Lieberman, J. A. (1992). Antipsychotic medication effects on neuropsychological functions. *Psychopharmacology Bulletin*, **28**, 353–66.

Bland, R. C. (1977). Demographic aspects of functional psychoses in Canada. *Psychiatrica Scandinavica*, **55**, 369–80.

Cadet, J. L., Lohr, J. B. & Jeste D. V. (1987). Tardive dyskinesia and schizophrenic burnout: the possible involvement of cytotoxic free radicals. In *Handbook of schizophrenia*, volume 2: *Neurochemistry and Pharmacology of Schizophrenia*, ed. F. A. Henns & L. E. DeLisi, Amsterdam: Elsevier Science Publishers.

Castle, D. J. & Murray, R. M. (1993). The epidemiology of late-onset schizophrenia. *Schizophrenia Bulletin*, **19**, 691–700.

Castner, S. A., Xiao, L. & Becker, J. B. (1993). Sex differences in striatal dopamine: in vivo microdialysis and behavioral studies. *Brain Research*, **610**, 127–34.

Ciompi, L. (1980). Catamnestic long-term study on the course of life and aging of schizophrenics. *Schizophrenia Bulletin*, **6**, 606–18.

Cowell, P. E., Kostianovsky, D. J., Gur, R. C., Turesky, B. I. & Gur, R. E. (1996). Sex differences in neuroanatomical and clinical correlations in schizophrenia. *American Journal of Psychiatry*, **153**(6), 799–805.

Crow, T. J. (1985). The two-syndrome concept: origins and current status. *Schizophrenia Bulletin*, **3**, 471–85.

Feinberg, I. (1983). Schizophrenia: caused by a fault in programmed synaptic elimination during adolescence? *Journal of Psychiatric Research*, **17**, 319–34.

Fenton, W.S. & McGlashan, T. H. (1991). Natural history of schizophrenia subtypes. II. Positive and negative symptoms and long-term course. *Archives of General Psychiatry*, 48, 978–86.

Flaum, M., Arndt, S. & Andreasen, N. C. (1990). The role of gender in studies of ventricle enlargement in schizophrenia: a predominantly male effect. *American Journal of Psychiatry*, 147, 1327–32.

Flaum, M., Swayze, V. W., O'Leary, D. S., Yuh, W. T. C., Ehrhardt, J. C., Arndt, S. V. & Andreasen, N. C. (1995). Effects of diagnosis, laterality, and gender on brain morphology in schizophrenia. *American Journal of Psychiatry*, 152(5), 704–14.

Flor-Henry, P. (1990). Influence of gender in schizophrenia as related to other psychopathological syndromes. *Schizophrenia Bulletin*, 16, 211–27.

Foulds, G. A. & Dixon, P. (1962). The nature of intellectual deficit in schizophrenia. *British Journal of Social Clinical Psychology*, 1, 199–207.

Gift, T. E., Harder, D. W., Ritzler, B. A. & Kokes, R. F. (1985). Sex and race of patients admitted for their first psychiatric hospitalizations: correlates and prognostic power. American Journal of Psychiatry, 142(12), 1447–9.

Gittelman-Klein, R. & Klein, D. F. (1969). Premorbid asocial adjustment and prognosis in schizophrenia. *Journal of Psychiatric Research*, 7, 35–53.

Goldberg, T. E., Berman, K. F. & Weinberger, D. R. (1995). Neuropsychology and neurophysiology of schizophrenia. *Current Opinions in Psychiatry*, 8, 34–40.

Goldstein, J. M. (1988). Gender differences in the course of schizophrenia. *American Journal of Psychiatry*, 145(6), 684–9.

Goldstein, J. M. & Link, B. G. (1988). Gender and the expression of schizophrenia. *Journal of Psychiatric Research*, 2, 141–55.

Goldstein, J. M. Santangelo, S. L., Simpson, J. C. & Tsuang, M. T. (1990). The role of gender in identifying subtypes of schizophrenia: a latent class analytic approach. *Schizophrenia Bulletin*, 16, 263–75.

Goldstein, J. M., Tsuang, M. T. & Faraone, S. V. (1989). Gender and schizophrenia: implications for understanding the heterogeneity of the illness. *Psychiatry Research*, 28, 243–53.

Gur, R. E., Mozley, P. D., Shtasel, D. L., Cannon, T. D., Gallacher, F., Turetsky, B., Grossman, R. & Gur, R. C. (1994). Clinical subtypes of schizophrenia: Differences in brain and CSF volume. *American Journal of Psychiatry*, 151(3) 343–50.

Gur, R. E., Petty, R. G., Turetsky, B. I. & Gur R. C. (1996). Schizophrenia throughout life: sex differences in severity and profile of symptoms. *Schizophrenia Research*, 21, 1–12.

Haas, G., Hein, D., Waked, W., Sweeney, J., Weiden, P. & Frances, A. (1989). Sex differences in schizophrenia. *Schizophrenia Research*, 2, 11.

Hafner, H., an der Heiden, W., Behrens, S., Gattaz, W. F., Hambrecht, M., Loffler, W., Maurer, K., Munk-Jorgensen, P., Nowotny, B., Riecher-Rossler, A. & Stein, A. (1998). Causes and consequences of the gender differences at onset of schizophrenia. *Schizophrenia Bulletin*, 24, 99–113.

Hafner, H., Reicher, A., Maurer, K., Loffler, K., Munk-Jorgensen, P. & Stromgren, E. (1989). How does gender influence age at first hospitalization for schizophrenia? *Psychological Medicine*, 19, 903–18.

Hafner, H., Riecher-Rossler, A., Maurer, K., Fatkenheuer B. & Loffler, W. (1992). First onset and early symptomatology of schizophrenia: a chapter of epidemiological and neurobiological research into age and sex differences. *European Archives of Psychiatry and Neurological Sciences,* 242, 109–18.

Hambrecht, M., Maurer, K., Hafner, H. & Sartorius, N. (1992). Transnational stability of gender differences in schizophrenia? An analysis based on the WHO study of determinants of outcome of severe mental disorders. *European Archives of Psychiatry and Clinical Neuroscience,* 242, 6–12.

Harris, M. J. & Jeste, D. V. (1988). Late-onset schizophrenia: an overview. *Schizophrenia Bulletin,* 14, 39–55.

Harrow, M., Westermeyer, J. F., Silverstein, M., Strauss, B. S. & Cohler, B. J. (1986). Predictors of outcome in schizophrenia: the process-reactive dimension. *Schizophrenia Bulletin,* 12, 195–207.

Heaton, R. K., Grant, I. & Matthews, C. G. (1991). *Comprehensive Norms for an Expanded Halstead-Reitan Battery: Demographic Corrections, Research Findings, and Clinical Applications.* Odessa, Florida: Psychological Assessment Resources, Inc.

Heaton, R. K., Paulsen, J., McAdams, L. A., Kuck, J., Zisook, S., Braff, D., Harris, M. J. & Jeste, D. V. (1994). Neuropsychological deficits in schizophrenia: relationship to age, chronicity and dementia. *Archives of General Psychiatry,* 51, 469–76.

Hoff, A. L., Neal, C., Kushner, M. & DeLisi, L. E. (1994). Gender differences in corpus callosum size in first-episode schizophrenics. *Biological Psychiatry,* 35, 913–19.

Hogarty, G. E., Goldberg, S. C., Schooler, N. A. & Ulrich, R. F. (1974). Drug and sociotherapy in the aftercare of schizophrenic patients: II. Two-year relapse rates. *Archives of General Psychiatry,* 31, 603–8.

Jeste, D. V. & Wyatt, R. J. (1982). *Understanding and Treating Tardive Dyskinesia.* New York: Guilford Press, Inc.

Jeste, D. V., Caligiuri, M. P., Paulsen, J. S., Heaton, R. K., Lacro, J. P., Harris, M. J., Bailey, A., Fell, R. L. & McAdams, L. A. (1995). Risk of tardive dyskinesia in older patients: a prospective longitudinal study of 266 outpatients. *Archives of General Psychiatry,* 52, 756–65.

Jeste, D. V., Symonds, L. L., Harris, M. J., Paulsen, J. S., Palmer, B. W., & Heaton, R. K. (1997). Non-dementia non-praecox dementia praecox?: late-onset schizophrenia. *American Journal of Geriatric Psychiatry,* 5, 302–17.

Lewine, R. R. J. (1981). Sex differences in schizophrenia: timing or subtype? *Psychological Bulletin,* 90, 432–44.

Lewine, R. R. J. (1985). Schizophrenia: an amotivational syndrome in men. *Canadian Journal of Psychiatry,* 30, 316–18.

Lewine, R. R. J., Gulley, L. R., Risch, S. C., Jewart, R. & Houpt, J. L. (1990). Sexual dimorphism, brain morphology, and schizophrenia. *Schizophrenia Bulletin,* 16(2), 195–203.

Lewine, R. R. J., Haden, C., Caudle, J. & Shurett, R. (1997). Sex-onset effects on neuropsychological function in schizophrenia. *Schizophrenia Bulletin,* 23, 51–61.

Lewine, R. R. J., Walker, E. F., Shurett, R., Caudle, J. & Haden, C. (1996). Sex differences in neuropsychological functioning among schizophrenic patients. *American Journal of Psychiatry,* 153, 1178–84.

Lindamer, L. A., Lohr, J. B., Harris, M. J. & Jeste, D. V. (1997). Gender, estrogen, and schizophrenia. *Psychopharmacology Bulletin,* 33, 221–8.

Lindamer, L. A., Lohr, J. B., Harris, M. J., McAdams, L. A. & Jeste, D. V. (1999). Gender-related clinical differences in older patients with schizophrenia. *Journal of Clinical Psychiatry*, 60, 61–7.

Loranger, A. W. (1984). Sex difference in age at onset of schizophrenia. *Archives of General Psychiatry*, 41, 157–61.

Loyd, D., Simpson, J. C. & Tsuang, M. T. (1985). Are there sex differences in the long-term outcome of schizophrenia? Comparison with mania, depression, and surgical controls. *Journal of Nervous and Mental Disease*, 173(11), 643–9.

Marneros, A. (1984). Frequency of occurrence of Schneider's first rank symptoms in schizophrenia. *European Archives of Psychiatry and Neurology Science*, 234, 78–82.

Marriott, P. & Hiep, A. (1978). Drug monitoring at an Australian depot phenothiazine clinic. *Journal of Clinical Psychiatry*, 39, 206–12.

McGlashan, T. H. & Bardenstein, K. K. (1990). Gender differences in affective, schizoaffective, and schizophrenic disorders. *Schizophrenia Bulletin*, 16, 319–29.

Mednick, S. A. & Cannon, T. D. (1991). Fetal development, birth, and the syndromes of adult schizophrenia. In *Fetal Neural Development and Adult Schizophrenia*, ed. S. A. Mednick, T. D. Cannon, C. E. Barr, M. Lyon, pp. 3–13. New York: Cambridge University Press.

Murray, R. M., Lewis, S. W., Owen, M. J., & Foerster, A. (1988). The neurodevelopmental origins of dementia praecox. In *Schizophrenia: The Major Issues*, ed. P. Bebbington & P. McGuffin, pp. 90–107. London: William Heinemann.

Nasrallah, H. A., Schwarzkopf, S. B., Olson, S. C. & Coffman, J. A. (1990). Gender differences in schizophrenia on MRI brain scans. *Schizophrenia Bulletin*, 16(2), 205–10.

National Institute of Mental Health. (1975). Abnormal Involuntary Movement Scale (AIMS). *Early Clinical Drug Evaluation Unit Intercom.*, 4, 3–6.

Nopoulos, P., Flaum, M. & Andreasen, N. C. (1997). Sex differences in brain morphology in schizophrenia. *American Journal of Psychiatry*, 154(12), 1648–54.

Nyman, A. K. & Jonsson, H. (1983). Differential evaluation of outcome in schizophrenia. *Acta Psychiatrica Scandinavica*, 68, 458–75.

Overall, J. E. & Gorham, D. R. (1988). The Brief Psychiatric Rating Scale (BPRS): recent developments in ascertainment and scaling. *Psychopharmacology Bulletin*, 24, 97–9.

Perlick, D., Mattis, S., Stastny, P. & Silverstein, B. (1992). Negative symptoms are related to both frontal and nonfrontal neuropsychologicl measure in chronic schizophrenia, *Archives of General Psychiaty*, 49, 2454–70.

Prudo, R. & Blum, H. M. (1987). Five-year outcome and prognosis in schizophrenia: a report from the London Field Research Centre of the International Pilot Study of Schizophrenia. *British Journal of Psychiatry*, 150, 345–54.

Reitan, R. M. & Wolfson, D. (1985). *The Halstead–Reitan Neuropsychological Test Battery*. Tuscon, Arizona: Neuropsychology Press.

Riecher-Rossler, A., Hafner, H., Stumbalum, M., Maurer, K. & Schmidt, R. (1994). Can estradiol modulate schizophrenic symptomatology? *Schizophrenia Bulletin*, 20, 203–13.

Runyon, N. W., Wagner, E. E. & Dambrot, F. H. (1985). Sex differences in acting out chronic undifferentiated schizophrenics. *Perceptual and Motor Skills*, 61, 631–5.

Salokangas, R. K. R. (1983). Prognostic implications of the sex of schizophrenic patients. *British Journal of Psychiatry*, 142, 145–51.

Saltz, B. L., Woerner, M. G., Kane, J. M., Leiberman, J. A., Alvir, J. M., Bergmann, K. J., Blank, K., Koblenzer, J. & Kahaner, K. (1991). Prospective study of tardive dyskinesa incidence in the elderly. *Journal of the American Medical Association*, 266, 2402–6.

The Scottish Schizophrenia Research Group. (1987). The Scottish first episode study. III. Cognitive performance. *British Journal of Psychiatry*, 150, 338–40.

Seeman, M. V. (1983). Interaction of sex, age, and neuroleptic dose. *Comprehensive Psychiatry*, 24(2), 125–8.

Seeman, M. V. (1985). Clinical and demographic correlates of neuroleptic response. *Canadian Journal of Psychiatry*, 30, 243–5.

Seeman, M. V. (1986). Current outcome in schizophrenia: women versus men. *Acta Psychiatrica Scandinavica*, 73, 609–17.

Shtasel, D. L., Gur R. E., Gallacher, F., Heimberg, C. & Gur, R. C. (1992). Gender differences in the clinical expression of schizophrenia. *Schizophrenia Research*, 7, 225–31.

Spitzer, R. L., Williams, J. B. W., Gibbon, M. & First, M. B. (1990). *User's Guide for the Structured Clinical Interview for DSM-III-R*. Washington, DC: American Psychiatric Press.

Szymanski, S., Lieberman, J. A., Alvir, J. M., Mayerhoff, D., Loebel, A., Geisler, S., Chakos, M., Koreen, A., Kane, J., Woerner, M. & Cooper, T. (1995). Gender differences in onset of illness, treatment response, course and biologic indexes in first-episode schizophrenic patients. *American Journal of Psychiatry*, 152, 698–703.

Tamminga, C. (1997). Gender and schizophrenia. *Journal of Clinical Psychiatry*, 58(suppl 15), 33–7.

Walter, B. J. & Keward, H. B. (1985). Gender differences in living conditions found among male and female schizophrenic patients: a follow-up study. *International Journal of Social Psychiatry*, 31, 205–61.

Wechsler, D. (1981). WAIS-R Manual. *Wechsler Adult Intelligence Scale-Revised*, 1st edn. New York: The Psychological Corporation.

Weinberger, D. R. (1987). Implications of normal brain development for the pathogenesis of schizophrenia. *Archives of General Psychiatry*, 44, 660–9.

Westermeyer, J. F. & Harrow, M. (1984). Prognosis and outcome using broad (DSM-II) and narrow (DSM-III) concepts of schizophrenia. *Schizophrenia Bulletin*, 10, 624–37.

Wong, D. F., Wagner, H. N. Jr., Dannals, R. F., Links, J. M., Frost, J. J., Ravert, H. T., Wilson, A. A. & Rosenbaum, A. E. (1984). Effects of age on dopamine and serotonin receptors measured by positron emission tomography in the living human brain. *Science*, 226, 1393–6.

Yassa, R. & Jeste, D. V. (1992). Gender differences in tardive dyskinesia: a critical review of the literature. *Schizophrenia Bulletin*, 18(4), 701–15.

Yassa, R., Uhr, S. & Jeste, D. V. (1991). Gender differences in chronic schizophrenia: need for further research. In *The Elderly With Chronic Mental Illness*, ed. E. Light & B. Lebowitz, pp. 16–31. New York: Springer.

Young, M. A. & Meltzer, H. Y. (1980). The relationship of demographic, clinical and outcome variables to neuroleptic treatment requirements. *Schizophrenia Bulletin*, 6, 88–101.

Zito, J. M., Craig, T. J. Wanderling, J. & Siegel, C. (1987). Pharmaco-epidemiology in 136 hospitalized schizophrenic patients. *American Journal of Psychiatry*, 144, 778–2.

11

Sex steroids and anxiety disorders

Teresa A. Pigott

Introduction

Anxiety disorders are much more prevalent in women than in men, perhaps due to the role of sex steroids in women. In addition to their purported role in the pathophysiology of anxiety, reproductive hormone cycles may also have a substantial impact on the clinical course of pre-existing anxiety conditions throughout the life cycle in women. With these issues in mind, this chapter will provide: (a) an overview of the potential impact of gender and aging on the epidemiology and clinical features of anxiety disorders; (b) a discussion of estrogen and progesterone's potential role in the pathogenesis and pathophysiology of anxiety disorders in females; and (c) a review of available data concerning the impact of reproductive transitions on the course of anxiety disorders throughout the female life cycle.

Anxiety disorder overview

Anxiety disorders represent the most common psychiatric disorders in the United States, with epidemiological surveys revealing that one out of four people will experience a lifetime anxiety disorder. Anxiety disorders affect more than 7% of adults in the United States. Female gender, age (<45 years), marital separation or divorce, and low socioeconomic status are all associated with a higher rate of anxiety disorders (Kessler et al., 1994; Regier et al., 1990).

Generalized anxiety disorder (GAD), panic disorder, agoraphobia, social phobia, obsessive–compulsive disorder (OCD), simple phobia, and Post-Traumatic Stress Disorder (PTSD) are all classified as anxiety disorders in DSM-IV (American Psychiatric Association, 1994). Women are two to three times as likely as men to have panic disorder (7.7% vs. 2.9%), agoraphobia (9.0% vs. 3.0%), simple phobia (13.9% vs. 7.2%), or PTSD (11.3% vs. 6.0%) during their lifetime. Although there is less of a gender difference, lifetime prevalence estimates suggest that women are also more likely to have OCD (3.1% vs. 2.0%) or social phobia (16.4% vs. 11.2%) during their lifetime than men (Bourdon et al., 1988; Breslau et al., 1990; Magee et al., 1996; Robins et al., 1984; Yonkers & Ellison, 1996). Unfortunately, data from these surveys also confirm that relatively few individuals who meet the full diagnostic criteria for an anxiety disorder receive any type of psychiatric treatment (Dick et al., 1994a, b; Kessler et al., 1994; Lindal & Stefansson, 1993; Weissman et al., 1994).

Anxiety disorders are typically associated with an early age of onset and chronic clinical course, and comorbid psychiatric conditions are very common. Depression is a particularly frequent complication of anxiety disorders, especially panic disorder, GAD, and OCD (Kessler et al., 1994; Keller & Hanks, 1993; Hollander et al., 1996; Breslau et al., 1995; Dick et al., 1994a; Regier et al., 1990; Weissman et al., 1994; Wittchen et al., 1994). Indeed, the presence of an anxiety disorder appears to increase the risk of subsequently developing a major depressive episode (Andrade et al., 1996; Boyd et al., 1990; Kessler et al., 1994; Robins et al., 1984). This finding has important implications since patients afflicted with complicated anxiety (anxiety disorder plus at least one comorbid psychiatric condition) appear to have more functional impairment and a poorer prognosis in comparison to uncomplicated anxiety disorder(s).

As a group, anxiety disorders are the most common psychiatric condition in the elderly (Blazer et al., 1991). Data from the largest reported community-based epidemiological studies of anxiety disorders in subjects aged 65 and over suggest that women continue to have a higher prevalence of anxiety disorders than men (Flint, 1994). The gender difference and overall prevalence of anxiety disorders, however, do appear to diminish with increasing age. In fact the majority of studies suggest that anxiety disorders are less common in the elderly than in younger adults. While it is unclear why this decrease in anxiety prevalence occurs in the elderly, it may in part reflect the difficulty accurately discriminating between symptoms of anxiety versus signs of chronic medical illnesses. This is a particularly vexing dilemma since most studies demonstrate that older patients with primary anxiety disorders often complain of diffuse systemic symptoms such as fatigue, malaise, muscle tension, and restlessness. More specific physiologic symptoms such as tachycardia or tachypnea are also not uncommon manifestations in the elderly (Livingston et al., 1997; Krasucki et al., 1998).

GAD and phobias account for most anxiety in late life, whereas panic disorder is rare. Agoraphobia, and possibly OCD in females, may emerge as a primary disorder in old age. Agoraphobia, which may represent as much as 80% of late-onset anxiety disorders, is often precipitated by stressful life events in older subjects. In contrast, the presence of simple phobia or panic disorder in elderly subjects, or OCD in geriatric males is most likely to represent either the persistence of the illness from younger years or a secondary condition or complication of a medical illness or pre-existing psychiatric disorder (Flint, 1994; Banazak, 1997; Livingston et al., 1997; Krasucki et al., 1998).

Follow-up studies conducted in subjects with anxiety disorders suggest that most pre-existing anxiety disorders do not remit during old age. Phobic anxiety is particularly persistent and refractory in geriatric females. Panic disorder and OCD exhibit a reduced likelihood of remission with increasing age in both sexes (Bland et al., 1997). The persistence of anxiety disorders into old age has a number of important consequences. Older subjects with anxiety continue to have substantial psychosocial impairment. Suicide in the elderly remains a major public health problem. The presence of an anxiety disorder appears to further enhance the risk of suicidal behavior in geriatric patients (Florio et al., 1997). In addition to an apparent increase in psychiatric morbidity, there is also evidence that the persistence of anxiety disorders into old age may be associated with medical complications and increased morbidity. For example, analysis of data collected during the large, long-term (32-year follow-up period) Normative Aging Study suggests that patients with anxiety disorders have an increased risk of fatal coronary artery disease, especially sudden cardiac death (Kawachi et al., 1994). These findings provide compelling support for the contention that anxiety disorders are associated with significant and life-long consequences (Flint, 1994; Banazak, 1997; Livingston et al., 1997; Krasucki et al., 1998).

The next section will review available data concerning the epidemiology and clinical features of the specific anxiety disorders with special attention to the potential impact of gender and age on the phenomenology and course of each anxiety disorder.

Specific anxiety disorders: Gender differences and aging effects

Generalized anxiety disorder (GAD)

GAD is one of the most common of the anxiety disorders. Data collected during the two largest community surveys conducted in the United States – the NIMH Epidemiological Catchment Area Study (ECA) and the National Comorbidity Survey (NCS) – estimate the lifetime prevalence rate for GAD at between 5% and 6% (Kessler et al., 1994; Boyd et al., 1990). Both studies also revealed that females were twice as likely as males to meet diagnostic criteria for GAD. In addition to a preponderance of females, data from the National Comorbidity Survey also found that GAD correlated with several other sociodemographic factors such as age (>24 years), marital status (separated, widowed, or divorced), and employment situation (unemployed or a homemaker). GAD was also significantly associated with severe functional impairment, increased utilization of medical and mental health services, and increased consumption of psychotropic medication (Wittchen et al., 1994). Usually chronic in course, GAD typically emerges during early adulthood. The presence of comorbid psychiatric conditions represents the rule in GAD, rather than the exception. Results from the NCS suggest that 90% of people with GAD will develop an additional psychiatric disorder during their lifetime. Depression, panic disorder, and social phobia are the most common comorbid psychiatric conditions that subsequently complicate GAD (Wittchen et al., 1994; Robins et al., 1984; Breslau et al., 1995).

Significant gender differences have been identified for GAD. Females are not only more likely to have GAD, but they are also more likely to have comorbid psychiatric disorder(s) (complicated GAD) in comparison to males with GAD. Mood disorders especially dysthymia are particularly common in GAD females (Wittchen et al., 1994). Genetic factors may be particularly instrumental in mediating the increased risk for comorbid depression in females with GAD. The interplay of various environmental factors is theorized to determine whether GAD or MDD develop as the phenotypic expression if the genotype is present and triggered within a susceptible individual (Kendler, 1996; Kendler et al., 1992b, 1995). The presence of comorbid conditions can have a substantial impact on the course of GAD. Complicated GAD appears to have a worse prognosis in comparison to the presence of GAD alone (Yonkers et al., 1996).

There is considerable evidence that the prevalence of GAD is maintained and may even increase with advancing age. This surprising finding likely reflects several factors. Individuals who develop GAD as adults often continue to have substantial symptoms throughout their geriatric years. In addition, the onset of GAD is not uncommon in the elderly. A recent systematic comparison of elderly subjects ($n = 44$) with persistent GAD and age-matched control subjects revealed that the GAD subjects had elevated levels of anxiety, worry, social fears, and depression. Interestingly, similar clinical features were present in the elderly GAD subjects regardless of whether the onset of GAD was in childhood or middle adulthood (Beck et al., 1996).

Panic disorder

Lifetime prevalence estimates for panic disorder in the ECA and NCS studies were 1.5% to 3.0%. Females were twice as likely as males to meet criteria for panic attacks and panic disorder (Regier et al., 1990; Eaton et al., 1991). Onset of panic is most often during early adulthood; onset after age 40 is rare. The mean age of onset for panic disorder is similar in males and females (Dick et al., 1994a). At least one-third of subjects with panic disorder in community surveys will also meet criteria for agoraphobia (Eaton et al., 1991; Joyce et al., 1989; Yonkers & Ellison, 1996). Panic disorder complicated by agoraphobia is associated with increased illness severity and a higher likelihood that comorbid psychiatric disorders will develop (Marshall, 1996).

Panic disorder is linked to a number of adverse consequences besides avoidance behavior. Increased utilization of medical and mental health services is consistently associated with a diagnosis of panic disorder (Hollifield et al., 1997; Katerndahl, 1990; Katerndahl & Realini, 1997). Subjects with panic disorder are at an increased risk for social impairment, relationship difficulties, and financial dependence. The NCS data indicated that panic disorder was associated with the most severe psychosocial impairment. Perhaps most surprising, panic disorder subjects have the worst outcome of the anxiety disorders, despite the finding that they have the highest utilization rates for all types of medical services, including mental health and general medical providers (Wittchen & Essau, 1993).

Panic disorder may also be linked to an additional and particularly ominous complication: suicidal behavior. ECA study results indicated that the presence of panic disorder, even in the absence of comorbid depression, was associated with an increased risk of suicide attempts (Weissman et al., 1989). More than 90% of individuals with panic disorder will develop a comorbid psychiatric disorder. Lifetime prevalence risks for major depressive episode (60% to 80%), alcohol abuse (40% to 50%), drug abuse (40% to 50%), and phobic disorders (40% to 50%) are all significantly elevated in subjects with primary panic disorder (Dick et al., 1994a; Yonkers & Ellison, 1996; Yonkers et al., 1998). Results from the largest prospective study of panic disorder to date (the HARP Study) estimate that almost half of panic patients will remain in treatment after a year and 20% to 40% will require maintenance treatment (Keller & Hanks, 1993).

Panic disorder has several important gender differences. Females with panic disorder endorse more individual symptoms of anxiety and more extensive phobic avoidance (Dick et al., 1994a). Data from the NCS reveal that the peak onset of panic disorder is earlier in females (age 20 to 30 years) than males (age 25 to 34 years; Wittchen & Essau, 1993). Comorbid psychiatric conditions, such as agoraphobia, depression, GAD, simple phobia, and somatization disorder, are significantly more likely to occur in females with panic disorder (Yonkers & Ellison, 1996; Yonkers et al., 1998; Marshall, 1996; Katerndahl, 1990; Andrade et al., 1996). In contrast, alcohol abuse and dependence is consistently reported more often in males with panic disorder (Cox et al., 1993). Although panic disorder males have a relatively greater incidence of comorbid alcohol abuse, comorbid alcohol abuse and dependence are not uncommon in women with panic disorder (Kessler et al., 1994; Otto et al., 1992). Gender differences in the course of panic disorder have also been reported. Multiple studies have demonstrated that panic disorder in females is characterized by relatively greater symptom severity, a more chronic course, and increased functional impairment in comparison to males with panic disorder

(Andrade et al., 1996; Boyd et al., 1990; Hollifield et al., 1997; Katerndahl & Realini, 1997; Joyce et al., 1989). Long-term follow-up data also suggest that females are more likely to have recurrence of panic symptoms after a period of remission occurs (Yonkers et al., 1998).

Although the overall prevalence of panic disorder decreases with increasing age, panic disorder generally persists into later life with similar symptomatology and enduring avoidance behaviors (Sheikh et al., 1991). Although relatively rare, panic disorder can also first present at an advanced age. Preliminary data suggest that a substantial portion of elderly subjects will endorse late-onset panic disorder (after age 60). Factors contributing to onset of panic in the elderly include stress, medical illness, and central nervous system disease (Raj et al., 1993). Characteristics associated with late-onset vs. early-onset panic disorder include fewer panic symptoms, less avoidance behaviors, frequent complaints of shortness of breath during panic attacks, and an elevated rate of comorbid medical disorders like chronic obstructive pulmonary disease, vertigo, and Parkinson's disease (Raj et al., 1993; Sheikh, 1993). Although a history of alcohol abuse or dependence predicts a significantly elevated panic disorder risk in younger individuals, this is not the case for panic disorder when it persists or emerges at an advanced age (Krystal et al., 1992). Unfortunately, the majority of elderly subjects with panic disorder have not received adequate treatment (Sheikh et al., 1991). Given the association of panic disorder with an elevated risk of suicide and an increased cardiovascular mortality rate, the lower prevalence of panic disorder in the elderly may partially result from panic patients not surviving into old age (Weissman et al., 1989; Coryell, 1988).

Simple phobia

According to the ECA and the National Comorbidity Survey, phobias (simple phobia, agoraphobia, and social phobia) represent the most common psychiatric disorders in the United States. Simple phobia and agoraphobia were significantly more likely to be identified in females, younger age groups, and in subjects with lower socioeconomic status (Boyd et al., 1990). Agoraphobia and simple phobia were frequently associated with comorbid depression, substance abuse, and OCD (Bourdon et al., 1988; Eaton et al., 1991; Kessler et al., 1994; Regier et al., 1990; Magee et al., 1996).

Community surveys estimate that simple phobias occur in 20% of adults; females are afflicted twice as often as males (Boyd et al., 1990; Bourdon et al., 1988; Dick et al., 1994b). Simple phobias can be classified into three distinct classes: (a) situational phobias (claustrophobia, acrophobia, etc.); (b) animal phobias (fear of spiders, insects, snakes, etc.); and (c) health-related phobias (fear of injections, blood, dental procedures, etc.). Situational phobias appear to be most prevalent, followed by animal and health-related phobias, respectively. Situational and animal phobias are reportedly two to three times more common in females, but health-related phobias are similar in gender prevalence (Fredrikson et al., 1996).

There is some evidence that the onset of simple phobia in females is earlier than in males (Dick et al., 1994b). Although agoraphobia and simple phobia tend to be chronic in course, only 20% to 25% of patients appear to enter treatment (Lindal & Stefansson, 1993; Boyd et al., 1990). Phobic disorders often aggregate in families. Results from female twin studies suggest that vulnerability for simple phobia is largely determined by environmental, rather than genetic influences. In contrast, the risk for agoraphobia is likely to arise primarily from genetic factors, with only a small contribution from nonspecific environmental influences (Kendler et al., 1992a).

Limited data are available concerning the impact of aging on the phenomenology or course of simple phobia or agoraphobia. Onset of agoraphobia has been described in elderly subjects, particularly after a debilitating physical illness. Phobic disorders are associated with increased medical and psychiatric morbidity in elderly subjects (Lindesay, 1991). Phobic fear of crime may be particularly prevalent among the elderly (Clarke & Lewis, 1982).

Social phobia

Although the ECA data suggested that social phobia was relatively rare at just 3% lifetime prevalence rate (Schneier et al., 1992; Boyd et al., 1990), subsequent community surveys including the NCS have demonstrated much higher lifetime prevalence rates of 13% (Kessler et al., 1994; Stein, 1997). Inadequate recognition of social phobia is likely to contribute to the discrepancies that have occurred in estimating the prevalence of social phobia, especially in the primary care setting where most of these patients are likely to initially present for evaluation. This issue is aptly demonstrated by the results of a recent large-scale study concerning the prevalence of social phobia in primary care settings. Less than 50% of the patients meeting criteria for social phobia were identified by their primary care physician as 'having a psychiatric illness' (Lecrubier & Weiller, 1997). Only a fourth of those patients were correctly identified as meeting criteria for social phobia. Instead, most of the patients meeting criteria for social phobia received a diagnosis of panic disorder, GAD, or depression. More than 85% of the social phobics with a co-existing psychiatric disorder were misdiagnosed (Lecrubier & Weiller, 1997; Bisserbe et al., 1996).

Women are estimated to be 1.5 times more likely than men to meet criteria for social phobia (Kessler et al., 1994; Dick et al., 1994b). Two social phobia subtypes (generalized and discrete) have been identified. The generalized subtype includes individuals with a broad range of social fears including performance and interactional anxiety, whereas the discrete subtype includes individuals with situational anxiety such as public speaking phobia or performance anxiety. Research data suggest that the two subtypes of social phobia are remarkably similar in terms of age of onset, family history, and certain sociodemographic correlates (Kessler et al., 1998; Stein, 1997). Discrete social phobia generally has an episodic course and only minor functional impairment (Stein, 1997). In contrast, generalized social phobia is more likely to be associated with a chronic clinical course, substantial functional impairment, and comorbid psychiatric conditions (Kessler et al., 1998).

The onset of social phobia is very early. Comorbid psychiatric disorders emerge in at least two-thirds of social phobics during their lifetime (Schneier et al., 1992; Stein, 1997; Kessler et al., 1998). Comorbid depression (60% to 90%) and alcohol abuse (30% to 40%) frequently complicate generalized social phobia (Kessler et al., 1994, 1998; Stein, 1997; Dick et al., 1994b). There is considerable evidence of overlap between generalized social phobia and avoidant personality disorder. That is, the vast majority of patients with generalized social phobia (70% to 90%) will also meet diagnostic criteria for avoidant personality disorder. The co-occurrence of social phobia and avoidant personality disorder may increase the risk of development of depressive disorder, especially atypical depression. Moreover, patients meeting criteria for both social phobia and avoidant personality disorder are more likely to have more severe impairment in comparison to patients with social phobia alone (Alpert et al., 1997). Although social phobia tends to be chronic in course, relatively few (20% to 25%) patients appear to enter treatment (Kessler et al., 1994; Boyd et al., 1990). This is a particularly surprising finding since social phobia is often associated with considerable disability and a diminished quality of life. In addition to an elevated rate of alcohol and drug abuse, social phobics appear to have an increased risk of prescription drug abuse (Bisserbe et al., 1996; Lecrubier & Weiller, 1997). Social phobia is also linked to an increased utilization of medical and health services, although apparently to a lesser degree than that associated with panic disorder (Stein, 1997). Initial analysis of the ECA data suggested that social phobia might be similar to panic disorder in terms of conveyance of an increased risk of suicidal behavior. However, further analyses revealed that the increase in suicide attempts in the social phobics was mainly attributable to the presence of comorbid conditions, especially depression. (Schneier et al., 1992).

There are relatively limited data available concerning potential gender differences in social phobia. Females with social phobia, in comparison to males with social phobia, may have an increased risk for developing agoraphobia (Dick et al., 1994b; Lecrubier & Weiller, 1997).

The effect of aging on social phobia is largely undetermined. A magnetic resonance imaging (MRI) study revealed evidence of structural brain differences with advancing age in social phobic subjects; greater age-related reductions in the volume of the putamen were detected in the social phobic vs. control subjects (Potts et al., 1994). However, the clinical relevance of this finding remains unclear. Preliminary investigations suggest that social phobia is chronic, unremitting, and persists into old age (Blazer et al., 1991). Elderly subjects with social phobia may be more likely to complain of distress associated with eating or writing in public, stressful situations that are further exaggerated by the increasing chance of tremors or wearing dentures with advancing age.

OCD

One of the most surprising findings from the ECA study was the relatively high life-time prevalence rate estimated for OCD (2% to 3%) in the United States (Karno et al., 1988). The subsequent Cross-National Collaborative Group Study that included six international sites also estimated the lifetime prevalence rate for OCD between 2.0% and 2.5% (Weissman et al., 1994). Results from most studies suggest that women are 1.5 times more likely than men to have OCD during their lifetime (Weissman et al., 1994).

OCD has been associated with a number of adverse psychosocial and economic consequences. Significant psychosocial difficulties and occupational dysfunction have been reported in 60% to 70% of OCD patients (Koran et al., 1996; Hollander et al., 1998). OCD is also associated with considerable morbidity as evidenced by relatively elevated utilization rates for medical and mental health services (Hollander et al., 1998; Kennedy & Schwab, 1997). The total yearly cost of OCD is estimated to exceed $8 billion dollars (Dupont et al., 1995). Most data suggest that OCD remains under-recognized and under-treated. In fact, results from a recent survey suggest that the average delay between onset of OCD and initial contact with a mental health or medical professional exceeds ten years (Hollander et al., 1998).

Most patients with OCD will have at least one additional lifetime psychiatric disorder. Major depressive disorder appears to be the most common co-existing (30% to 50%) and lifetime (60% to 85%) diagnosis in OCD, but coexisting anxiety disorders are also very prevalent (40%; Antony et al., 1998; Pigott et al., 1994; Weissman et al., 1994; Rasmussen & Eisen, 1992). Panic disorder and social phobia represent the most frequent anxiety diagnoses complicating OCD (Pigott et al., 1994; Rasmussen & Eisen, 1992). Substance abuse, schizophrenia, body dysmorphic disorder, hypochondriasis, Tourette's Syndrome, and anorexia nervosa are other comorbid conditions routinely reported in OCD patients (Pigott et al., 1994; Rasmussen & Eisen, 1992; Antony et al., 1998; Weissman et al., 1994). As illustrated by these results, relatively few patients with OCD will be free of co-existing psychiatric conditions. Comorbid panic disorder, obsessions about aggressive impulses, and cleaning compulsions are reported to occur more frequently in females than males with OCD (Noshirvani et al., 1991; Lensi et al., 1996; Castle et al., 1995). Interestingly, the presence of comorbid anxiety disorders or specific OCD symptom constellations appear to have little impact on the course, prognosis, or treatment response in patients with OCD (Steketee et al., 1997; Demal et al., 1993).

Several studies have systematically investigated the potential impact of gender on

OCD. Community surveys suggest that the onset of OCD is later in females (mean age 25 years) than in males (mean age 20 years; Neziroglu et al., 1994; Thomsen & Mikkelsen, 1995). A greater history of perinatal trauma, a higher frequency of intrusive thoughts about sex, exactness, and symmetry obsessions, and an increased rate of atypical rituals have all been associated with males with early onset OCD. In the same study, females with OCD were reported to have a later onset, an elevated rate of comorbid panic, and a higher frequency of aggressive obsessions (Lensi et al., 1996).

A particular fascinating finding is that prior to puberty, three times as many boys as girls are diagnosed with OCD. After puberty, the incidence of OCD markedly increases in females and eventually surpasses males (Weissman et al., 1994; Karno et al., 1988). This finding, in particular, has elicited considerable interest in the potential impact of sex steroids in the pathophysiology of OCD.

These observations have elicited considerable speculation concerning the role of genetic vs. hormonal influences in determining propensity for OCD. Genetic factors are often implicated in boys who develop OCD, since it is often characterized by a prepubertal onset, greater familial loading, and an increased risk of comorbid tic disorders. Females who develop OCD, in contrast, may be more likely to have a relatively late (postmenarche) onset and a more episodic clinical course (Hantouche & Lancrenon, 1996; Thomsen & Mikkelsen, 1995). As a result, neuro-endocrine factors such as the sex steroids may play an important role in determining risk for OCD development in females. Sex steroids are also often implicated in the underlying pathophysiology of anorexia and bulimia nervosa. Interestingly, both anorexia nervosa and bulimia nervosa are reported to frequently coexist in females with OCD (Rubenstein et al., 1992).

OCD, as has previously been noted in panic disorder, has a decreased likelihood of remission with increasing age (Bland et al., 1997). The onset of OCD can also, on rare occasions, occur in the elderly. Follow-up data from subjects that initially participated in the ECA survey revealed a relatively high rate of new cases of OCD in elderly females, although this finding may in part reflect differences in diagnostic classification systems used (Nestadt et al., 1998). A systematic comparison of the clinical features of elderly vs. younger OCD patients revealed relatively few differences. The elderly OCD patients were noted to have a later age at onset, more frequent hand-washing rituals and obsessions about sin, and relatively less symmetry obsessions and counting rituals (Kohn et al., 1997).

PTSD

Although many individuals are exposed to trauma, only one out of four will develop PTSD (Breslau et al., 1990). Community surveys consistently report that the lifetime prevalence rate for PTSD is greater in females (12.5%) than males

(6.2%; Drummond, 1993). Although many individuals are exposed to trauma, only one out of four will develop PTSD (Breslau et al., 1990). The most common cause of PTSD in men is combat exposure. In contrast, women are most likely to develop PTSD as a consequence of a physical and/or sexual assault or threat, a life-threatening experience, or witnessing a life-threatening event. PTSD is often complicated by comorbid conditions such as depression and alcohol abuse (Breslau et al., 1997).

The gender difference in prevalence of PTSD has been linked to a differential rate of exposure to trauma. However results from several studies suggest that women are not more likely than men to be exposed to trauma (Breslau et al., 1990, 1995, 1997; Kessler & McLeod, 1984). Instead, men appear to be less likely to develop PTSD as a sequelae of trauma. These issues are illustrated by a recent study reported by Breslau and colleagues (1997). Despite the lack of gender differences in the amount or rate of exposure to traumatic events in a sample of over 1000 young adults, substantially more of the women than the men met criteria for PTSD (Breslau et al., 1997). They also carefully examined potential confounding factors such as the increased prevalence of pre-existing anxiety or major depressive disorders in females, but such factors contributed relatively little to the observed sex difference in PTSD. Instead, the females appeared to have a markedly increased susceptibility to develop PTSD after a traumatic experience. Moreover, females were particularly vulnerable to PTSD development if the traumatic exposure occurred prior to age 15 (Breslau et al., 1997).

Major depression and generalized anxiety disorder are common comorbid disorders in PTSD regardless of gender, whereas coexisting somatoform pain disorder is more common only in females with PTSD. There is also evidence of gender differences in neuroendocrine function between males and females with PTSD. Although male combat veterans with PTSD display elevated norepinephrine-to-cortisol ratios, females with PTSD do not display this pattern. Instead, females with PTSD demonstrate significantly elevated daily levels of urinary norepinephrine, epinephrine, dopamine, and cortisol (Lemieux & Coe, 1995).

PTSD is frequently a chronic disorder that persists into old age. Moreover, accumulating evidence suggests that PTSD can develop in old age. Preliminary data from survivors of the 1988 Armenian earthquake reveal that the overall severity of PTSD is independent of age of exposure. The elderly survivors reported less re-experiencing symptomatology but more signs of hyperarousal when compared to younger survivors (Goenjian et al., 1994).

PTSD has also been investigated in elderly subjects who were exposed to combat or war-related atrocities in early adulthood. Almost 25% of US men over the age of 55 are combat veterans. More than 40 years after exposure to moderate or heavy combat in World War II, veterans were 13 times more likely to have PTSD symptoms than noncombat veterans in a recent study conducted in aging men (Spiro et al., 1994). Elderly subjects who were former World War II prisoners of war (POWs) had greatly elevated rates of PTSD and a moderately elevated lifetime prevalence rate for depressive disorders in comparison to age-matched control subjects. POWs who lost more than 35% of their body weight during captivity were particularly symptomatic. They had higher rates of PTSD, depressive disorders, and schizophrenia compared with the other POWs (Eberly & Engdahl, 1991). Examinations of elderly subjects who are survivors of the Holocaust have provided important information concerning the impact of factors such as age at exposure and cumulative life stressors on PTSD occurrence and phenomenology. Results from these studies suggest that the earlier the age of trauma exposure, the more likely that psychogenic amnesia, hypervigilence, and emotional detachment will occur as manifestations of PTSD. In contrast, a positive correlation between age and intrusive thoughts was observed. Cumulative lifetime stress was positively associated with symptoms of avoidance (Yehuda et al., 1997).

Significant gender differences have been identified in the prevalence, phenomenology, and course of anxiety disorders. In addition, a growing body of evidence suggests that anxiety disorders often persist and can even emerge during old age. Considerable research efforts have recently focused on the potential role of female sex hormones in the development and persistence of anxiety disorders in women across the life cycle. With this in mind, the next section will review the purported neurobiological actions associated with estrogen and progesterone and their potential role in the pathophysiology of pathological anxiety states.

Sex steroids and neurotransmission

Dysregulation of noradrenergic, serotonergic, GABAergic, and dopaminergic pathways have all been implicated in the pathophysiology of anxiety disorders. Data from functional imaging studies such as positron emission tomography (PET) scans have also revealed abnormal patterns of cortical and subcortical activity in anxiety patients (Johnson et al., 1998). Several lines of evidence support the role of the sex steroids estrogen and progesterone in the synthesis, release, turnover, and metabolism of neurotransmitters critical in the mediation of anxiety and the regulation of the stress response. The changing levels of sex steroids during menstruation and after menopause may substantially impact the relative risk for development and clinical course of anxiety disorders in women.

Estrogen

Estrogen can influence monoamine synthesis and metabolism, as well as the responsiveness of various monoamine receptors within the brain (Halbreich,

1997b). Estrogen inhibits monoamine oxidase (MAO), the major enzyme responsible for metabolizing norepinephrine. As a result of the inhibition of MAO, norepinephrine concentrations are increased within the brain (Chakravorty & Halbreich, 1997). Estrogen also influences norepinephrine function by its effect on the α_2-adrenergic receptor. The α_2-adrenergic receptor, an autoreceptor, acts as a 'brake' for the norepinephrine system. That is, rising norepinephrine concentrations within the synaptic cleft stimulate the α_2-adrenergic receptor to respond. Stimulation of the α_2-adrenergic receptor results in inhibition of further norepinephrine release from the pre-synaptic neuron into the synapse. Estrogen is able to diminish the responsiveness of the α_2-adrenergic receptor when it is stimulated (Etgen & Karkanias, 1994; Stahl, 1997; Schmidt et al., 1997).

Estrogen's effects on norepinephrine via the α_2-adrenergic receptor are implicated in the gender differences identified in the stress response between males and females. After administration of a pharmacological agent that selectively blocks the α_2-adrenergic receptor, males have a much greater release of norepinephrine in comparison to females (Schmidt et al., 1997; Etgen & Karkanias, 1994). Results from a recent PET scan study demonstrate gender differences in brain activity when subjects are administered agents that block the α_2-adrenergic receptor. Global increases in brain metabolism were detected in females, whereas no detectable change in global brain metabolism was identified in males (Schmidt et al., 1997). While estrogen appears to blunt the stress-induced response via its actions on the α_2-adrenergic receptor, it has also been implicated in the exaggerated physiological stress response that occurs during estrogen withdrawal states. For example, the increased risk of cardiovascular disease in postmenopausal women has been linked in part to the loss of estrogen's purported restraint of the stress response (Fink et al., 1996; Etgen & Karkanias, 1994).

Estrogen also influences dopamine. Estrogen reduces the primary enzyme responsible for metabolism of dopamine: tyrosine hydroxylase. Several lines of evidence suggest that estrogen may possess some anti-dopaminergic or neuroleptic-like action. Estrogen is associated with a significant increase in dopamine-2 (D_2) receptors in the striatum in animal studies (Fink et al., 1996). Moreover, the later age of onset of schizophrenia in females has been linked to estrogen's actions on dopamine and there is some evidence that estrogen replacement therapy (ERT) may enhance neuroleptic response in female schizophrenics (Lindamer et al., 1997). Estrogen's anti-dopaminergic actions have also been implicated in the pathophysiology of postpartum psychosis (Halbreich & Tworek, 1993; Vinogradov & Csernansky, 1990).

Estrogen's impact on serotonin may be particularly critical to the development of anxiety disorders. Estrogen enhances serotonin function by increasing serotonin transporter sites and decreasing monoamine oxidase enzyme activity (Stahl, 1997;

Chakravorty & Halbreich, 1997). Estrogen also appears to be integral to maintaining optimal serotonin function. Data from pharmacological challenge studies reveal that post-menopausal women display evidence of a reduced serotonin response. However, addition of estrogen via ERT has been reported to effectively 'normalize' serotonin responsiveness in postmenopausal women (Halbreich et al., 1995). Estrogen may also have a role in the down-regulation of serotonin receptors that is felt to be critical to the onset of antidepressant action. Animal studies have long suggested that estrogen must be present before the serotonin receptor adaptations associated with antidepressant action can occur (Kendall et al., 1982). Reanalysis of data from a multicenter geriatric depression study of fluoxetine revealed that elderly, depressed women were more likely to respond if they were also receiving ERT (Schneider et al., 1997).

Progesterone

Relatively less information is available concerning progesterone's purported actions within the brain. Progesterone has been associated with well-documented dysphoric effects and more recently has been linked to anxiolytic-like effects (Sherwin, 1991; Halbreich, 1997a). The purported dysphoric and anxiolytic-like actions are linked to progesterone's actions at the GABA–benzodiazepine receptor complex (GBRC; Kroboth & McAuley, 1997; Majewska et al., 1986; Majewska, 1992).

GABA is one of the major inhibitory neurotransmitters in the brain. The GBRC refers to the receptor complex comprising the GABA-A receptor, an adjoining chloride channel, and in close proximity, a benzodiazepine receptor site. The GABA-A receptor acts as a gatekeeper for the chloride channel. Binding of the neurotransmitter, GABA, to the GABA-A receptor site results in conductance of chloride through the channel. If GABA is not bound to the GABA-A receptor, the channel will remain closed to chloride conductance. Binding of a benzodiazepine to the benzodiazepine receptor will not result in chloride conduction through the channel unless GABA is also bound to its receptor. However, the benzodiazepine receptor can act as an allosteric modulator for GABA. That is, if GABA is present at the GABA-A receptor, subsequent binding of a benzodiazepine will result in enhanced chloride conductance (Stahl, 1996). Progesterone may also function as an allosteric modulator of GABA, although its effect is relatively weak in comparison to a benzodiazepine (Jensvold et al., 1996; Janowsky et al., 1996). These allosteric modulating functions at the GBRC complex are thought to mediate the anxiolytic and sedating properties associated with benzodiazepine, and perhaps progesterone, administration in humans.

Progesterone's actions at the GBRC may help to explain the finding that women taking oral contraceptive medication appear to have enhanced sedation, increased amnestic effects, and greater psychomotor impairment when administered benzodiazepine medication (Kroboth & McAuley, 1997). This finding may have important implications for the treatment of anxiety symptoms in women. It suggests that women taking oral contraceptives may require benzodiazepine dose reduction. In addition, this data suggest that HRT or adjunctive progesterone therapy should be considered in women with anxiety disorders who fail, or only partially respond to, benzodiazepine or other anxiolytic medication strategies.

Many of progesterone's neurobiological effects appear to oppose the actions of estrogen. For example, progesterone enhances MAO enzyme activity (Chakravorty & Halbreich, 1997). Progesterone is also responsible for dismantling synapses within the myometrium that were initially constructed under the influence of estrogen at the beginning of the menstrual cycle. Progesterone's role in increasing monoamine catabolism, disrupting synapses, and enhancing GABA-ergic tone all contribute to the anxiolytic and mood de-stabilizing effects associated with progesterone (Jensvold et al., 1996; McEwen & Parsons, 1987; Janowsky et al., 1996; Sherwin, 1991). Progesterone's impact on mood and anxiety can have important clinical ramifications. Adding progesterone to estrogen replacement therapy may effectively neutralize the mood-enhancing effects associated with estrogen administration. (Stahl, 1997; Holst et al., 1989; McEwen, 1991; Sherwin, 1996; Yen & Jaffe, 1986; Jensvold et al., 1996; Janowsky et al., 1996). In addition, estrogen's ability to alter the stress response in postmenopausal women may be attenuated by the addition of progesterone (Lindheim et al., 1994). It is, however, important to note that progesterone has an extremely complex metabolism. Multiple metabolic pathways have been identified for progesterone and many of progesterone's metabolites also possess biological activity. As a result, the specific metabolic pathway utilized largely determines the net biological effect associated with progesterone (Majewska et al., 1986; Majewska, 1992).

In summary, estrogen's neurobiological actions include enhancement of serotonin neurotransmission, neuroleptic-like activity via dopamine receptor blockade, and restraint of the stress response through modulation of adrenergic pathways. In contrast, progesterone's actions largely oppose estrogen's effects. Serotonergic and noradrenergic neurotransmission are attenuated by progesterone's promotion of MAO activity. Moreover, progesterone's complex effects at the GBRC result in enhanced GABA-ergic tone. The biological basis of anxiety is most often linked to dysfunction of the serotonergic and noradrenergic pathways, the GABA-ergic system, and/or dysregulation of the HPA axis-catecholamine stress response. The considerable overlap between the sex steroids' identified biological actions within the brain and the neural pathways that mediate anxiety provides at least circumstantial evidence implicating sex steroids in the development of anxiety states. Examination of data on the relationship between hormones and anxiety symptoms may give us insight into the relationships of sex steroids and anxiety in aging.

Female reproductive cycles impact on course of anxiety

Complaints of increased anxiety, dysphoria, and affective lability are relatively common in females during the premenstrual phase. These symptoms are thought to arise from the precipitous drop in circulating estrogen and progesterone concentrations that occurs in the four to five days prior to onset of menstruation. Preliminary evidence suggests that females who present with severe menstrual-related symptoms have an increased risk of later developing anxiety disorders (Yonkers, 1997). Given their multiple neurobiological actions, it is likely that relatively large fluctuations in sex steroids associated with the normal female menstrual cycle may trigger momentary changes in neurotransmission. The precipitous, premenstrual drop in estrogen is likely to result in diminished serotonergic responsiveness and loss of restraint upon the stress response on at least a transitory basis. In addition, decreased GABA-ergic tone may briefly occur as a consequence of the declining progesterone concentrations during the premenstrual phase. These transient, menstrual phase-induced alterations in neurotransmitter function might have a substantial impact in the context of ongoing pathological anxiety states.

Several case reports have suggested that panic patients experience an increase in anxiety and frequency of panic attacks during the premenstrual phase (Yonkers et al., 1998; Cohen et al., 1994; Altshuler et al., 1998). Preliminary evidence also suggests premenstrual worsening in OCD symptoms (Yaryura Tobias et al., 1995; Williams & Koran, 1997).

Menopause and the perimenopause have been associated with an increased risk of depressive and anxiety symptoms, presumably due to estrogen withdrawal. Relatively few women, however, will meet full criteria for a mood (13% to 20%) or an anxiety disorder (7% to 14%) during menopause or peri-menopause (Sherwin, 1996). The relatively gradual and protracted time of transition into menopause may serve to attenuate the risk of new onset anxiety disorders during this time period. There is some evidence that the perimenopausal in comparison to postmenopausal period may be associated with relatively greater levels of anxiety and/or psychological distress. Relatively high levels of FSH during the perimenopause may be associated with a subsequent increase in risk for depressive or anxiety disorders (Huerta et al., 1995).

Rapid or substantial changes in estrogen and/or progesterone availability have been linked to the emergence of anxiety and anxiety disorders, as well as to substantial changes in pre-existing anxiety states (Yonkers et al., 1998; Yen & Jaffe, 1986; Warnock & Bundren, 1997; Vliet & Davis, 1991; Weiss et al., 1995; Dembert et al., 1994; Deci et al., 1992; Chung et al., 1995; Arpels, 1996). There is a surprising lack of reported studies that have systematically or prospectively examined the course of specific anxiety disorders during the time of perimenopause and menopause.

As previously discussed, increasing evidence indicates that gender differences in the anxiety disorders diminish with increasing age. A confluence of hormonal and age-related changes in neural function are likely to contribute to this finding. Cessation of ovarian production of the sex steroids after menopause results in a transition in the predominating circulating estrogen from ovarian-secreted estradiol to estrone. Estrone arises from peripheral conversion of adrenally produced androstenedione and is a much weaker steroid than estradiol (Longscope, 1981). These factors suggest that the absence of ovarian-produced estradiol as well as cessation of the female reproductive cycle-induced fluctuations in sex steroid concentrations may well abolish the sex difference. In addition, several neurobiological changes have been identified that occur with the aging process. Serotonergic responsivity appears to diminish with increasing age (Lawlor et al., 1989). Advanced age is also associated with impairment of the stress response (DeSouza, 1995) and attenuation of noradrenergic responsiveness (Flint et al., 1998). These factors may further reduce the risk of emergence of anxiety disorders in the elderly and may also contribute to some of the phenomenological differences between younger and older subjects with anxiety disorders.

The results from research studies summarized throughout this chapter suggest that important gender and age differences are present in the epidemiology and phenomenology of anxiety disorders. Sex steroids have multiple and complex neurobiological actions that are likely to be involved in the pathophysiology of pathological anxiety states. Moreover, sex steroids may play a critical role in explaining the gender and age differences associated with anxiety disorders.

REFERENCES

Affonso, D. D., Lovett, S., Paul, S. M. & Sheptak, S. (1990). A standardized interview that differentiates pregnancy and postpartum symptoms from perinatal clinical depression. *Birth*, 17, 121–30.

Alpert, J. E., Uebelacker, L. A., McLean, N. E., Nierenberg, A. A., Pava, J. A., Worthington, J. J. 3rd, Tedlow, J. R., Rosenbaum, J. F. & Fava, M. (1997). Social phobia, avoidant personality disorder and atypical depression: co-occurrence and clinical implications. *Psychological Medicine*, 27, 627–33.

Altshuler, L. L., Hendrick, V. & Cohen, L. S. (1998). Course of mood and anxiety disorders during pregnancy and the postpartum period. *Journal of Clinical Psychiatry*, 2, 29–33.

American Psychiatric Association. (1994). *Diagnostic and Statistical Manual of Mental Disorders, Fourth Edition*. Washington, DC: American Psychiatric Association.

Andrade, L., Eaton, W. W. & Chilcoat, H. D. (1996). Lifetime co-morbidity of panic attacks and major depression in a population-based study: age of onset. *Psychological Medicine*, 26, 991–6.

Antony, M., Downie, F. & Swinson, R. (1998). Diagnostic issues and epidemiology in OCD. In

OCD: Theory, Research, and Treatment, ed. R. Swinson, M. Antony, S. Rachman & M. Richter, pp. 3–32. New York: The Guilford Press.

Arpels, J. C. (1996). The female brain hypoestrogenic continuum from the premenstrual syndrome to menopause. A hypothesis and review of supporting data. *Journal of Reproductive Medicine*, 41, 633–9.

Banazak, D. A. (1997). Anxiety disorders in elderly patients. *Journal of the American Board of Family Practitioners*, 10(4), 280–9.

Battaglia, M., Bernardeschi, L., Politi, E., Bertella, S. & Bellodi, L. (1995). Comorbidity of panic and somatization disorder: a genetic–epidemiological approach. *Comprehensive Psychiatry*, 36, 411–20.

Beck, J. G., Stanley, M. A. & Zebb, B. J. (1996). Characteristics of generalized anxiety disorder in older adults: a descriptive study. *Behavior Research Therapeutics*, 34(3), 225–34.

Bisserbe, J. C., Weiller, E., Boyer, P., Lepine, J. P. & Lecrubier, Y. (1996). Social phobia in primary care: level of recognition and drug use. *International Clinical Psychopharmacology*, 3, 25–8.

Bland, R. C., Newman, S. C. & Orn, H. (1997). Age and remission of psychiatric disorders. *Canadian Journal of Psychiatry*, 42(7), 722–9.

Blazer, D., George, L. K. & Hughes, D. (1991). The epidemiology of anxiety disorders: an age comparison. In *Anxiety in the Elderly*, ed. C. Salzman & B. D. Lebowitz, pp. 17–30. New York, Springer Publishing.

Bourdon, K., Boyd, J. & Rae, D.(1988). Gender differences in phobias: results of the ECA community survey, *Journal of Anxiety Disorders*, 2, 227–41.

Boyd, J. H., Rae, D. S., Thompson, J. W., Burns, B. J., Bourdon, K., Locke, B. Z. & Regier, D. A. (1990). Phobia: prevalence and risk factors. *Society of Psychiatry and Psychiatric Epidemiology*, 25, 314–23.

Breslau, N., Davis, G. & Andreski, P. (1990). Traumatic events and traumatic stress disorder in an urban population of young adults. *Archives of General Psychiatry*, 48, 218–22.

Breslau, N., Davis, G. C., Andreski, P., Peterson, E. L. & Schultz, L. R. (1997). Sex differences in posttraumatic stress disorder. *Archives of General Psychiatry*, 54, 1044–8.

Breslau, N., Schultz, L. & Peterson, E. (1995). Sex differences in depression: a role for pre-existing anxiety. *Psychiatry Research*, 58, 1–12.

Bromet, E., Sonnega, A. & Kessler, R. C. (1998). Risk factors for DSM-III-R posttraumatic stress disorder: findings from the National Comorbidity Survey. *American Journal of Epidemiology*, 147, 353–61.

Cameron, O., Kuttesch, D., McPhee, K. & Curtis, G. C. (1988). Menstrual fluctuation in the symptoms of panic anxiety. *Journal of Affective Disorders*, 15, 169–74.

Castle, D. J., Deale, A. & Marks, I. M. (1995). Gender differences in obsessive compulsive disorder. *Australian and New Zealand Journal of Psychiatry*, 29, 114–17.

Chakravorty, S. G. & Halbreich, U. (1997). The influence of estrogen on monoamine oxidase activity. *Psychopharmacology Bulletin*, 33, 229–33.

Chung, C., Remington, N. & Suh, B. (1995). Estrogen replacement therapy may reduce panic symptoms [letter; comment]. *Journal of Clinical Psychiatry*, 56, 533.

Clarke, A. H. & Lewis, M. J. (1982). Fear of crime among the elderly. *British Journal of Criminology*, 22, 49–62.

Cohen, L. S., Sichel, D. A., Dimmock, J. A. & Rosenbaum, J. F. (1994). Impact of pregnancy on panic disorder: a case series [see comments]. *Journal of Clinical Psychiatry*, 55, 284–8.

Cook, B., Noyes, R., Garvey, M., Beach, V., Sobotka, J. & Chaudhry, D. (1990). Anxiety and the menstrual cycle in panic disorder. *Journal of Affective Disorders*, 19, 221–6.

Coryell, W. (1988). Mortality of anxiety disorders. In *Handbook of Anxiety, Vol 2: Classification, Etiological Factors and Associated Disturbances*, ed. R. Noyes Jr, M. Roth & G. D. Burrows, pp. 311–20. Amsterdam: Elsevier Science Publishers.

Cox, B. J., Swinson, R. P., Shulman, I. D., Kuch, K. & Reichman, J. T. (1993). Gender effects and alcohol use in panic disorder with agoraphobia. *Behavior Research Therapeutics*, 31, 413–16.

Deci, P. A., Lydiard, R. B., Santos, A. B. & Arana, G. W. (1992). Oral contraceptives and panic disorder. *Journal of Clinical Psychiatry*, 53, 163–5.

Demal, U., Lenz, G., Mayrhofer, A., Zapotoczky, H. G. & Zitterl, W. (1993). Obsessive-compulsive disorder and depression. A retrospective study on course and interaction, *Psychopathology*, 26, 145–50.

Dembert, M., Dinneen, M. & Opsahl, M. (1994). Estrogen-induced panic disorder [letter; comment] [see comments]. *American Journal of Psychiatry*, 151, 1246.

DeSouza, E. B. (1995). Corticotropin-releasing factor receptors physiology, pharmacology, biochemistry and role in central nervous system and immune disorders. *Psychoneuroendocrinology*, 20(8), 789–819.

Dick, C. L., Bland, R. C. & Newman, S. C. (1994a). Epidemiology of psychiatric disorders in Edmonton. Panic disorder. *Acta Psychiatrica Scandinavica*, 376(Suppl), 45–53.

Dick, C. L., Sowa, B., Bland, R. C. & Newman, S. C. (1994b). Epidemiology of psychiatric disorders in Edmonton. Phobic disorders. *Acta Psychiatrica Scandinavica*, 376(Suppl), 36–44.

Drummond, L. (1993). The treatment of severe, chronic, resistant, OCD. An evaluation of an inpatient programme using behavioural psychotherapy in combination with other treatments. *British Journal of Psychiatry*, 163, 223–9.

Dupont, R., Rice, D., Shiraki, S. & Rowland, C. (1995). Pharmacoeconomics: economic costs of obsessive–compulsive disorder. *Medical Interface*, 4, 102–9.

Eaton, W., Dryman, A. & Weissman, M. (1991). Panic and phobia. In *Psychiatric Disorders in America: The Epidemiologic Catchment Area Study*, ed. L. Robins & D. Regier, pp. 53–80. New York: Free Press.

Eberly, R. E. & Engdahl, B. E. (1991). Prevalence of somatic and psychiatric disorders among former prisoners of war. *Hospital and Community Psychiatry*, 42(8), 807–13.

Etgen, A. M. & Karkanias, G. B. (1994). Estrogen regulation of noradrenergic signaling in the hypothalamus. *Psychoneuroendocrinology*, 19, 603–10.

Fava, G. A., Grandi, S., Michelacci, L., Saviotti, F., Conti, S., Bovicelli, L., Trombini, G. & Orlandi, C. (1990). Hypochondriacal fears and beliefs in pregnancy. *Acta Psychiatrica Scandinavica*, 82, 70–2.

Fink, G., Sumner, B. E., Rosie, R., Grace, O. & Quinn, J. P. (1996). Estrogen control of central neurotransmission: effect on mood, mental state, and memory. *Cellular and Molecular Neurobiology*, 16, 325–44.

Flint, A. J. (1994). Epidemiology and comorbidity of anxiety disorders in the elderly. *American Journal of Psychiatry*, 151(5), 640–9.

Flint, A. J., Koszycki, D., Vaccarino, F. J., Ladieux, A., Boulenger, J. P. & Bradwejn, J. (1998). Effect of aging on cholecystokinin-induced panic. *American Journal of Psychiatry*, 155(2), 283–5.

Florio, E. R., Hendriyx, M.S., Jensen, J. E., Rockwood, T. H., Raschko, R., Dyck, D. G. (1997). A comparison of suicidal and consuicidal elders referred to a community mental health centre programme. *Suicide and Life-threatening Behavior*, 27(2), 182–93.

Foa, E. B. (1997). Trauma and women: course, predictors, and treatment, *Journal of Clinical Psychiatry*, 9, 25–8.

Fredrikson, M., Annas, P., Fischer, H. & Wik, G. (1996). Gender and age differences in the prevalence of specific fears and phobias. *Behavior Research Therapeutics*, 34, 33–9.

Fyer, A. J., Mannuzza, S., Chapman, T. F., Lipsitz, J., Martin, L. Y. & Klein, D. F. (1996). Panic disorder and social phobia: effects of comorbidity on familial transmission. *Anxiety*, 2, 173–8.

Goenjian, A. K., Najorian, L. M., Pynoos, R. S., Steinberg, A. M., Manoukian, G., Tavosian, A. & Fairbanks, L. A., (1994). PTSD in elderly and younger adults after the 1988 earthquake in Armenia. *American Journal of Psychiatry*, 151,(6), 895–901.

Griez, E., Hauzer, R. & Meijer, J. (1995). Pregnancy and estrogen-induced panic [letter; comment]. *American Journal of Psychiatry*, 152, 1688.

Halbreich, U. (1997a). Hormonal interventions with psychopharmacological potential: an overview. *Psychopharmacology Bulletin*, 33, 281–6.

Halbreich, U. (1997b). Role of estrogen in postmenopausal depression. *Neurology*, 48, 516–19.

Halbreich, U. & Tworek, H. (1993). Altered serotonergic activity in women with dysphoric premenstrual syndromes. *International Journal of Psychiatry and Medicine*, 23, 1–27.

Halbreich, U., Rojansky, N., Palter, S., Tworek, H., Hissin, P. & Wang, K. (1995). Estrogen augments serotonergic activity in postmenopausal women. *Biological Psychiatry*, 37, 434–41.

Hantouche, E. G. & Lancrenon, S. (1996). [Modern typology of symptoms and obsessive–compulsive syndromes: results of a large French study of 615 patients]. *Encephale*, 22(Spec No. 1), 9–21.

Hollander, E., Greenwald, S., Neville, D., Johnson, J., Hornig, C. & Weissman, M. (1996). Uncomplicated and comorbid obsessive–compulsive disorder in an epidemiologic sample. *Journal of Depression and Anxiety*, 4, 111–19.

Hollander, E., Stein, D., Kwon, J., Rowland, C., Wong, C., Broatch, J. & Himelein, C. (1998). Psychosocial function and economic costs of obsessive-compulsive disorder. *CNS Spectrums*, 3, 48–58.

Hollifield, M., Katon, W., Skipper, B., Chapman, T., Ballenger, J. C., Mannuzza, S. & Fyer, A. J. (1997). Panic disorder and quality of life: variables predictive of functional impairment. *American Journal of Psychiatry*, 154, 766–72.

Holst, J., Blackstrom, T. & Hammerback, S. (1989). Progestin addition during oestrogen replacement therapy – effects on vasomotor symptoms and mood. *Maturitas*, 11, 13–20.

Huerta, R., Mena, A., Malacara, J. & Diaz-deLeon, J. (1995). Symptoms at perimenopausal period: its association with attitudes toward sexuality, life-style, family function, and FSH levels. *Psychoneuroendocrinology*, 20, 135–48.

Janowsky, D., Halbreich, U. & Rausch, J. (1996). Association between ovarian hormones, other hormones, emotional disorders and neurotransmitters. In *Psychopharmacology and Women: Sex, Gender, and Hormones*, ed. M. Jensvold, U. Halbreich & J. Hamilton, pp. 85–106. Washington, DC: American Psychiatric Press Inc.

Jensvold, M., Halbreich, U. & Hamilton, J. (eds.) (1996). *Psychopharmacology and Women: Sex, Gender, and Hormones*. Washington, DC: American Psychiatric Press Inc.

Johnson, M., Marazziti, D., Brawman-Mintzer, O., Emmanuel, N., Ware, M., Morton, W., Rossi, A., Cassano, G. & Lydiard, R. (1998). Abnormal peripheral benzodiazepine receptor density associated with generalized social phobia. *Biological Psychiatry*, **43**, 306–9.

Joyce, P. R., Bushnell, J. A., Oakley Browne, M. A., Wells, J. E. & Hornblow, A. R. (1989). The epidemiology of panic symptomatology and agoraphobic avoidance. *Comprehensive Psychiatry*, **30**, 303–12.

Karno, M., Golding, J., Sorenson, S. & Burnam, M. (1988). The epidemiology of obsessive–compulsive disorder in five U.S. communities. *Archives of General Psychiatry*, **45**, 1094–9.

Katerndahl, D. A. (1990). Factors associated with persons with panic attacks seeking medical care. *Family Medicine*, **22**, 462–6.

Katerndahl, D. A. & Realini, J. P. (1997). Quality of life and panic-related work disability in subjects with infrequent panic and panic disorder. *Journal of Clinical Psychiatry*, **58**, 153–8.

Kawachi, I., Sparrow, D., Vokonas, P. S. & Weiss, S. T. (1994). Symptoms of anxiety and risk of coronary heart disease. The Normative Aging Study [see comments]. *Circulation*, **90**(5), 2225–9.

Keller, M. B. & Hanks, D. L. (1993). Course and outcome in panic disorder. *Progress in Neuropsychopharmacology and Biological Psychiatry*, **17**, 551–70.

Kendall, D., Stancel, G. & Enna, S. (1982). The influence of sex hormones on antidepressant-induced alterations in neurotransmitter receptor binding. *Journal of Neurosciences*. **2**, 354–60.

Kendler, K. S. (1996). Major depression and generalized anxiety disorder. Same genes, (partly) different environments – revisited. *British Journal of Psychiatry*, **30**(Suppl.), 68–75.

Kendler, K. S., Neale, M. C., Kessler, R. C., Heath, A. C. & Eaves, L. J. (1992a). The genetic epidemiology of phobias in women. The interrelationship of agoraphobia, social phobia, situational phobia, and simple phobia. *Archives of General Psychiatry*, **49**, 273–81.

Kendler, K. S., Neale, M. C., Kessler, R. C., Heath, A. C. & Eaves, L. J. (1992b). Major depression and generalized anxiety disorder. Same genes, (partly) different environments? *Archives of General Psychiatry*, **49**, 716–22.

Kendler, K. S., Walters, E. E., Neale, M. C., Kessler, R. C., Heath, A. C. & Eaves, L. J. (1995). The structure of the genetic and environmental risk factors for six major psychiatric disorders in women. Phobia, generalized anxiety disorder, panic disorder, bulimia, major depression, and alcoholism. *Archives of General Psychiatry*, **52**, 374–83.

Kennedy, B. & Schwab, J. (1997). Utilization of medical specialists by anxiety disorder patients. *Psychosomatics*, **38**, 109–12.

Kessler, R. & McLeod, J. (1984). Sex differences in vulnerability to undesirable life events, *Sociological Review*, **49**, 620–31.

Kessler, R. C., McGonagle, K. A., Zhao, S., Nelson, C. B., Hughes, M., Eshleman, S., Wittchen, H. U. & Kendler, K. S. (1994). Lifetime and 12-month prevalence of DSM-III-R psychiatric disorders in the United States. Results from the National Comorbidity Survey. *Archives of General Psychiatry*, **51**, 8–19.

Kessler, R. C., Stein, M. B. & Berglund, P. (1998). Social phobia subtypes in the National Comorbidity Survey. *American Journal of Psychiatry*, **155**, 613–19.

Kohn, R., Westlake, R. J., Rasmussen, S. A., Marsland, R. T., & Norman, W. H. (1997). Clinical features of OCD in elderly patients. *American Journal of Geriatric Psychiatry*, 5(3), 211–15.

Koran, L., Thieneman, M. & Davenport, R. (1996). Quality of life for patients with obsessive–compulsive disorder. *American Journal of Psychiatry*, 153, 783–8.

Krasucki, C., Howard, R. & Mann, A. (1998). The relationship between anxiety disorders and age. *International Journal of Geriatric Psychiatry*, 13(2), 79–99.

Kroboth, P. & McAuley, J. (1997). Progesterone: does it affect response to drug? *Psychopharmacology Bulletin*, 33, 297–301.

Krystal, J. H., Leaf, P. J., Bruce, M. L. & Charney, D. S. (1992). Effects of age and alcoholism on the prevalence of panic disorder. *Acta Psychiatrica Scandinavica*, 85(1), 77–82.

Lawlor, B. A., Sunderland, T., Hill, J. L., Mellow, A. M., Molchan, S. E., Mueller, E. A., Jacobsen, F. M. & Murphy, D. L. (1989). Evidence for a decline with age in behavioral responsivity to the serotonin agonist, M-CPP, in healthy human subjects. *Psychiatric Research*, 29(1), 1–10.

Leckman, J. F., Goodman, W. K., North, W. G., Chappell, P. B., Price, L. H., Pauls, D. L., Anderson, G. M., Riddle, M. A., McDougle, C. J., Barr, L. C. & et al. (1994). The role of central oxytocin in obsessive compulsive disorder and related normal behavior. *Psychoneuroendocrinology*, 19, 723–49.

Lecrubier, Y. & Weiller, E. (1997). Comorbidities in social phobia. *International Clinical Psychopharmacology*, 12, 517–21.

Lemieux, A. & Coe, C. (1995). Abuse-related posttraumatic stress disorder: evidence for chronic neuroendocrine activation in women. *Psychosomatic Medicine*, 57, 105–15.

Lensi, P., Cassano, G. B., Correddu, G., Ravagli, S., Kunovac, J. L. & Akiskal, H. S. (1996). Obsessive–compulsive disorder. Familial-developmental history, symptomatology, comorbidity and course with special reference to gender-related differences. *British Journal of Psychiatry*, 169, 101–7.

Leonard, H., Lenane, M., Swedo, S., Rettew, D., Gershon, E. & Rapaport, J. (1992). Tics & Tourette's syndrome: a two to seven year follow-up of 54 OCD children. *American Journal of Psychiatry*, 149, 1244–51.

Lindal, E. & Stefansson, J. G. (1993). The lifetime prevalence of anxiety disorders in Iceland as estimated by the US National Institute of Mental Health Diagnostic Interview Schedule, *Acta Psychiatrica Scandinavica*, 88, 29–34.

Lindamer, L. A., Lohr, J. B., Harris, M. J. & Jeste, D. V. (1997). Gender, estrogen, & schizophrenia. *Psychopharmacology Bulletin*, 33, 221–8.

Lindesay, J. (1991). Phobic disorders in the elderly. *British Journal of Psychiatry*, 159, 531–41.

Lindheim, S. R., Legro, R. S., Morris, R. S., Wong, I. L., Tran, D. Q., Vijod, M. A., Stanczyk, F. Z. & Lobo, R. A. (1994). The effect of progestins on behavioral stress responses in postmenopausal women. *Journal of the Society for Gynecologic Investigation*, 1, 79–83.

Livingston, G., Watkin, V. Milne, B., Manela, M. V. & Katona, C. (1997). The natural history of depression and the anxiey disorders in older people: the Islington community study. *Journal of Affective Disorders* 46(3), 255–62.

Longscope, C. (1981). Metabolic clearance and blood production rates in postmenopausal women. *American Journal of Obstetrics and Gynecology*, 111, 779–85.

Magee, W., Eaton, W., Wittchen, H., McGonagle, K. & Kessler, R. (1996). Agoraphobia, simple phobia, and social phobia in the National Comorbidity Survey. *Archives of General Psychiatry,* 53, 159–68.

Majewska, M. (1992). Neurosteroids: endogenous bimodal modulators of the GABA-A receptor mechanism of action and physiological significance. *Progress in Neurobiology,* 38, 379–95.

Majewska, M., Harrison, N., Schwartz, R., Barker, J. L. & Paul, S. M. (1986). Steroid hormone metabolites are barbiturate-like modulators of the GABA receptors. *Science,* 232, 1004–7.

Marshall, J. R. (1996). Comorbidity and its effects on panic disorder. *Bulletin of the Menninger Clinic,* 60, 9225–84.

McCauley, J., Kern, D. E., Kolodner, K., Dill, L., Schroeder, A. F., DeChant, H. K., Ryden, J., Derogatis, L. R. & Bass, E. B. (1997). Clinical characteristics of women with a history of child-hood abuse: unhealed wounds [see comments]. *Journal of the American Medical Association,* 277, 1362–8.

McEwen, B. (1991). Nongenomic and genomic effects of steroids on neural activity. *Trends in Pharmacological Science,* 12, 141–7.

McEwen, B. & Parsons, B. (1987). Gonadal steroid action on the brain: neurochemistry and neuropharmacology. *Annual Review of Pharmacology and Toxicology,* 22, 555–98.

McLeod, D. R., Hoehn Saric, R., Foster, G. V. & Hipsley, P. A. (1993). The influence of premen-strual syndrome on ratings of anxiety in women with generalized anxiety disorder. *Acta Psychiatrica Scandinavica,* 88, 248–51.

Nestadt, G., Bienvenu, O. J., Cal, G., Samuels, J. & Eaton, W. W. (1998). Incidence of OCD in adults. *Journal of Nervous Mental Disorders,* 186(7), 401–6.

Neziroglu, F., Anemone, R. & Yaryura-Tobias, J. (1992). Onset of obsessive-compulsive disorder in pregnancy. *American Journal of Psychiatry,* 149, 947–50.

Neziroglu, F. A., Yaryura Tobias, J. A., Lemli, J. M. & Yaryura, R. A. (1994). [Demographic study of obsessive compulsive disorder]. *Acta Psiquiatrica y Psicologica de America Latina,* 40, 217–23.

Noshirvani, H. F., Kasvikis, Y., Marks, I. M., Tsakiris, F. & Monteiro, W. O. (1991). Gender-diver-gent aetiological factors in obsessive-compulsive disorder. *British Journal of Psychiatry,* 158, 260–3.

Otto, M. W., Pollack, M. H., Sachs, G. S., O'Neil, C. A. & Rosenbaum, J. F. (1992). Alcohol depen-dence in panic disorder patients. *Journal of Psychiatric Research,* 26, 29–38.

Pauls, D., Alsobrook, J., Goodman, W., Rasmussen, S. & Leckman, J. (1995). A family study of obsessive–compulsive disorder. *American Journal of Psychiatry,* 152, 76–84.

Pigott, T., L'Heureux, F., Dubbert, B., Bernstein, S. & Murphy, D. (1994). Obsessive–compulsive disorder: comorbid conditions. *Journal of Clinical Psychiatry,* 55, 15–27.

Potts, N. L., Davidson, J. R., Krishnan, K. R. & Doraiswamy, P. M. (1994). Magnetic resonance imaging in social phobia. *Psychiatric Research,* 52(1), 35–42.

Raj, B. A., Corvea, M. H. & Dagon, E. M. (1993). The clinical characteristics of panic disorder in the elderly: a retrospective study. *Journal of Clinical Psychiatry,* 54, 150–5.

Rasmussen, S. & Eisen, J. (1992). The epidemiology and clinical features of obsessive–compul-sive disorder. *Psychiatric Clinics of North America,* 15, 743–58.

Regier, D. A., Narrow, W. E. & Rae, D. S. (1990). The epidemiology of anxiety disorders: the Epidemiologic Catchment Area (ECA) experience. *Journal of Psychiatric Research,* 2, 3–14.

Robins, L., Helzer, J., Weissman, M., Orvaschel, H., Gruenberg, E., Burke, J. D. Jr & Regier, D. A. (1984). Lifetime prevalence of specific psychiatric disorders in three sites. *Archives of General Psychiatry*, 41, 949–58.

Rubenstein, C., Pigott, T., L'Heureux, F., Hill, J. & Murphy, D. (1992). A preliminary investigation of the lifetime prevalence rate of anorexia and bulimia nervosa in patients with OCD. *Journal of Clinical Psychiatry*, 53, 309–14.

Schmidt, M. E., Matochik, J. A., Goldstein, D. S., Schouten, J. L., Zametkin, A. J. & Potter, W. Z. (1997). Gender differences in brain metabolic and plasma catecholamine responses to alpha 2-adrenoceptor blockade. *Neuropsychopharmacology*, 16, 298–310.

Schneider, L., Small, G., Hamilton, S., Bystritsky, A., Nemeroff, C. & Meyers, B. (1997). Estrogen replacement and response to fluoxetine in a multi-center geriatric depression trial. *American Journal of Geriatric Psychiatry*, 5, 97–106.

Schneier, F. R., Johnson, J., Hornig, C. D., Liebowitz, M. R. & Weissman, M. M. (1992). Social phobia. Comorbidity and morbidity in an epidemiologic sample. *Archives of General Psychiatry*, 49, 282–8.

Sheikh, J. I. (1993). Is late-onset panic disorder a distinct syndrome? In *Proceedings of the 196th Annual Scientific Meeting of the American Psychiatric Association*, San Francisco.

Sheikh, J. I., King, R. J. & Taylor, C. B. (1991). The comparative phenomenology of early-onset versus late-onset panic attacks: a pilot survey. *American Journal of Psychiatry*, 148(9), 1231–3.

Sherwin, B. (1991). The impact of different doses of estrogen and progestin on mood and sexual behavior in post-menopausal women. *Journal of Clinical Endocrinology and Metabolism*, 72, 336–43.

Sherwin, B. (1996). Menopause, early aging and elderly women. In *Psychopharmacology and Women: Sex, Gender, and Hormones*, ed. M. Jensvold, U. Halbreich & J. Hamilton. Washington, DC: American Psychiatric Press Inc.

Sholomskas, D. E., Wickamaratne, P. J., Dogolo, L., O'Brien, D. W., Leaf, P. J. and Woods, S. W. (1993). Postpartum onset of panic disorder: a coincidental event? [see comments]. *Journal of Clinical Psychiatry*, 54, 476–80.

Sichel, D., Cohen, L., Dimmock, J. and Rosenbaum, J. (1993). Postpartum obsessive compulsive disorder: a case series. *Journal of Clinical Psychiatry*, 54, 156–9.

Spiro, A., Schnurr, P. P. & Aldwin, C. M. (1994). Combat-related PTSD symptoms in older men. *Psychology of Aging*, 9(1), 17–26.

Stahl, S. (1997). Reproductive hormones as adjuncts to psychotropic mediation in women. *Essential Psychopharmacology*, 2, 147–64.

Stahl, S. M. (1996). *Essential Psychopharmacology*. New York: Cambridge University Press.

Stein, D., Hollander, E., Simeon, D., Cohen, L. & Hwang, M. (1993). Pregnancy and OCD. *American Journal of Psychiatry*, 150, 1131–2.

Stein, M. B. (1997). Phenomenology and epidemiology of social phobia. *International Journal of Clinical Psychopharmacology*, 12, 1268–315.

Stein, M. B., Chartier, M. J., Hazen, A. L., Kozak, M. V., Tancer, M. E., Lander, S., Furer, P., Chubaty, D. & Walker, J. R. (1998). A direct-interview family study of generalized social phobia. *American Journal of Psychiatry*, 155, 90–7.

Stein, M. B., Schmidt, P. J., Rubinow, D. R. & Uhde, T. W. (1989). Panic disorder and the menstrual cycle: panic disorder patients, healthy control subjects, and patients with premenstrual syndrome. *American Journal of Psychiatry*, **146**, 1299–303.

Steketee, G., Eisen, J., Dyck, I., Warshaw, M. & Rasmussen, S. (1997). Course of Illness in OCD. In *Review of Psychiatry*, volume 16, ed. L. Dickstein, M. Riba, M. & J. Oldham, pp. 73–95. Washington, DC: American Psychiatric Association.

Sutherland, C., Bybee, D. & Sullivan, C. (1998). The long-term effects of battering on women's health. *Women's Health*, **4**, 41–70.

Thomsen, P. H. & Mikkelsen, H. U. (1995). Course of obsessive-compulsive disorder in children and adolescents: a prospective follow-up study of 23 Danish cases. *Journal of the American Academy of Child and Adolescent Psychiatry*, **34**, 1432–40.

Vinogradov, S. & Csernansky, J. G. (1990). Postpartum psychosis with abnormal movements: dopamine supersensitivity unmasked by withdrawal of endogenous estrogens? *Journal of Clinical Psychiatry*, **51**, 365–6.

Vliet, E. L. & Davis, V. L. (1991). New perspectives on the relationship of hormone changes to affective disorders in the perimenopause. *NAACOGS' Clinical Issues in Perinatal and Womens Health Nursing*, **2**, 453–71.

Warnock, J. & Bundren, J. (1997). Anxiety and mood disorders associated with gonadotropin-releasing hormone agonist therapy. *Psychopharmacology Bulletin*, **33**, 311–16.

Weiss, M., Baerg, E., Wisebord, S. & Temple, J. (1995). The influence of gonadal hormones on periodicity of obsessive–compulsive disorder. *Canadian Journal of Psychiatry*, **40**, 205–7.

Weissman, M., Klerman, G., Markowitz, J. & Ouellette, R. (1989). Suicidal ideation and suicide attempts in panic disorder and attacks, *New England Journal of Medicine*, **321**, 1209–14.

Weissman, M. M., Bland, R. C., Canino, G. J., Greenwald, S., Hwu, H. G., Lee, C. K., Newman, S. C., Oakley Browne, M. A., Rubio Stipec, M., Wickramaratne, P. J. et al., (1994). The cross national epidemiology of obsessive compulsive disorder. The Cross National Collaborative Group. *Journal of Clinical Psychiatry*, **55**, 5–10.

Williams, K. E. & Koran, L. M. (1997). Obsessive–compulsive disorder in pregnancy, the puerperium, and the premenstruum, *Journal of Clinical Psychiatry*, **58**, 330–4.

Wisner, K. L., Peindl, K. S. & Hanusa, B. H. (1996). Effects of childbearing on the natural history of panic disorder with comorbid mood disorder. *Journal of Affective Disorders*, **41**, 173–80.

Wittchen, H. N. & Essan C. A. (1993). Epidemiology of panic disorder: progress and unresolved issues. *Journal of Psychiatric Research*, **27**(1), 47–68.

Wittchen, H. U., Zhao, S., Kessler, R. C. & Eaton, W. W. (1994). DSM-III-R generalized anxiety disorder in the National Comorbidity Survey. *Archives of General Psychiatry*, **51**, 355–64.

Yaryura Tobias, J. A., Neziroglu, F. A. & Kaplan, S. (1995). Self-mutilation, anorexia, and dysmenorrhea in obsessive compulsive disorder. *International Journal of Eating Disorders*, **17**, 33–8.

Yehuda, R., Schmeidler, J., Siever, L. J., Binder-Brynes, K. & Elkin, A. (1997). Individual differences in PTSD symptom profiles in Holocaust survivors in concentration camps or in hiding. *Journal of Trauma and Stress*, **10**(3), 453–63.

Yen, S. & Jaffe, R. (eds.) (1986). *Reproductive Endocrinology, Physiology, Pathophysiology and Clinical Management*. Philadelphia: W.B. Saunders.

Yonkers, K. & Ellison, J. (1996). Anxiety disorders in women and their pharmacological treatment. In *Psychopharmacology and Women: Sex, Gender, and Hormones*, ed. M. Jensvold, U. Halbreich & J. Hamilton, pp. 261–85. Washington, DC: American Psychiatric Press Inc.

Yonkers, K. A. (1997). Anxiety symptoms and anxiety disorders: how are they related to premenstrual disorders? *Journal of Clinical Psychiatry*, 3, 62–7.

Yonkers, K. A., Warshaw, M. G., Massion, A. O. & Keller, M. B. (1996). Phenomenology and course of generalised anxiety disorder. *British Journal of Psychiatry*, 168, 308–13.

Yonkers, K. A., Zlotnick, C., Allsworth, J., Warshaw, M., Shea, T. & Keller, M. B. (1998). Is the course of panic disorder the same in women and men? *American Journal of Psychiatry*, 155, 596–602.

12

Gender and hormonal factors in pain and pain inhibition

Wendy F. Sternberg

Introduction

Much recent research has focused on differences between the sexes in both physiology and behavior. The idea that differences between men and women can be attributable to biological factors that do not result from rearing or sociocultural variables is intriguing for many reasons, not the least of which is that it can help to explain sex differences in important health-related endpoints. One such endpoint is the experience of pain.

A consideration of the hormonal basis for gender differences in pain perception is relevant to a volume on the neuroendocrine aspects of aging for several reasons. One of the foremost observations of health care practitioners is the enormous degree of individual variability that exists among patients with respect to pain and analgesia. For example, some individuals continue to report pain following substantial doses of morphine (Lasagna & Beecher, 1954), while others exhibit significant pain relief following treatment with placebo (Beecher, 1959). As health care providers face aging populations, in whom chronic pain conditions and painful disease are increasingly prevalent, it is essential to understand the factors that contribute to such variability in order to effectively treat pain. Gender is one such factor.

Furthermore, a likely contributing factor to gender variability in pain experience is hormonal status, as will be discussed later in this chapter. Widespread changes in gonadal hormone levels, particularly in females, are characteristic of the aging process and may play a role in painful experience. Therefore, a consideration of sex differences in pain and analgesia across age cohorts is useful for understanding the rôle of hormones, gender, and aging in susceptibility to painful disease. Lastly, insofar as pain is stressful, and stress can alter the experience of pain (to be discussed at length later), the differences in the neuroendocrine stress response that accompany aging can also alter the experience of pain.

Several converging lines of evidence suggest that males and females experience pain differently. First, sex differences exist in laboratory and psychophysical measures of pain sensitivity. Such laboratory studies, however, often produce inconsistent results, biased by numerous influencing variables, and the difficulty inherent in collecting self-report data where gender-related sociocultural factors might be expected to play a role. Second, females seek medical care for relief from pain more frequently, data which are also potentially confounded by sociocultural influences like report bias. Third, there is a significant over-representation of female patients among chronic pain sufferers, particularly for illnesses with no known underlying pathology. Human sex differences such as these are supported by findings of sex differences in pain-related behaviors in laboratory experiments using animal subjects, where the confounds associated with sociocultural variables are not present. Sex differences also exist in laboratory animals (as well as in human subjects) with respect to analgesic drug responses and the expression of analgesia in response to stressful encounters.

Many of these findings related to sex differences in pain or analgesia can be explained by the different hormonal makeup of males and females, as evidenced by gonadectomy and hormone replacement studies in animals, and by the existence of variation in pain responses across the menstrual cycle in human females. Each of these lines of evidence will be considered below.

Sex differences in the response to noxious stimuli in the laboratory

Sex differences exist in sensitivity to stimuli in nearly every sensory modality. Females have a greater acuity than males for a variety of tastes, odors, auditory frequencies and intensities, and tactile stimuli (tested by two point discrimination), although males exhibit greater visual acuity than females (for review see Valle, 1987). Not surprisingly, tolerance to sensory stimuli is inversely related to sensitivity; females have a lower tolerance for certain auditory and tactile stimuli while they are more light tolerant than men (McGuiness, 1972, 1976; Notermans & Tophoff, 1967). Sex hormones appear to play a role in the expression of these sex differences, as they are usually not noted until after puberty, and thresholds to some types of sensory stimuli exhibit cyclicity across the menstrual cycle in females (e.g. Doty et al., 1981). Often, explanations of sex differences such as these emphasize the differing environmental pressures facing males and females throughout the course of evolution (Valle, 1987). It is interesting to note that although sensitivity to some sensory stimuli shows an overall decline with age, sex differences are still maintained (Valle, 1987).

Considered in this context, it is not surprising to learn that sex differences exist in tests of pain sensitivity. This section examines the experimental literature establishing that sex differences exist in the response to noxious stimuli in laboratory experiments, and considers some of the factors that often make uncovering such sex differences difficult in the laboratory setting. Experimental investigations

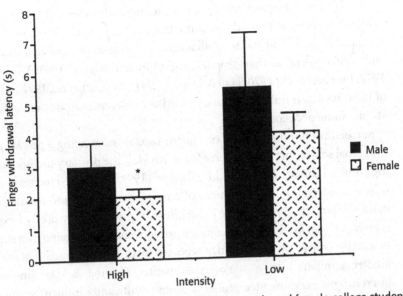

Figure 12.1. Sex differences in pain response latency among male and female college students. Males exhibited longer latencies to finger withdrawal from a noxious radiant heat source, particularly to the high intensity stimulus (*, t(8) = 2.83; P = 0.02). At the lower intensity, the difference approached significance (t(8) = 1.91; P = 0.09).

generally seem to indicate that, as in other sensory realms, women exhibit greater sensitivity to noxious stimuli (e.g. Feine et al., 1991) and lower pain tolerance than men (e.g. Notermans & Tophoff, 1967). Although experimental pain responses do show age-related alterations in the laboratory (with inconsistent results), no definitive studies have specifically examined sex differences in human experimental pain across age cohorts.

One hallmark of the literature investigating sex differences is the large number of experimental models that have been employed to address this question, and the different results that have been obtained across laboratories. In recent extensive reviews of the literature, Fillingim and Maixner (1995) and Berkley (1997) summarize these findings. Many different types of noxious stimuli have been studied: pressure applied to different parts of the body; electrical cutaneous stimulation; thermal stimulation from radiant heat, lasers, or contact probes; ischemia (tourniquet pain); and cold stimuli. The overwhelming consistency is that when sex differences are seen, females exhibit more pain behavior than males, particularly for stimuli of high intensity (Ellermeier & Westphal, 1995). Preliminary findings from my laboratory using a radiant heat stimulus at several intensities support this general trend in the literature (see Fig. 12.1). However, sex differences are not always reliably demonstrated (Bush et al., 1993; Neri & Agazzani, 1984).

Of all the experimental models applied to the study of sex differences in pain sensitivity, mechanical pressure, radiant heat, and noxious cold stimuli appear to produce the most reliable sex differences, with males displaying lower sensitivity and higher tolerance than females (e.g. Otto & Dougher, 1985; Woodrow et al., 1972; Procacci et al., 1970; Hall & Davies, 1991; Westcott et al., 1977). However, all of the noxious stimuli tested have yielded sex differences in this same direction on at least some occasions.

Sociocultural influences are one factor capable of exerting a powerful effect on the verbal self-report of pain perception, which is the primary method for measuring pain in humans. Levine and DeSimone (1991) attempted to create conditions of sexual interest in the assessment of pain report in male and female subjects by manipulating the gender of the experimenter (provocatively dressed experimenters were chosen on the basis of physical attractiveness) and found, not surprisingly, that male college students under-reported pain to an attractive female experimenter compared to a male experimenter (Levine & De Simone, 1991). Interestingly, experimenter gender did not significantly influence pain report in female students. These findings suggest that social context is an important factor that can contribute to the existence of sex differences in pain report, particularly in males. In this study, pain report did not differ between males and females when both groups were tested by same sex experimenters. However, striking sex differences in pain report were seen simply by manipulating the gender of the experimenter.

It would be misleading to believe that experimenter gender could explain all of the sex differences in pain that have been reported by other groups. In carefully controlled studies that account for experimenter gender, males continue to be less sensitive to noxious thermal stimuli than females (Feine et al., 1991; Otto & Dougher, 1985). Females also show greater two point discriminability for noxious stimuli suggesting that sensory factors are at the basis of the observed sex differences (Feine et al., 1991).

Other factors also exist that may influence the ability to detect sex differences in pain perception in experimental situations. Differences in the hormonal milieu between the sexes are often implicated as being responsible for sex differences in pain perception (discussed later). Also, circadian influences (Procacci et al., 1970), tobacco use (Mueser et al., 1984), sugar and fat consumption (Frye et al., 1994; Krahn et al., 1994), presence of psychiatric conditions (Davis et al., 1979), and oral contraceptive use (Goolkasian, 1980) are potentially confounding factors that must be controlled in such investigations.

Given the large number of factors that can lead to inconsistencies in the experimental literature and the statistical nature of the sex differences that are seen (i.e.

small and statistically significant rather than practically important differences) other investigators have indicated that an overall *lack* of sex differences in human pain perception is the overwhelming conclusion that must be drawn from an examination of the literature (Berkley, 1995, 1997). My interpretation of this body of literature focuses on the similarities in the findings, rather than the differences among these studies. Sex differences in the response to noxious stimuli must be particularly robust if they are seen so frequently, in the same direction every time, despite the large number of potentially influencing factors (Sternberg, 1997).

Sex differences in health care utilization and chronic pain conditions

Clearly, laboratory experiments of sex differences in pain perception do not represent a clinical problem, but they may give insight into the mechanisms underlying well-established sex differences in clinical pain conditions. Many reports indicate that women suffer more chronic pain than men (e.g., Margolis et al., 1984). The incidence of painful illness varies considerably across sex, and sex differences in some pain conditions are dependent on subject age. For example, migraine with aura, some types of headache, Raynaud's disease, fibromyalgia syndrome, irritable bowel syndrome, and rheumatoid arthritis are more prevalent in women than in men, whereas postherpetic neuralgia, coronary artery disease, and duodenal ulcer are more prevalent in men than women (Berkley, 1997). In addition, somatization disorder (characterized by unexplained physical symptoms) is far more prevalent in women than in men (e.g. Golding et al., 1991). Low back pain is believed to be a primarily male disorder (Horton, 1984), whereas facial pain sufferers are generally female (Vallerand, 1995).

Clinical studies of sex differences in pain arising from endogenous origin have yielded some interesting results. A study examining pain perceptions related to headache among the general population found that women reported a higher level of pain associated with their most recent headache than men (Celentano et al., 1990). In addition, women consistently report headaches of longer duration, a greater frequency of headaches, and a greater utilization of medical care for treatment of headaches than men. In contrast, Tait et al. (1990) report that, among chronic pain patients currently seeking treatment at a multidisciplinary pain center, women report less disability, psychological distress and pain severity than men. These apparently conflicting findings can be explained by considering that women may simply be more likely to report pain than men (Hibbard & Pope, 1986). When men do seek help for chronic pain conditions, they may be in a more severely disabled state. In fact, given the heightened sensitivity women appear to have to somatic sensations (previous section) and their increased level of body awareness compared to men (e.g. Fucci & Petrosino, 1983), these findings do not at all seem unlikely.

Sex differences in responses to analgesic drugs

Several studies have addressed sex differences in the response to analgesic drugs and administration practices of such drugs in human clinical populations. Male and female patients have been shown to differ in their response to analgesics in the clinical setting, although as characteristic of some of this literature, the findings have been equivocal. Following orthopedic surgery, female patients request analgesia earlier than males (McQuay et al., 1988). In contrast, fewer female than male cancer patients required a strong opiate analgesic (Twycross, 1977), although more women than men were prescribed anxiolytics, a possible confound in this study. Clearly, the sociocultural factors discussed above are relevant when considering that administration of analgesic drugs in the clinical setting is usually dependent on the patient's verbal report of pain and requests for pain relief. Women demanded less of an opiate analgesic following hip replacement surgery than men in a patient-controlled analgesia (PCA) condition (McQuay et al., 1980). This finding is particularly interesting in that PCA administration removes some of the barriers to pain relief that may be influenced by sociocultural variables.

Females have recently been reported to experience greater analgesia resulting from κ-opiate agonist drugs than males when these drugs are administered for postoperative dental pain (Gordon et al., 1995; Gear et al., 1996a,b). These quantitative differences in analgesic magnitude are clinically relevant, as they suggest different dosage requirements for achieving sufficient analgesia in a clinical setting. Research into sex differences in the mechanisms of κ-analgesia reported in the animal literature (discussed later) may shed some light on the reasons for these observed differences in humans.

Interestingly, sex differences in analgesic requirements may also be a result of the attitudes of the health care practitioner regarding the needs of male and female patients in pain. Physicians may approach the treatment of their complaints differently, based on their gender. For example, when presented with identical case studies of a hypothetical patient with only the gender of the patient altered, physicians (both male and female) judged the female patient's complaints as more emotional than the male's (identical) complaints (Colameco et al., 1983). In addition, Calderone (1990) found that female coronary artery bypass graft patients were more likely to receive sedative medication and less likely to receive pain medication, than males matched for age and surgical procedure. Other studies confirm the undermedication of female pain patients compared to male pain patients

(Vallerand, 1995). These studies indicate that physicians' and nurses' attitudes toward the patient based on gender can be a factor influencing role expectations of men and women in pain.

Hormonal factors in human pain sensitivity

Several studies indicate that pain perception among females varies as a function of the ovulatory cycle, although some conflicting reports do exist as to the presence and direction of the phase differences. For example, Goolkasian (1980) found that pain sensitivity was increased during the ovulation phase in normally cycling women, and that pain perception in this phase was significantly different from males and from females taking oral contraceptives (who were not significantly different from males). Other studies, however, indicate that the greatest period of pain sensitivity is directly before menstruation, while the lowest pain sensitivity occurs during the ovulation phase (Herren, 1933; Tedford et al. 1977). Herren (1933) reported that premenstrual pain thresholds in normal cycling women were significantly lower than those in either the postmenstrual phases or the intermenstrual phases. Furthermore, Tedford et al. (1977) noted a similar pattern of results in normally cycling women, and found that this cyclicity of pain perception disappeared in women taking oral contraceptives.

Conversely, other investigators have failed to find a relationship between menstrual cycle phase and pain perception (Amodei & Nelson-Gray, 1989; Kuczmierczyk et al., 1986; Kuczmierczyk & Adams, 1986). The inconsistencies in the literature with respect to hormonal factors in experimental pain perception likely result from a dependence on studying hormonal fluctuations associated with the menstrual cycle. Further insight into hormonal contributors to sex differences in human experimental pain perception can be obtained by studying sex differences in pain sensitivity across a wide range of age cohorts, from prepubescence to postmenopause. Studies assessing pain sensitivity across varying age cohorts provide little evidence for consistent changes in pain processing in older adults (increases, decreases, and no changes have all been reported; Harkins & Price, 1992), however, no systematic studies of sex differences in laboratory pain perception across the lifespan have been carried out.

Evidence has been reported for the cyclical nature of some chronic pain conditions in females, such as migraine headache (Edelson, 1985). Following puberty, females are four to eight times more likely than males to experience migraine headache (the variety without aura). Furthermore, about 60% of women with migraine can relate a periodicity of their headaches to the menstrual cycle. Thus, migraine headache is an example of a chronic pain condition that is more prevalent in females, and it is highly dependent on circulating hormone levels. However, among female sufferers of migraine, patients do not report changes in symptoms post-menopausally (Whitty & Hockaday, 1968) when changes in circulating hormones would be expected to result in alterations of headache symptoms.

Given this evidence that fluctuations in ovarian hormones in some way contribute to (or at least explain part of) the variability in human pain responsiveness between men and women, one would expect that there would be fewer differences between aged men and aged women with respect to painful disorders. However, this does not seem to be the case. For some painful disorders, sex differences persist throughout the lifespan, whereas in other conditions, sex differences are age-dependent. For example, sex differences in osteoarthritis are dependent on the age of the patient; females suffer from this condition more than males after age 45, whereas males are afflicted more often before age 45 (Berkley, 1997). The same trend is noted in gout sufferers, where males are afflicted more frequently before age 60 and females more often afflicted after that age (Berkley, 1997). So, although there is little, if any, data regarding human sex differences in experimental pain in aged populations, the clinical picture suggests that painful disorders associated with aging do not occur with equal frequency between the sexes. The continued prevalence of sex differences in painful disorders in aged populations, coupled with the appearance of sex differences in some conditions post-menopausally, suggests that circulating or fluctuating gonadal hormones in the female cannot be the sole causal factor for differences between the sexes in chronic pain in humans.

Sex differences and hormonal factors in pain sensitivity in animal subjects

Much of what we have learned about mechanisms underlying sex differences in pain is derived from studies using animals. Working with animals has obvious benefits, as the physiological determinants of sex differences may be studied without the confounds of report biases and sex role appropriate behaviors. Furthermore, since the lifespan of the typical laboratory rodent is on the order of two years, studies of sex differences in varying age cohorts are more manageable.

Sex differences are apparent between male and female rodents (rats and mice) on a wide range of pain tests. Some authors have observed sex differences in pain thresholds, with females displaying more sensitivity to shock (Beatty & Beatty, 1970) and to noxious thermal stimuli on both the hot-plate (Kavaliers & Innes, 1987a) and tail-flick (Kepler et al., 1989; Romero & Bodnar, 1986) tests. Kepler et al. (1989) reported that females display shorter tail-flick latencies (time until tail is vigorously flicked following tail-immersion in hot water, or application of a noxious heat stimulus to the tail) than males, although there were no differences between the sexes reported in jump test latencies (time until both hind paws leave the surface of a grid through which electrical shock is delivered). In contrast, Romero & Bodnar (1986) found that there were no significant sex differences with respect to tail-flick latencies, whereas females displayed shorter jump latencies. Other stimulus characteristics, such as duration, and the tonic vs. phasic nature of the pain-producing agent, may play a role in the existence and direction of sex differences in pain behavior (Sternberg et al., 1993). While there have been inconsistencies reported across test of basal nociception, the results seem to indicate that females are more sensitive to noxious stimuli. These findings are consistent with the most well controlled of the human studies (Feine et al., 1991).

These sex differences in pain sensitivity can be reversed when gonadectomies are performed (Beatty & Fessler, 1976; Forman et al., 1989), thus indicating that the underlying difference in male and female pain perception are likely to be hormonal in nature in some paradigms. Forman et al. (1989) demonstrated that gonadal steroid replacement therapy in castrated male and female rats resulted in a reinstatement of the natural response pattern. With age, pain thresholds tend to decrease, however, and this effect was noted in rats of both sexes (Islam et al., 1993), suggesting that, as in human studies, fluctuations in gonadal hormones cannot be the only mediator of such sex differences.

As in humans, the ovulatory cycle may have a modest effect on pain sensitivity in rodents. The estrous cycle is on the order of 4 to 5 days long, and consists of two stages of sexual non-receptivity (metestrous and diestrous) and two phases of sexual receptivity (proestrous and estrous). Female rodents have been shown to display differential pain sensitivity across the estrous cycle (e.g. Leer et al., 1988), although, as in human studies, these differences are sensitive to the pain test employed, and a great deal of conflicting evidence exists. Leer et al. (1988) report that sexually receptive female rats (in proestrous) display an elevated footshock threshold compared to non-sexually receptive rats (in metestrous). In contrast, Kepler et al. (1989) demonstrated a significantly higher pain sensitivity in proestrous females compared to met/diestrous groups, making conclusions regarding estrogen modulation of pain sensitivity across the ovulatory cycle difficult.

Since female animals are subject to different evolutionary pressures across the ovulatory cycle, it would be reasonable to expect that pain sensitivity varies somewhat across the cycle. For instance, most animals (excluding humans and some non-human primates) copulate only during phases of the cycle when conception is likely. Therefore, if hormonal variation influenced pain sensitivity, then copulation would be more likely during these times of sexual receptivity. Indeed, hormonal changes across the estrous cycle have been linked to changes in receptive field size of peripheral afferents (Bereiter & Barker, 1980), suggesting a peripheral mechanism for estrous cycle effects on pain sensitivity.

Animal sex differences and hormonal factors in the analgesic responses to environmental stress and pharmaceuticals

The experience of pain in any individual in a given situation is due not just to an ascending sensory component from nociceptor (peripheral pain receptor) to cerebral cortex, but also depends on a descending, or modulatory, input from the brain that could potentially alter the activity of peripheral afferents. The first empirical demonstration of the brain's modulatory influences on pain sensation was reported in 1969, when Reynolds discovered that electrical stimulation of certain regions of the rat brainstem could result in profound analgesia. It is now believed that endogenous analgesia mechanisms exist for the inhibition of pain during stressful circumstances, when the beneficial or adaptive nature of pain as a warning signal may in fact interfere with important survival behaviors. The ability of stressful environmental events to inhibit pain perception has been studied extensively in the laboratory.

Early studies of 'stress-induced analgesia' (SIA) focused on the opioid peptides as the neurochemical mediators of the analgesic effect. It is believed that morphine and other opiate analgesics produce their pain inhibitory effects by binding to receptors for endogenous opiates in the SIA pathway. Once it was demonstrated that SIA could be elicited that did not meet the three criteria for opioid mediation (reduction or elimination of analgesia by the opiate antagonist naloxone, tolerance development, and cross tolerance to morphine), the search for the non-opioid neurochemical mediators was initiated. Several monoaminergic neurotransmitters are believed to play a role in SIA, and recent evidence implicates excitatory amino acids such as glutamate and aspartate binding at NMDA receptors in the production of non-opioid SIA (as determined by antagonism by the NMDA-antagonist MK-801; Marek et al., 1992).

Understanding sex differences in these descending analgesia pathways is important for a number of reasons. First, magnitudinal sex differences in SIA (or analgesia produced by pharmacological activation of these pathways – see below) can help us to understand the differences in the response to analgesics in human populations, and to help clinicians predict whether analgesics may be effective at the same doses between the sexes. It is also important to ascertain whether pain inhibitory pathways in males and females employ the same neurochemical mediators, information which is essential for the development of novel analgesic agents which activate non-opioid analgesia pathways in a mechanism analogous to that of morphine analgesia. In addition, examining sex differences in endogenous analgesia pathways may help to shed light on the observed sex differences in pain behavior in the laboratory and the clinic.

Magnitudinal differences in analgesia between the sexes

With respect to opioid forms of SIA (those reversible by naloxone), it has been reported that males manifest more SIA than females after a variety of stressors including restraint (Kavaliers & Innes, 1987b), footshock (Maier et al., 1980), and forced swim (Romero & Bodnar, 1986). There has also been one report of quantitative sex differences in a non-opioid form of SIA wherein females exhibit more analgesia than males after a brief exposure to a natural predator (Kavaliers & Colwell, 1991). Thus, many reports indicate that males display more and females display less SIA, although there is some conflicting evidence.

It is also possible to study sex differences in descending analgesia pathways by activating the neural substrates with analgesic pharmaceuticals which bind to receptors in the SIA pathway. Some studies report that female rodents display less analgesia resulting from morphine (which binds preferentially to μ-opioid receptors) than males when administered systemically (e.g. Baamonde et al., 1989; Cicero et al., 1996) or centrally (e.g. Boyer et al., 1998). This finding indicates that females may have fewer receptors for opioid peptides and can also help to explain the observed magnitudinal sex differences in the expression of opioid SIA. Differences in analgesic responsiveness have also been noted across the estrous cycle in female rats (Banerjee et al., 1983; Kepler et al., 1989; Frye et al., 1992).

Attempts to account for sex differences in both basal nociception and endogenous analgesia have centered around consideration of opioid peptide levels, opiate receptor levels, and the influence of circulating gonadal steroids on these levels. Receptors for gonadal steroids have been localized to many brain areas particularly relevant to the pathways mediating pain and analgesia (Pfaff & Keiner, 1973), suggesting an interplay of hormones and opiates. Female rodents have been found to have lower levels than males of the natural opioid peptides (Hong et al., 1982), which may also explain their higher pain sensitivity and lower pain thresholds. There is also direct evidence linking gonadal steroids, leuteinizing hormone, and opioids (Ferin et al., 1984), a link which may be responsible, in part, for the differences noted in pain and analgesia between the sexes, and across the estrous cycle.

Analgesic responses to opiate drugs also change across the lifespan, and the developmental profile of aging effects on opioid analgesia differs between the sexes. Age-related changes in analgesic magnitude resulting from morphine administration have been observed in female rats, with reductions in analgesia occurring at 14-, 19-, and 24-month time points compared to rats aged 4 and 9 months (Kramer & Bodnar, 1986). Likewise, Islam et al. (1993) demonstrated that female rats displayed significant decreases in morphine analgesia with aging, although male rats exhibited increases in morphine analgesia at 18 and 24 months as compared with young (6 months) animals. Therefore, a sex difference exists in the effects of aging on morphine analgesia.

Similar patterns of aging effects emerge in studies of stress-induced analgesia (SIA), which is insensitive to naloxone antagonism and is therefore considered to be non-opioid in nature. In studies assessing the analgesic effects of non-opioid cold-water swim stress and 2–DG administration, Bodnar and colleagues demonstrated a significant reduction in analgesic magnitudes with increasing age in female rats (Kramer & Bodnar, 1986). However, male rats display age-related increases in analgesia resulting from hormonally mediated (Hamm & Knisely, 1985), but not neurally mediated non-opioid swim SIA paradigms.

With respect to opioid-mediated SIA paradigms, there does not appear to be a sex difference in the effect of aging on analgesia. Consistent with findings on the decline of opioid-mediated SIA noted in female rats (Kramer et al., 1985), electric shock to the front paws produces an opioid-mediated analgesia that declines in magnitude in older male rats (Hamm & Knisely, 1985). These decrements in opioid SIA are likely to be due to the decline in activity of the endogenous opioid system that occurs with aging (e.g. Messing et al. 1980), although the mechanism underlying the increase in morphine analgesia seen in aged male rats is less readily explainable.

That aging may influence the magnitude of SIA responses differentially in males and females is not entirely surprising when considering the interplay between gonadal hormones (that are well known to fluctuate with aging) and stress hormones, in general. Estrogen stimulates the hypothalamic–pituitary–adrenal (HPA) axis – the hormonal substrate of stressful experience (Kirschbaum et al., 1996). Since HPA activation is accompanied by analgesia, hormone replacement therapy may serve a protective function in preventing chronic pain conditions following menopause. However, the equivocal nature of menstrual cycle studies on pain perception makes drawing conclusions like this tentative at best. More research is needed to fully understand the role of sex hormones in painful experience in men and women across the lifespan.

Qualitative differences in analgesia between the sexes

Differences in the neurochemical nature of SIA between the sexes have also been reported. Romero and colleagues (1986) found that SIA induced by intermittent cold water swimming, previously reported to be opioid mediated in male rats, is in fact not attenuated by naloxone in female rats (signifying non-opioid mediation in females). In contrast, Wong (1987) reported that SIA induced by brief warm water swim is attenuated by naloxone in female, but not male mice in a test of visceral pain sensitivity (abdominal constriction test).

Whereas much of the literature concerning sex differences in SIA focuses on differences in opioid analgesia, a striking qualitative sex difference exists between male and female mice on tests of non-opioid analgesia (that analgesia not attenuated by naloxone). Previous research suggests that the NMDA-receptor antagonist MK-801 selectively blocks cold-water swim analgesia, while naloxone is ineffective at attenuating SIA resulting from 3 minute swims at this temperature (Marek et al., 1992). However, this characterization appears to be specific to males. We (Mogil et al., 1993) found that MK-801 (the NMDA-receptor blocker) antagonizes non-opioid swim SIA in males only, whereas in females, cold water swim SIA is insensitive to both naloxone and MK-801 antagonism. Thus, swim SIA in intact females is neither opioid, nor mediated by the excitatory amino acids, yet it is of similar magnitude to the SIA displayed by intact males. In gonadectomized females MK-801 blocks non-opioid SIA (as it does in males), and estrogen replacement in gonadectomized females reinstates the normal 'female' pattern of insensitivity to this drug. These findings suggest the existence of a novel, female-specific, estrogen-dependent mechanism of swim SIA (Mogil et al., 1993). Additional evidence for sex differences in NMDA-mediation of SIA has been provided by studies utilizing different stressors (e.g. Kavaliers & Galea, 1996; Kavaliers & Choleris, 1997) suggesting that this effect is not specific to swim stress. Since exposure of female mice to testosterone early during ontogeny can partially reverse these sex difference seen in adult mice (Sternberg et al., 1995), it is believed that absence of testosterone during a critical period is necessary for the development of estrogen-sensitive, female-specific analgesia. Furthermore, these sex differences do not appear until animals reach reproductive age, although they persist well past the age of female reproductive capacity (Sternberg et al., 1993).

It is these qualitative, rather than quantitative, differences in analgesia processes that are most likely to result in inadequate or inappropriate treatment of pain in the clinical setting. The young adult male rodent is the typical research subject in the laboratory setting, findings from which often form the basis for experimental pharmaceutical development. If sex differences in the neurochemical mediation of analgesia exist in humans, we would expect that drugs developed on the basis of single-sex studies would not be equally effective in both sexes and across age groups.

This point is made clear when considering the effectiveness of κ-opiate analgesics. Converging lines of evidence suggest that κ-opioid agonists activate an NMDA-mediated analgesia system, as evidenced by the effectiveness of NMDA antagonists in inhibiting analgesia resulting from the κ-agonists U-50488 and U-69593 (Kest et al., 1992; Kavaliers & Choleris, 1997). However, as in NMDA-mediated stress-induced analgesia, this characterization is true for male subjects only (Kavaliers & Choleris, 1997). NMDA antagonists are ineffective in blocking κ-analgesia in female subjects. That an analgesic pharmaceutical operates by a neurochemically distinct mechanism in male and female subjects may provide some insight into the observed sex differences in the clinical efficacy of κ-opiates in human subjects (reported by Gordon et al., 1995; Gear et al., 1996a,b). The magnitudinal sex difference observed by these authors may reflect output of neurochemically distinct substrates, rather than different degrees of activation of the same system (Mogil & Kest, 1999). Further research is certainly needed to determine the root of such sex differences for the optimal treatment of pain in patients of both sexes.

Conclusions

The literature review provided in this chapter leads to several general conclusions. First, it should be clear that sex and hormonal factors can play a role in explaining some of the variability in pain responsiveness. However, the contribution of gender-related factors to pain in any given individual is dependent on many additional factors, which can make the gender differences seem insignificant by comparison. By reducing the inter-individual variability by controlling for rearing and eliminating sociocultural influences, the comparative (cross-species) approach to the study of sex differences in pain and pain inhibition can put these findings into perspective.

The striking sex differences that are seen in animal subjects with respect to pain modulation can help us to re-evaluate our view of sex differences in chronic pain conditions and experimental pain by focusing on the descending component of the pain pathway. One way to understand sex differences in chronic pain (e.g. as in painful joint or gastrointestinal conditions, which are usually more prevalent in females) is to look to sex differences in descending pain modulatory circuitry that may normally inhibit these pain messages from reaching the brain. Perhaps a tonically active pain inhibition mechanism that normally acts to inhibit nociceptive information from the joints or gut is disturbed in patients suffering from these syndromes.

Understanding the nature of sex differences in pain (both chronic and acute) and related phenomena is essential to the successful treatment of clinical pain problems. Of obvious importance is the recognition that females experience pain in a different manner than males and across the menstrual cycle. These factors must be taken into consideration when assessing the nature of chronic pain symptoms. Furthermore, researchers must be aware of these differences as the typical subject in experiments on pain is the male rat. Information obtained from these studies may not be generalizable to females. Lastly, the exciting possibility that females may have a novel analgesia system may serve as an impetus to research that focuses on alleviating pain problems specific to women.

REFERENCES

Amodei, N. & Nelson-Gray, R. O. (1989). Reactions of dysmenhorreic and non- dysmenhorreic to experimentally induced pain throughout the menstrual cycle. *Journal of Behavioral Medicine,* 12(4), 373–85.

Baamonde, A. I., Hidalgo, A. & Andres-Trelles, F. (1989). Sex-related differences in the effects of morphine and stress on visceral pain. *Neuropharmacology,* 28(9), 967–70.

Banerjee, P., Chatterjee, T. K. & Ghosh, J.J. (1983). Ovarian steroids and modulation of morphine-induced analgesia and catalepsy in female rats. *European Journal of Pharmacology,* 96, 291–4.

Beatty, W.W. & Beatty, P.A. (1970). Hormonal determinants of sex differences in avoidance behavior and reactivity to electric shock in the rat. *Journal of Comparative Physiological Psychology,* 16, 413–17.

Beatty, W. W. & Fessler, R. G. (1976). Ontogeny of sex differences in open field behavior and sensitivity to electric shock in the rat. *Physiology and Behavior,* 16 413–17.

Beatty, W. W. & Fessler, R. G. (1977). Gonadectomy and sensitivity to electric shock in the rat. *Physiology and Behavior,* 19, 1–6.

Beecher, H.K. (1959). *Measurement of Subjective Responses.* New York: Oxford University Press.

Bereiter, D. A. & Barker, D. J. (1980). Hormone-induced enlargements of receptive fields in trigeminal mechanoreceptive neurons: 1. Time course, hormone, sex, and modality specificity. *Brain Research,* 184, 395–410.

Berkley, K. (1995). From psychophysics to the clinic? Take caution. *Pain Forum,* 4(4), 225–7.

Berkley, K. (1997). Sex differences in pain. *Behavioral and Brain Sciences,* 20(3) 371–80.

Boyer, J.S., Morgan, M.M. & Craft, R.M. (1998). Microinjection of morphine into the rostroventral medulla produces greater antinociception in male compared to female rats. *Brain Research,* 796, 315–18.

Bush, F. M., Harkins, S. W., Harrington, W. G. & Price, D. D. (1993). Analysis of gender effects on pain perception and symptom presentation in temporomandibular joint pain. *Pain,* 53, 73–80.

Calderone, K. L. (1990). The influence of gender on the frequency of pain and sedative medication administered to postoperative patients. *Sex Roles,* 23(11/12), 713–25.

Celentano, D. D., Linet, M. S. & Stewart, W. F. (1990). Gender differences in the experience of headache. *Social Science and Medicine,* 30(12), 1289–95.

Cicero, T.J., Nock, B. & Meyer, E.R. (1996). Gender-related differences in the antinociceptive properties of morphine. *Journal of Pharmacology and Experimental Therapeutics,* 279, 767–73.

Colameco, S., Becker, L. A. & Simpson, M. (1983). Sex bias in the assessment of patient complaints. *The Journal of Family Practice,* 16(6), 1117–21.

Davis, G. C., Buchsbaum, M. S. & Bunney, W. E. (1979). Analgesia to painful stimuli in affective illness. *American Journal of Psychiatry,* 136, 1148–51.

Doty, R. L., Snyder, P., Huggins, G. & Lowry, L.D. (1981). Endocrine, cardiovascular and psychological correlates of olfactory sensitivity changes during human menstrual cycle. *Journal of Comparative Physiological Psychology,* 95, 45–60.

Edelson, R. N. (1985). Menstrual migraine and other hormonal aspects of migraine. *Headache* 25, 376–9.

Ellermeier, W. & Westphal, W. (1995). Gender differences in pain ratings and pupil reactions to painful pressure stimuli. *Pain*, 61, 435–9.

Feine, J. S., Bushnell, M. C., Miron, D. & Duncan, G. H. (1991). Sex differences in the perception of noxious heat stimuli. *Pain*, 44, 255–62.

Ferin, M., Van Vugt, D. A. & Wardlaw, S. L. (1984). The hypothalamic control of the menstrual cycle and the role of endogenous opioid peptides. *Recent Progress in Hormone Research*, 40, 441–85.

Fillingim, R. B. & Maixner, W. (1995). Gender differences in the response to noxious stimuli. *Pain Forum*, 4(4), 209–21.

Forman, L. J., Tingle, V., Estilow, S. & Cater, J. (1989). The response to analgesia testing is affected by gonadal steroids in the rat. *Life Sciences*, 45, 447–54.

Frye, C. A., Bock, B. C. & Kanarek, R. B. (1992). Hormonal milieu affects tailflick latency in female rats and may be attenuated by access to sucrose. *Physiology and Behavior*, 52, 699–706.

Frye, C. A., Crystal, S., Ward, K. D. & Kanarek, R. B., (1994). Menstrual cycle and dietary restraint influence taste preferences in young women. *Physiology and Behavior*, 55, 561–7.

Fucci, D. & Petrosino, L. (1983). Lingual vibrotactile sensation magnitudes: Comparison of suprathreshold responses in men and women. *Perception-and-Psychophysics*, 33, 93–5.

Gear, R. W., Gordon, N. C., Heller, P. H., Paul, S., Miaskowski, C. & Levine, J. D. (1996a). Gender differences in analgesic response to the kappa-opioid pentazocine. *Neuroscience Letters*, 205, 207–9.

Gear, R. W., Miaskowski, C., Gordon, N. C., Paul, S., Heller, P. H. & Levine, J. D. (1996b). Kappa-opioids produce significantly greater analgesia in women than in men. *Nature Medicine*, 2, 1248–50.

Golding, J. M., Smith, G. R. & Kashner, M. (1991). Does somatization disorder occur in men? Clinical characteristics of women and men with multiple unexplained somatic symptoms. *Archives of General Psychiatry*, 48, 231–5.

Goolkasian, P. (1980). Cyclic changes in pain perception: an ROC analysis. *Perception and Psychophysics*, 27, 499–504.

Goolkasian, P. (1983). Phase and sex effects in pain perception: a critical review. *Psychology of Women Quarterly*, 9(1), 15–28.

Gordon, N. C., Gear, R. W., Heller, P. H., Paul, S., Miaskowski, C. & Levine, J. D. (1995). Enhancement of morphine analgesia by the GABA$_B$ agonist baclofen, *Neuroscience*, 69, 345–9.

Hall, E. G. & Davies, S. (1991). Gender differences in perceived intensity and affect of pain between athletes and non-athletes. *Perceptual and Motor Skills*, 73, 779–86.

Hamm, R. J. & Knisely, J. S. (1985). Environmentally induced analgesia: an age related decline in an endogenous opioid system. *Journal of Gerontology*, 40, 268–74.

Harkins, S. W. & Price, D. D. (1992). Assessment of pain in the elderly. In *Handbook of Pain Assessment*, ed. D. C. Turk & R. Melzack. Guilford Press: New York.

Herren, R. G. (1933). The effect of high and low female sex hormone concentration on the two-point threshold of pain and touch upon tactile sensitivity. *Journal of Experimental Psychology*, **16**, 324–7.

Hibbard, J. H. & Pope, C. R. (1986). Another look at sex differences in the use of medical care: illness orientation and the types of morbidities for which services are used. *Women and Health*, **11**, 21.

Hong, J. S., Yoshikawa, K. & Lamartinere, C. A. (1982). Sex-related differences in the rat pituitary met-enkephalin level altered by gonadectomy. *Brain Research*, **251**, 380–3.

Horton, C. F. (1984). Women have headaches, men have backaches: patterns of illness in an Appalachian community. *Social Science Medicine*, **19**(6), 647–54.

Islam, A. K., Cooper, M. L. & Bodnar, R. J. (1993). Interactions among aging, gender and gonadectomy effects upon morphine antinociception in rats. *Physiology and Behavior*, **54**, 45–53.

Kavaliers, M. & Innes, D. (1987a). Stress-induced opioid analgesia and activity in deer mice: sex and population differences. *Brain Research*, **425**, 49–56.

Kavaliers, M. & Innes, D. G. L. (1987b). Sex and day–night differences in opiate-induced responses of insular wild deer mice, *Peromyscus maniculatus triagularis*. *Pharmacology, Biochemistry and Behavior*, **27**, 477–82.

Kavaliers, M. & Colwell, D. D. (1991). Sex differences in opioid and non-opioid mediated predator-induced analgesia in mice. *Brain Research*, **568**, 173–7.

Kavaliers, M. & Galea, L. A. M. (1996). Sex differences in the expression and antagonism of swim stress-induced analgesia in deer mice vary with the breeding season. *Pain*, **63**, 327–34.

Kavaliers, M. & Choleris, E. (1997). Sex differences in N-methyl-D-aspartate involvement in κ-opioid and non-opioid predator-induced analgesia in mice. *Brain Research*, **768**, 30–6.

Kepler, K. L., Kest, B., Kiefel, J. M., Cooper, M. L. & Bodnar, R. J. (1989). Roles of gender, gonadectomy and estrous phase in the analgesic effects of intracerebroventricular morphine in rats. *Pharmacology, Biochemistry and Behavior*, **34**, 119–27.

Kest, B., Marek, P. & Liebeskind, J. C. (1992). The specific N-methyl-D-asparate (NMDA) receptor antagonist MK-801 blocks U-50488, but not morphine antinociception, *Brain Research*, **589**, 139–42.

Kirschbaum, C., Schommer, N., Federenco, I., Gaab, J., Nermann, O., Oellers, M., Rohleder, N., Untiedt, A., Hanker, J., Pirke, K. M. & Hellhammer, D. H. (1996). Short-term estradiol treatment enhances pituitary–adrenal axis and sympathetic responses to psychological stress in healthy young men. *Journal of Clinical Endocrinology and Metabolism*, 39–43.

Krahn, D., Gosnell, B., Redmond, L. & Bohn, M. (1994). Effects of palpable food intake on response to pain. *Biological Psychiatry*, **35**, 736.

Kramer, E. & Bodnar, R. J. (1986). Age related decrements in morphine analgesia: a parametric analysis. *Neurobiology of Aging*, **7**, 185–91.

Kramer, E., Sperber, E. S. & Bodnar, R. J. (1985). Age related decrements in the analgesic and hyperphagic reponses to 2 deoxy-D-glucose. *Physiology and Behavior*, **35**, 929–34.

Kuczmierczyk, A. R. & Adams, H. E. (1986). Autonomic arousal and pain sensitivity in women with premenstrual syndrome at different phases of the menstrual cycle. *Journal of Psychosomatic Research*, **30**(4), 421–8.

Kuczmierczyk, A. R., Adams, H. E., Calhoun, K. S., Naor, S., Giombetti, R., Cattalini, M. &

McCann, P. (1986). Pain responsivity in women with premenstrual syndrome across the menstrual cycle. *Perceptual and Motor Skills*, 63, 387–93.

Lasagna, L. & Beecher, H.K. (1954). The optimal dose of morphine. *Journal of the American Medical Association*, 156, 230–4.

Leer, M. N., Bradbury, A., Maloney, J. C. & Stewart, C. N. (1988). Elevated shock threshold in sexually receptive female rats. *Physiology and Behavior*, 42, 617–20.

Levine, F. M. & De Simone, L. L. (1991). The effects of experimenter gender on pain report in male and female subjects. *Pain*, 44, 69–72.

Maier, S. F., Davies, S., Grau, J. W., Jackson, R. L., Morrison, D. H., Moye, T., Madden, J. & Barchas, J. D. (1980). Opiate antagonists and long- term analgesic reaction induced by inescapable footshock. *Journal of Comparative Physiological Psychology*, 94, 1172–83.

Marek, P., Mogil, J. S., Sternberg, W. F., Panocka, I. & Liebeskind, J., C. (1992). N-Methyl-D-aspartic acid (NMDA) receptor antagonist MK-801 blocks non-opioid stress-induced analgesia. II. Comparison across three swim stress paradigms in selectively bred mice. *Brain Research*, 578, 197–203.

Margolis, R. B., Zimny, G. H., Miller, D. & Taylor, J. M. (1984). Internists and the chronic pain patient. *Pain*, 20, 151–6.

McGuiness, D. (1972). Hearing: individual differences in perceiving. *Perception*, 1, 465–73.

McGuiness, D. (1976). Away from a unisex psychology: individual differences in visual sensory and perceptual processes. *Perception*, 5, 279–94.

McQuay, H. J., Bullingham, R. E., Paterson, G. M. & Moore, R. A. (1980). Clinical effects of buprenorphine during and after operation. *British Journal of Anaesthesiology*, 52, 1013–19.

McQuay, H. J., Carroll, D. & Moore, R. A. (1988). Postoperative orthopaedic pain- the effect of opiate premedication and local anaesthetic blocks. *Pain*, 33, 291–5.

Messing, R. B., Vasquez, B. J., Spiehler, V. R., Martinez, J. L., Jenson, R. A., Rigter, H. & McGaugh, J. L. (1980). H-dihydomorphine binding in brain regions of young and aged rats. *Life Sciences*, 26, 921–7.

Mogil, J.S. & Kest, B. (1999). Sex differences in opioid analgesia: of mice and women. *Pain Forum*, 8, 48–50.

Mogil, J. S., Sternberg, W. F., Marek, P., Kest, B. & Liebeskind, J. C. (1993). Sex differences in the antagonism of non-opioid swim stress-induced analgesia by the NMDA receptor antagonist MK-801: effects of gonadectomy and estrogen replacement. 53, 17–25.

Mueser, K., Waller, D., Levander, S. & Schalling, D. (1984). Smoking and pain: a method of limits and sensory decision theory analysis. *Scandinavian Journal of Psychology*, 25, 289–96.

Neri, M. & Agazzani, E. (1984). Aging and right–left asymmetry in experimental pain measurement. *Pain*, 19, 43–8.

Notermans, S. L. H. & Tophoff, M. (1967). Sex differences in pain tolerance and tolerance and pain apperception. *Psychiatria, Neurologia, Neurochirugia*, 70, 23–9.

Otto, M. W. & Dougher, M. J. (1985). Sex differences and personality factors in responsivity to pain. *Perceptual and Motor Skills*, 61, 383–90.

Pfaff, D. W. & Keiner, M. (1973). Atlas of estradiol-concentrating cells in the central nervous system of the female rat. *Journal of Comparative Neurology*, 151, 121–58.

Procacci, P., Bozza, G., Buzzelli, G. & Della Corte, M. (1970). The cutaneous pricking threshold in old age. *Gerontology Clinic*, **12**, 213–18.

Reynolds, D. V. (1969). Surgery in the rat during electrical analgesia induced by focal brain stimulation. *Science*, **164**, 444–5.

Romero, M. T. & Bodnar, R. J. (1986). Gender differences in two forms of cold-water swim analgesia. *Physiology and Behavior*, **37**, 893–7.

Sternberg, W. F. (1997). Sex differences in descending pain modulatory pathways may clarify sex differences in pain. *Behavioral and Brain Sciences*, **20**(3), 466.

Sternberg, W. F., Kest, B., Mogil, J. S. & Liebeskind, J. C. (1993). Female mice display less pain behavior following acetic acid or formalin administration. *Society for Neuroscience Abstracts*, **19**, 1572.

Sternberg, W. F., Mogil, J. S., Kest, B., Page, G. G., Leong, Y., Yam, V. & Liebeskind, J. C. (1995). Neonatal testosterone exposure influences neurochemistry of non-opioid swim stress-induced analgesia in adulthood. *Pain*, **63**, 321–6.

Tait, R. C., Chinball, J. T. & Krause, S. (1990). The pain disability index: psychometric properties. *Pain*, **40**(2), 171–82.

Tedford, W. H., Warren, D. E. & Flynn, W. E. (1977). Alteration of shock aversion thresholds during the menstrual cycle. *Perception and Psychophysics*, **21**, 193–6.

Twycross, R. G. (1977). Choice of strong analgesics in terminal cancer: diamorphine or morphine? *Pain*, **3**, 93–104.

Valle, W. (1987). Sex differences in sensory function. *Perspectives in Biology and Medicine*, **30**, 491–522.

Vallerand, A. H. (1995). Gender differences in pain. *IMAGE: Journal of Nursing Scholarship*, **27**(3), 235–7.

Westcott, T. B., Huesz, L., Boswell, D. & Herold, P. (1977). Several variables of importance in the use of the cold pressor as a noxious stimulus in behavioral research. *Perceptual and Motor Skills*, **44**, 401–2.

Wong, C-L. (1987). Sex difference in naloxone antagonism of swim stress induced antinociception in mice. *Methods and Findings in Experimental Clinical Pharmacology*, **9**, 275–8.

Woodrow, K. M., Friedman, G. D., Siegelaub, A. B. & Collen, M. F. (1972). Pain tolerance: differences according to sex and race. *Psychosomatic Medicine*, **34**, 548–56.

Whitty, C. W. & Hockaday, J. M. (1968). Migraine: a follow-up study of 92 patients. *British Medical Journal*, **1**, 735–36.

Part III

Effects of hormones and behavior on immune function

13

Estrogens, stress, and psychoneuroimmunology in women over the lifespan

Mary H. Burleson, Susan Robinson-Whelen, Ronald Glaser and Janice K. Kiecolt-Glaser

Stress, sex hormones, and psychoneuroimmunology

Studies of relationships among the central nervous system (CNS), the immune system, and the endocrine system have shown that the systems interact through multiple pathways. The 'stress' hormones have received the greatest attention in the neuroimmunology literature, particularly cortisol and the catecholamines; sex hormones have not been studied as intensively. In this chapter we first briefly review estrogen's immunomodulatory effects. Next we discuss estrogen-related differences in cardiovascular and neuroendocrine reactivity to brief stressors. In the last section we discuss research regarding the effects of estrogen on immune reactivity to stress, and speculate about the possibility that estrogen may moderate hormonal and immunological responses to stress through alterations in sympathetic nervous system reactivity, as well as through regulation of corticotropin-releasing hormone (CRH; Vamvakopoulos & Chrousos, 1993).

Estrogen and immune function

Estrogens, androgens, and progestogens can serve as regulators of immune function; in turn, the circulating levels of these hormones can be modulated by the immune system. Many of these interactions between the immune system and gonadal steroids appear to be mediated through feedback loops in the hypothalamic–pituitary–gonadal–thymic axis, with thymic factors playing a key role (Erbach & Bahr, 1991; Grossman, 1985). In addition, there are at least two types of estrogen receptors in human immune cells: low-affinity high-capacity (Type II) binding sites found in peripheral blood mononuclear cells (Ranelletti et al., 1988), and high-affinity low-capacity (Type I) receptors that appear to be restricted to CD8+ cells both in blood (Cohen et al., 1983; Stimson, 1988; but see Weusten et al., 1986) and in synovial tissue (Cutolo et al., 1993). Receptors for estrogen also have been found in other immune cells and tissues including macrophages (e.g.

Gulshan et al., 1990), cytosol from human thymus (e.g. Nilsson et al., 1984; Weusten et al., 1986), and spleen (e.g. Danel et al., 1983). Gonadectomy typically leads to hypertrophy of the thymus, spleen, and lymph nodes (see Forsberg, 1984; Grossman, 1984).

Estrogen effects on immune function are complex. The nature of the reported effects may depend on many factors, including the concentration of estrogens relative to androgens or progestogens, the hormone dosage and route of administration, the state of the host being investigated (e.g. age, reproductive status, autoimmune disease condition), and the aspect of immune function being measured. For the most part, however, estrogens appear to enhance humoral immune function (Ansar Ahmed et al., 1985; Grossman, 1984, 1985; Schuurs & Verheul, 1990), although they likely suppress B cell lymphopoeisis during pregnancy in mice (Medina & Kincade, 1994; Smithson et al., 1998). Apparent effects on cellular immune function depend on the method of investigation, with both suppression and enhancement reported (Ansar Ahmed et al., 1985; Grossman, 1984, 1985; Schuurs & Verheul, 1990).

Antibody production can be enhanced by estrogens both in vitro and in vivo. For example, the addition of physiological levels of estradiol to pokeweed mitogen-stimulated human peripheral blood lymphocytes (PBL) increased the number of B cells secreting immunoglobulin M (IgM; Paavonen et al., 1981). This effect was apparently mediated by inhibition of CD8+ T-lymphocytes; because these T-cells down-regulate antibody production by B cells, constraints on CD8+ T-cell function can promote antibody production. Illustrating the importance of dosage, enhanced immunoglobulin G (IgG) production was found after stimulation of human PBL with physiological levels of estradiol, whereas supraphysiological levels inhibited IgG production (Weetman et al., 1981). An in vitro study of human tonsillar lymphocytes demonstrated that the presence of intact T-cells was obligatory for the enhancing effect of estradiol on production of both IgG and IgM by B cells (Evagelatou & Farrant, 1994). In vivo studies suggest that estrogen-related amplification of humoral immunity appears to require the presence of thymic factors. For example, Erbach and Bahr (1991) demonstrated in mice that exogenous estradiol led to increased antibody titers to fluorescein only in mice with intact thymus glands or in thymectomized mice receiving thymosin fraction 5 replacement.

The effects of estrogens on cellular immune responses appear primarily to be inhibitory, although stimulatory effects also have been reported (for review see Ansar Ahmed et al., 1985; Grossman, 1984, 1985; Schuurs & Verheul, 1990). Estrogens have well-established down-regulatory effects on the thymus (see Grossman, 1985), and estradiol appears to regulate the production of thymic factors that influence cell-mediated immunity. For example, serum from castrates enhanced rat thymocyte blastogenesis in response to the mitogens phytohemagglutinin (PHA) and concanavalin A (Con A), but serum from castrated rats that were treated with physiological levels of estradiol depressed the blastogenic response back to pre-castrate levels (Grossman et al., 1982). Estradiol added in vitro also can inhibit the stimulation of human PBL by PHA and Con A (Herrera et al., 1992; Mendelsohn et al., 1977; Neifeld & Tormey, 1979; Wyle & Kent, 1977). The suppression of CD8+ lymphocyte function described above (Paavonen et al., 1981) is another example of a down-regulatory effect of estradiol on one aspect of cellular immune function. On the other hand, enhancement may be illustrated by the effects of in vitro culture of tonsillar T-lymphocytes with a wide range of estradiol concentrations. Without mitogenic stimulation, all levels of estradiol led to increased proliferation, whereas when cells were stimulated with PHA, only the higher concentrations of estradiol enhanced proliferation (Evagelatou & Farrant, 1994).

Estrogens have potent regulatory effects on both developmental and effector functions in macrophages and monocytes (for review see Miller & Hunt, 1996). For example, depending on the dose, estradiol can either enhance or suppress cytokine production. Interleukin-1 (IL-1) was increased in rat peritoneal macrophages incubated with low concentrations of estradiol (Hu et al., 1988), whereas the addition of increasing concentrations of estradiol led to a graded reduction of both IL-1 (Polan et al., 1988) and IL-1β mRNA (Polan et al., 1989) production in lipopolysaccharide (LPS)-activated cultured human peripheral monocytes. Estradiol treatment in vitro also inhibited the LPS-stimulated expression of mRNA for monocyte chemoattractant protein-1 by murine peritoneal macrophages, an effect that was reversed by the addition of tamoxifen (Frazier-Jessen & Kovacs, 1995).

Numerous animal studies have documented enhancement of cellular immunity resulting from gonadectomy, including suppression of tumor development and more rapid tissue rejection responses (see Grossman, 1984). In these models, sex steroid replacement typically restores presurgical function. For example, both male and female mice infected with the parasitic protozoan *Toxoplasma gondii* showed decreased mortality following gonadectomy; in contrast, implantation of a hexo-estrol (a synthetic estrogen) pellet in half the animals led to increased mortality (Kittas & Henry, 1980). Similar enhancement of cellular immune function has been found in women undergoing surgical menopause. For example, Pacifici et al. (1991) showed that surgically induced menopause in 15 healthy premenopausal women led to increases in phytohemagglutinin (PHA)-induced secretion of granulocyte-macrophage colony-stimulating factor, as well as elevations in spontaneous secretion of IL-1 and tumor necrosis factor a (TNF-a). Nine women in their study subsequently began estrogen replacement therapy 4 weeks after surgery; cytokine secretion returned to presurgical levels among these women following estrogen replacement.

Modulation of immune function by estrogen has health consequences. In general, immune function in females tends to be higher than that in males. Females have higher levels of immunoglobulins, a stronger in vitro response to mitogens, and better resistance to the induction of immune tolerance (for review see Ansar Ahmed et al., 1985; Lahita, 1997; Schuurs & Verheul, 1990). This higher level of immune function can be beneficial, as in the case of better resistance in females to a variety of infections. On the other hand, females are far more prone to autoimmune diseases, and sex hormones appear to be a factor in this susceptibility (Ansar Ahmed et al., 1985; Beeson, 1994). For example, estrogens accelerate murine lupus erythematosus, while androgens decelerate the disease process (Roubinian et al., 1979). In humans, postmenopausal estrogen replacement therapy has been associated with a slightly higher relative risk for systemic lupus erythematosus (Sanchez-Guerrero et al., 1995). Oral contraceptives containing estrogens can exacerbate the symptoms of lupus (Garovich et al., 1980). On the other hand, estrogen-containing oral contraceptives reduce, rather than enhance, the characteristic joint inflammation of rheumatoid arthritis in many patients (Vandenbroucke et al., 1982), illustrating the complexity of sex hormone-immune interactions.

Estrogen-related differences in physiological reactivity to brief stressors

Individual differences in cardiovascular and neuroendocrine reactivity to brief stressors, such as verbal subtraction and speech preparation and delivery, have been studied extensively because they appear to be risk factors for coronary heart disease. These stressors typically lead to activation of the sympathetic-adrenal medullary (SAM) axis, as indicated by increases in heart rate, blood pressure, and catecholamine levels, and less consistently to activation of the hypothalamic–pituitary–adrenal (HPA) axis, as indexed by increases in adrenocorticotrophic hormone (ACTH) and cortisol (Cacioppo et al., 1995). However, relatively little research has assessed cardiovascular and endocrine reactivity in women, while a broad literature exists on men's stress responses (Manuck & Polefrone, 1987; Saab, 1989). Limited evidence suggests that women typically show smaller blood pressure and epinephrine stress responses than men, indicating lower SAM activation (Frankenhaeuser, 1983; Matthews & Stoney, 1988; Stoney et al., 1987), and female reproductive hormones, especially estrogens, are thought to be possible contributors to these gender differences (Matthews, 1989; Saab et al., 1989).

Studies investigating the effects of the menstrual cycle on SAM reactivity to psychological stress are contradictory; overall, the weight of the evidence suggests that hormonal fluctuations during a normal menstrual cycle may be insufficient in either magnitude or duration to cause detectable estrogen effects on SAM reactivity (e.g. Stoney et al., 1990; Litschauer et al., 1998; for review see Light et al., 1998). Studies that include both pre- and postmenopausal women are thus of particular interest in exploring the influence of estrogens on cardiovascular and neuroendo-crine responses. For example, Saab et al. (1989) compared the responses of 15 pre-menopausal and 16 postmenopausal women to two stressors, mental arithmetic and a speech stressor. Postmenopausal women showed greater heart rate increases than premenopausal women on both tasks, with the largest differences during the speech stressor. In addition, postmenopausal women also showed greater increases in epinephrine and systolic blood pressure (SBP) than premenopausal women during the speech stressor only. Similarly, Blumenthal et al. (1991) documented greater epinephrine reactivity for postmenopausal compared to premenopausal women in response to a speech task. In a third study, Owens et al. (1993) compared the cardiovascular and neuroendocrine function of pre- and postmenopausal women and of men in response to brief psychological stressors. Postmenopausal women had higher stress-reactive increases in both SBP and diastolic blood pres-sure (DBP) than did either premenopausal women or men. Finally, Stoney et al. (1997) prospectively compared premenopausal women who had either hysterec-tomy or bilateral salpingo oophorectomy (BSO). Before surgery, there were no differences in stress responses; after surgery, marginally higher stress-induced increases in SBP and DBP were found in the BSO group. These results support the idea that estrogens ameliorate SAM responses to brief stressors, but are not conclu-sive because of their non-experimental nature.

To address this issue, Lindheim et al. (1992) conducted a two-part investigation of cardiovascular and neuroendocrine responses to brief speech and math stres-sors. First, a cross-sectional comparison between 13 premenopausal and 36 post-menopausal women showed that postmenopausal women produced larger stress-reactive elevations in SBP and smaller increases in cortisol than premeno-pausal women. After this baseline testing, the postmenopausal women were ran-domly assigned to either a placebo or a transdermal estradiol treatment condition. Six weeks later, stress reactivity was reassessed and the researchers compared the maximum percent change in women who received estradiol with those who received placebo. Although there were no pre-existing differences between the groups, the estradiol treatment eliminated significant cardiovascular (SBP and DBP) and neuroendocrine (ACTH, cortisol, norepinephrine, and androstenedi-one) responses to laboratory stressors. In a later study, Lindheim et al. (1994) tested the effects on stress reactivity of adding a progestin to estradiol treatment. Stress-induced increases in DBP, ACTH, and cortisol did not differ between the two treat-ment groups, although both were lower than in the placebo group. However, stress effects on SBP and norepinephrine were similar in the placebo group and the estradiol plus progestin group, indicating that progestin may reverse some of the ameliorating effects of estradiol on the stress response.

In an experimental test of acute effects of transdermal estradiol on stress responses in menopausal women, Del Rio et al. (1998) demonstrated higher stress-induced SBP and epinephrine increases in the placebo group, suggesting that some of the effects of estradiol may occur through non-genomic pathways. A randomized, double blind, placebo-controlled, cross-over experiment carried out in young men also found reduced heart rate, SBP, epinephrine, and norepinephrine reactivity to brief psychological stressors after transdermal treatment with estradiol (Del Rio et al., 1994).

These data strongly support a role for estrogens in modulating both SAM and HPA reactivity to stress. However, one recent report provides somewhat contradictory evidence (Matthews et al., 1998). In this study, a sample of young women had their ovarian hormones temporarily suppressed using an agonist to gonadotropin releasing hormone. Although the suppression of estradiol was accompanied by typical menopause symptoms, cardiovascular and neuroendocrine responses did not differ from their pre-suppression levels. Thus, factors in addition to estrogen level may contribute to the reduction in physiological effects of stress seen in post-menopausal women after estradiol treatment.

Estrogen-related differences in immune reactivity to stress: possible pathways

Recent studies of the immunological consequences of brief experimental stressors have provided preliminary evidence that individuals who exhibited the largest sympathetically mediated increases in cardiovascular reactivity also showed the largest catecholaminergic increases and immune changes (Cacioppo et al., 1995; Kiecolt-Glaser et al., 1992; Manuck et al., 1991; Sgoutas-Emch et al., 1994). These same individuals also may show the highest increases in ACTH and cortisol (Cacioppo et al., 1995), and very preliminary work in our laboratory suggests that individuals who demonstrated the greatest cortisol changes in response to brief stressors also showed poorer responses to influenza vaccine, as measured by the IL-2 response of T-lymphocytes to virus-specific antigens in vitro (Cacioppo, 1994). In addition, Mills et al. (1995a) showed that cellular immune responses were best predicted by lower basal norepinephrine, higher stress-induced norepinephrine, and higher sensitivity of $\beta2$–adrenergic receptor on lymphocytes. Thus, if estrogen dampens SAM activity or reactivity, it could have implications for immune reactivity to stress.

Alterations in SAM function could be particularly important in older adults because SAM activity can inhibit antigen processing and presentation (Heilig et al., 1993). Infectious diseases exact a high toll in morbidity and mortality among the elderly; together, pneumonia and influenza are the fourth leading cause of death in individuals over the age of 75 (Yoshikawa, 1983).

The question of estrogen effects on immune reactivity to brief stressors has been addressed in past research by investigating the possible effects of menstrual cycle stage on stress-related changes in leukocyte subsets (Mills et al., 1995a) and in the proliferative response of PBLs to PHA (Caggiula et al., 1990). Neither study found any differences in immune reactions that could be attributed to menstrual cycle phase. Given that menstrual phase effects on SAM reactivity are negligible (Stoney et al., 1990; Litschauer et al., 1998), this lack of findings is not surprising, and may be explained by the fact that the duration of action of estrogens can be maintained for up to 13 weeks (Gangar et al., 1991). Thus, the time window afforded by changes in menstrual cycle phase may be too short to detect estrogen effects (Mills et al., 1995b). Postmenopausal women provide a population in which estrogen effects can be more closely controlled, through the comparison of women using estrogen replacement therapy (ERT) with women not using any hormone treatment.

Two studies from our laboratory provide information relevant to the issue of ERT effects on stress reactivity in older women. In the first, 22 postmenopausal women carried out brief math and speech stressors (Cacioppo et al., 1995). As in other populations, the stressors heightened SAM activity, as indexed by cardiac activation and elevated plasma catecholamine concentrations, and reduced cellular immune function, as indexed by mitogen-stimulated blastogenesis of PBLs. The subset of women on ERT had lower plasma epinephrine, consistent with other studies, but we found no significant interactions between use of estrogen supplements and physiological changes induced by the stressors. However, only 6 of the 22 women in the study were taking estrogen supplements, severely limiting power for detecting estrogen differences.

The second study was designed specifically to evaluate possible effects of long-term ERT (longer than two years) on stress reactivity. Three groups of postmenopausal women carried out laboratory speech and math tasks: women who did not use ERT; women who were taking estrogen alone; and women who were taking both estrogen and progestin. Cardiovascular, neuroendocrine, and immune variables were measured prior to and after the stress protocols, providing us with estimates of baseline function and stress reactivity (Burleson et al., 1998).

In contrast to many previous studies of brief stress effects on immune function in which mitogen-stimulated blastogenesis declined post-stress (e.g. Cacioppo et al., 1995; Sgoutas-Emch et al., 1994), we did not find significant main effects of the stress tasks on Con A- or PHA-stimulated lymphocyte proliferation. Closer examination of our data, however, revealed that among the women who were not using ERT, the expected stress-related declines in blastogenesis did occur. Only in the two groups of women using ERT was mitogen-stimulated blastogenesis unaffected by the stress tasks. If stress-related changes in cellular immune function result from activation of the SAM system, as proposed by Manuck et al. (1991), then these findings would be consistent with reduced sympathetic reactivity in the women using ERT. Although our data provide no direct evidence of reduced SAM responsiveness with ERT, previous research described above has found both premenopausal status and exogenous estrogen treatment to be associated with reduced stress reactivity in the SAM system.

Along with the difference in immune reactivity, the women using ERT had significantly higher baseline and overall levels of both Con A- and PHA-induced blastogenesis than the women who did not use hormones. Because the level of mitogen-stimulated blastogenesis is considered an index of the ability of lymphocytes to respond to a pathogen, this finding supports a tonic stimulatory effect of long-term ERT on cellular immune function in this sample. Previous studies of estrogen effects on mitogen-stimulated blastogenesis typically have shown either no effect (e.g. Grossman et al., 1982) or a suppressive effect (e.g. Morishima & Henrich, 1974); however, ours is the first reported study in this population using long-duration estrogen treatment.

In addition to modulating SAM or HPA stress reactivity, recent research suggests another pathway through which estrogen may influence immune reactivity to stress. Vamvakopoulos and Chrousos (1993) provided evidence for direct estrogenic enhancement of human CRH gene expression. Through its central role in the activity of the HPA axis, CRH plays an important role in the regulation of both stress responses and immune and inflammatory reactions. Thus, these findings also may help to explain sexual dimorphism in the stress response and in immune regulation.

Our understanding of the roles that the sex hormones play in the complex interactions among the central nervous system, the SAM and HPA axes, and the immune system is still in its infancy. The limited evidence available to date suggests the effects could be very important.

REFERENCES

Ansar Ahmed, S., Penhale, W. J. & Talal, N. (1985). Sex hormones, immune responses, and auto-immune diseases: mechanisms of sex hormone action. *American Journal of Pathology*, 121, 531–51.

Beeson, P. B. (1994). Age and sex association of 40 autoimmune diseases. *American Journal of Medicine*, 96, 457–62.

Blumenthal, J. A., Fredrikson, M., Matthews, K. A., Kuhn, C. M., Schneibolk, S., German, D., Rifai, N., Steege, J. & Rodin, J. (1991). Stress reactivity and exercise training in premenopausal and postmenopausal women. *Health Psychology*, 10, 384–91.

Burleson, M. H., Malarkey, W. B., Cacioppo, J. C., Poehlmann, K. M., Kiecolt-Glaser, J. K., Berntson, G. G. & Glaser, R. (1998). Postmenopausal hormone replacement: effects on autonomic, neuroendocrine, and immune reactivity to brief psychological stressors. *Psychosomatic Medicine*, 60, 17–25.

Cacioppo, J. T. (1994). Social neuroscience: autonomic, neuroendocrine, and immune response to stress. *Psychophysiology*, 31, 113–28.

Cacioppo, J. T., Malarkey, W. B., Kiecolt-Glaser, J. K., Uchino, B. N., Sgoutas-Emch, S. A., Sheridan, J. F., Berntson, G. G. & Glaser, R. (1995). Heterogeneity in neuroendocrine and immune responses to brief psychological stressors as a function of autonomic cardiac activation. *Psychosomatic Medicine*, 57, 154–64.

Caggiula, A. R., Stoney, C. M., Matthews, K. A., Owens, J. F., Davis, M. C. & Rabin, B. S. (1990). T-lymphocyte reactivity during the menstrual cycle in women. *Clinical Immunology and Immunopathology*, 56, 130–4.

Cohen, J. H. M., Danel, L., Cordier, G., Saez, S. & Revillard, J-P. (1983). Sex steroid receptors in peripheral T-cells: absence of androgen receptors and restriction of estrogen receptors to OKT8–positive cells. *Journal of Immunology*, 131, 2767–71.

Cutolo, M., Accardo, S., Villaggio, B., Clerico, P., Bagnasco, M., Coviello, D. A., Carruba, G., lo Casto, M. & Castagnetta, L. (1993). Presence of estrogen-binding sites on macrophage-like synoviocytes and CD8+, CD29+, CD45RO+ T-lymphocytes in normal and rheumatoid synovium. *Arthritis and Rheumatism*, 36, 1087–97.

Danel, L., Souweine, G., Monier, J. C. & Saez, S. (1983). Specific estrogen binding sites in human lymphoid cells and thymic cells. *Journal of Steroid Biochemistry*, 18, 559–63.

Del Rio, G., Velardo, A., Zizzo, G., Avogaro, A., Cipolli, C., Della Casa, L., Marrama, P. & MacDonald, I. A. (1994). Effect of estradiol on the sympathoadrenal response to mental stress in normal men. *Journal of Clinical Endocrinology and Metabolism*, 79, 836–40.

Del Rio, G., Velardo, A., Menozzi, R., Zizzo, G., Tavernari, V., Venneri, M. G., Marrama, P. & Petraglia, F. (1998). Acute estradiol and progesterone administration reduced cardiovascular and catecholamine responses to mental stress in menopausal women. *Neuroendocrinology*, 67, 269–74.

Erbach, G.T & Bahr, J.M. (1991). Enhancement of in vivo humoral immunity by estrogen: permissive effect of a thymic factor. *Endocrinology*, 128, 1352–8.

Evagelatou, M. & Farrant, J. (1994). Effect of 17β-estradiol on immunoglobulin secretion by human tonsillar lymphocytes *in vitro*. *Journal of Steroid Biochemistry and Molecular Biology*, 48, 171–7.

Forsberg, J-G. (1984). Short-term and long-term effects of estrogen on lymphoid tissues and lymphoid cells with some remarks on the significance for carcinogenesis. *Archives of Toxicology*, 55, 79–90.

Frankenhaeuser, M. (1983). The sympathetic–adrenal and pituitary–adrenal response to challenge: comparison between the sexes. In *Biobehavioral Basis of Coronary Artery Disease*, ed. T. M. Dembroski, T. H. Schmidt & G. Blumchen, pp. 91–103. New York: Karger.

Frazier-Jessen, M. R. & Kovacs, E. J. (1995). Estrogen modulation of JE/monocyte chemoattractant protein-1 mRNA expression in murine macrophages. *Journal of Immunology*, 154, 1838–45.

Gangar, K. F., Vyas, S., Whitehead, M., Crook, D., Meire, H. & Campbell, S. (1991). Pulsatility index in internal carotid artery in relation to transdermal oestradiol and time since menopause. *Lancet*, 338, 839–42.

Garovich, M., Agudelo, C. & Pisko, E. (1980). Oral contraceptives and systemic lupus erythematosus. *Arthritis and Rheumatism*, **23**, 1396–8.

Grossman, C. J. (1984). Regulation of the immune system by sex steroids. *Endocrine Reviews*, **5**, 435–55.

Grossman, C. J. (1985). Interactions between the gonadal steroids and the immune system. *Science*, **227**, 257–60.

Grossman, C. J., Sholiton, L. J. & Roselle, G. (1982). Estradiol regulation of thymic lymphocyte function in the rat: mediation by serum thymic factors. *Journal of Steroid Biochemistry*, **16**, 683–6.

Gulshan, S., McCruden, A. B. & Stimson, W. H. (1990). Oestrogen receptors in macrophages. *Scandinavian Journal of Immunology*, **31**, 691–7.

Heilig, M., Irwin, M., Grewal, I. & Sercarz, E. (1993). Sympathetic regulation of T-helper cell function. *Brain, Behavior, and Immunity*, **7**, 154–63.

Herrera, L. A., Montero, R., Leon-Casares, J. M., Rojas, E., Gonsebatt, M. & Ostrosky-Wegman, P. (1992). Effects of progesterone and estradiol on the proliferation of PHA-stimulated human lymphocytes. *Mutation Research*, **270**, 211–18.

Hu, S. K., Mitcho, Y. L. & Rath, N. (1988). Effect of estradiol in interleukin 1 synthesis by macrophages. *International Journal of Immunopharmacology*, **10**, 247–52.

Kiecolt-Glaser, J. K., Cacioppo, J. T., Malarkey, W. B. & Glaser, R. (1992). Acute psychological stressors and short-term immune changes: what, why, for whom, and to what extent? *Psychosomatic Medicine*, **54**, 680–5.

Kittas, C. & Henry, L. (1980). Effect of sex hormones on the response of mice to infection with *Toxoplasma gondii*. *British Journal of Experimental Pathology*, **61**, 590–600.

Lahita, R. G. (1997). Effects of gender on the immune system: implications for neuropsychiatric systemic lupus erythematosus. *Annals of the New York Academy of Sciences*, **823**, 247–51.

Light, K. C., Girdler, S. S., West, S. & Brownley, K. A. (1998). Blood pressure response to laboratory challenges and occupational stress in women. In *Women, Stress, and Heart Disease*, ed. K. Orth-Gomer, M. Chesney & N. K. Wenger, pp. 237–61. Mahwah, NJ: Lawrence Erlbaum Associates, Inc.

Lindheim, S. R., Legro, R. S., Bernstein, L., Stanczyk, F. Z., Vijod, M. A., Presser, S. C. & Lobo, R. A. (1992). Behavioral stress responses in premenopausal and postmenopausal women and the effects of estrogen. *American Journal of Obstetrics and Gynecology*, **167**, 1831–6.

Lindheim, S. R., Legro, R. S., Morris, R. S., Wong, I. L., Tran, D. Q., Vijod, M. A., Stanczyk, F. Z. & Lobo, R. A. (1994). The effect of progestins on behavioral stress responses in postmenopausal women. *Journal of the Society for Gynecologic Investigation*, **1**, 79–83.

Litschauer, B., Zauchner, S., Huemer, K. H. & Kafra-Luetzow, A. (1998). Cardiovascular, endocrine, and receptor measures as related to sex and the menstrual cycle phase. *Psychosomatic Medicine*, **60**, 219–26.

Manuck, S. B. & Polefrone, J. (1987). Psychophysiologic reactivity in women. In *Coronary Heart Disease in Women*, ed. E. D. Eaker, B. Packard & N. K. Wenger, pp. 164–71. New York: Haymarket Doyna.

Manuck, S. B., Cohen, S., Rabin, B. S., Muldoon, M. F. & Bachen, E. A. (1991). Individual differences in cellular immune response to stress. *Psychological Science*, **2**, 111–15.

Matthews, K. A. (1989). Interactive effects of behavior and reproductive hormones on sex differences in risk for coronary heart disease. *Health Psychology*, 8, 373–87.

Matthews, K. A. & Stoney, C. M. (1988). Influences of sex and age on cardiovascular responses during stress. *Psychosomatic Medicine*, 50, 46–56.

Matthews, K. A., Berga, S. L., Owens, J. F. & Flory, J. D. (1998). Effects of short-term suppression of ovarian hormones on cardiovascular and neuroendocrine reactivity to stress in women. *Psychoneuroendocrinology*, 23, 307–22.

Medina, K. L. & Kincade, P. W. (1994). Pregnancy-related steroids are potential negative regulators of B lymphopoeisis. *Proceedings of the National Academy of Sciences, USA*, 91, 5382–6.

Mendelsohn, J., Multer, M. M. & Bernheim, J. L. (1977). Inhibition of human lymphocyte stimulation by steroid hormones: cytokinetic mechanisms. *Clinical and Experimental Immunology*, 27, 127–34.

Miller, L. & Hunt, J. S. (1996). Sex steroid hormones and macrophage function. *Life Sciences*, 59, 1–14.

Mills, P. M., Berry, C. C., Dimsdale, J. E., Ziegler, M. G., Nelesen, R. A. & Kennedy, B. P. (1995a). Lymphocyte subset redistribution in response to acute experimental stress: effects of gender, ethnicity, hypertension, and the sympathetic nervous system. *Brain, Behavior, and Immunity*, 9, 61–9.

Mills, P. M., Ziegler, M. G., Dimsdale, J. E. & Parry, B. L. (1995b). Enumerative immune changes following acute stress: effect of the menstrual cycle. *Brain, Behavior and Immunity*, 9, 190–5.

Morishima, A. & Henrich, R. (1974). Lymphocyte transformation and oral contraceptives. *Lancet*, Sept 14, 646.

Neifeld, J. P. & Tormey, D. C. (1979). Effects of steroid hormones on PHA-stimulated human PBL. *Transplantation*, 27, 309–14.

Nilsson, B., Carlsson, S., Damber, M-G., Lindblom, D., Sodergaed, R. & von Schoulz, B. (1984). Specific binding of 17β-estradiol in the human thymus. *American Journal of Obstetrics and Gynecology*, 149, 544–7.

Owens, J. F., Stoney, C. M. & Matthews, K. A. (1993). Menopausal status influences ambulatory blood pressure levels and blood pressure changes during mental stress. *Circulation*, 88, 2784–802.

Paavonen, T., Andersson, L. C. & Adlercreutz, H. (1981). Sex hormone regulation of in vitro immune response. Estradiol enhances human B cell maturation via inhibition of suppressor T-cells in pokeweed mitogen-stimulated cultures. *Journal of Experimental Medicine*, 154, 1935–45.

Pacifici, R., Brown, C., Puscheck, E., Friedrich, E., Slatopolsky, E., Maggio, D., McCracken, R. & Avioli, L. V. (1991). Effect of surgical menopause and estrogen replacement on cytokine release from human blood mononuclear cells. *Proceedings of the National Academy of Sciences, USA*, 88, 5134–8.

Polan, M. L., Daniele, A. & Kuo, A. (1988). Gonadal steroids modulate human monocyte interleukin-1 (IL-1) activity. *Fertility and Sterility*, 49, 964–8.

Polan, M. L., Loukides, J., Nelson, P., Carding, S., Diamond, M., Walsh, A. & Bottomly, K. (1989). Progesterone and estradiol modulate interleukin-1β messenger ribonucleic acid levels in cultured human peripheral monocytes. *Journal of Clinical Endocrinology and Metabolism*, **89**, 1200–6.

Ranelletti, F. O., Piantelli, M., Carbone, A., Rinelli, A., Scambia, G., Panici, P. B. & Mancuso, S. (1988). Type II estrogen-binding sites and 17β-hydroxysteroid dehydrogenase activity in human peripheral blood monocuclear cells. *Journal of Clinical Endocrinology and Metabolism*, **67**, 888–92.

Roubinian, J. R., Talal, N., Siiteri, P. K. & Sadakian, J. A. (1979). Sex hormone modulation of autoimmunity in NZB/NZW mice. *Arthritis and Rheumatism*, **22**, 1162.

Saab, P. G. (1989). Cardiovascular and neuroendocrine responses to challenge in males and females. In *Handbook of Research Methods in Cardiovascular Behavioral Medicine* ed. N. Schneiderman, S. M. Weiss & P. G. Kaufman. New York: Plenum.

Saab, P. G., Matthews, K. A., Stoney, C. M. & McDonald, R. H. (1989). Premenopausal and post-menopausal women differ in their cardiovascular and neuroendocrine responses to behavioral stressors. *Psychophysiology*, **26**, 270–80.

Sanchez-Guerrero, J., Liang, M. H., Karlson, E. W., Hunter, D. J. & Colditz, G. A. (1995). Postmenopausal estrogen therapy and the risk for developing systemic Lupus erythematosus. *Annals of Internal Medicine*, **122**, 430–3.

Schuurs, A. H. & Verheul, H. A. (1990). Effects of gender and sex steroids on the immune response. *Journal of Steroid Biochemistry*, **35**, 157–72.

Sgoutas-Emch, S.A., Cacioppo, J. T., Uchino, B., Malarkey, W., Pearl, D., Kiecolt-Glaser, J. K. & Glaser, R. (1994). The effects of an acute psychological stressor on cardiovascular, endocrine, and cellular immune response: a prospective study of individuals high and low in heart reactivity. *Psychophysiology*, **31**, 264–71.

Smithson, G., Couse, J. F., Lubahn, D. B., Korach, K. S. & Kincade, P. W. (1998). The role of estrogen receptors and androgen receptors in sex steroid regulation of B lymphopoiesis. *Journal of Immunology*, **161**, 27–34.

Stimson, W. H. (1988). Oestrogen and human T-lymphocytes: presence of specific receptors in the T suppressor/cytotoxic subset. *Scandinavian Journal of Immunology*, **28**, 345–50.

Stoney, C. M., Davis, M. C. & Matthews, K. A. (1987). Sex differences in physiological responses to stress and in coronary heart disease: a causal link? *Psychophysiology*, **24**, 127–31.

Stoney, C. M., Owens, J. F., Guzick, D. S. & Matthews, K. A. (1997). A natural experiment on the effects of ovarian hormones on cardiovascular risk factors and stress reactivity: bilateral salpingo oophorectomy versus hysterectomy only. *Health Psychology*, **16**, 349–58.

Stoney, C. M., Owens, J. F., Matthews, K. A., Davis, M. C. & Caggiula, A. R. (1990). Influences of the normal menstrual cycle on physiologic functioning during behavioral stress. *Psychophysiology*, **27**, 125–35.

Vamvakopoulos, N. C. & Chrousos, G. P. (1993). Evidence of direct estrogenic regulation of human corticotropin-releasing hormone gene expression: potential implications for the sexual dimorphism of the stress response and immune/inflammatory reaction. *Journal of Clinical Investigation*, **92**, 1896–902.

Vandenbroucke, J. P., Valkenburg, H. A. & Boersma, J. W. (1982). Oral contraceptives and rheumatoid arthritis: further evidence for a preventive effect. *Lancet*, **2**(8303), 839–42.

Weetman, A. P., McGregor, A. M., Rees Smith, B. & Hall, R. (1981). Sex hormones enhance immunoglobulin synthesis by human peripheral blood lymphocytes. *Immunology Letters*, 3, 343–6.

Weusten, J. J. A. M., Blankenstein, M. A., Gmelig-Meyling, F. H. J., Schuurman, H. J., Kater, L. & Thijssen, J. H. H. (1986). Presence of oestrogen receptors in human blood mononuclear cells and thymocytes. *Acta Endocrinologica*, 112, 409–14.

Wyle, F. A. & Kent, J. R. (1977). Immunosuppression by sex steroid hormones. *Clinical and Experimental Immunology*, 27, 407–15.

Yoshikawa, T. T. (1983). Geriatric infectious diseases: an emerging problem. *Journal of the American Geriatrics Society*, 31, 34–9.

14

Gender differences in immune function at the cellular level

Eva Redei and Suresh G. Shelat

Introduction

Over the past 15 years, it has become increasingly apparent that, to achieve homeo-stasis, the immune system interacts and communicates through soluble signals with other major systems of the body, such as the nervous and the endocrine systems. Through the finely tuned modulation of the neuroendocrine system, the organism can cope with stress and similarly, through the finely tuned modulation of the immune system, pathogens are eliminated without injury to the host. Excessive activation of the neuroendocrine system leads to stress-related disorders including affective disorders, and excessive activation of the immune system can lead to autoimmune diseases, allergies, hypersensitivity, and anaphylaxis. In con-trast, hypoactivation or suppression of the neuroendocrine stress-response can lead to fatigue and certain mood disorders, and hypoactivation of the immune system can promote infectious diseases and neoplasia.

A number of autoimmune illnesses have a female prevalence. The question arises whether there is a common biological etiology in these illnesses since mood disor-ders known to be precipitated or worsened by stress, such as depression, rapid cycling bipolar disorder and certain types of anxiety disorders, have much higher prevalence among women. The most frequently examined biological parameter, resting plasma cortisol levels, shows a biphasic distribution in affective disorders: hypercortisolemia in melancholic depression and hypocortisolemia in atypic depression. In contrast, hypocortisolemia is frequently found in autoimmune ill-nesses, and the most common treatment for these illnesses is pharmacological doses of glucocorticoids used as immunosuppressants. Thus, it seems to be appar-ent that in pathophysiology characterized by increased levels of glucocorticoids the immune system is suppressed. Furthermore, female sex hormones, particularly estrogen, may interfere with the glucocorticoid response to prolonged stress that can precipitate depression or the glucocorticoid response to inflammation, as occurs in some autoimmune inflammatory illnesses. Therefore, estrogen can inter-fere with inflammatory responses directly, or via altering the efficacy of glucocorticoids to change the expressions of genes involved in an immune or inflammatory response.

In this chapter, we propose the hypothesis that common genes are involved in certain autoimmune diseases and mood disorders. Aging and hormone replacement therapy may affect the expression of these genes, since many of them are known to be directly or indirectly regulated by estrogen. Next, we elaborate on the possible cellular and molecular mechanisms of the female prevalence in autoimmune illnesses as a model for understanding the role of sex hormones in immune function. Since animal models of autoimmune illnesses have implicated the T-helper cells as the primary mediators of autoimmune disease, we are also focusing on mediators of T-helper cell function and their relationship to sex steroids.

Sex differences in the neuroendocrine stress response: the role of glucocorticoids and their receptors.

Sex differences in basal cortisol levels and/or in the secretion of plasma glucocorticoids in response to environmental stressors or corticotropin releasing factor have been established in humans, with levels tending to be higher in women (Zumoff et al., 1974, Luisi et al., 1998). In rats, basal plasma corticosterone levels and corticosterone responses to stress are generally higher in females than in males (for review see Redei et al., 1994). During the normal menstrual cycle, basal secretion of cortisol follows a cyclic pattern that approximates the changes found in plasma estradiol (E_2) and progesterone (P) levels (Genazzani et al., 1975). In the normal female rat, increased or unchanged basal plasma corticosterone levels were reported at about the time of proestrus. During proestrus, corticosterone stress-responses have exceeded those seen during diestrus and estrus (Viau & Meaney, 1991). However, the corticosterone response to endotoxin stimulation did not vary during the cycle (Spinedi et al., 1992). The removal of gonadal hormones by gonadectomy increased the amount of corticosterone secreted in response to IL-1β (Rivier, 1994), and estrogen replacement in ovariectomized animals reduced plasma corticosterone responses to footshock stress (Redei et al., 1994). Thus it seems that during the reproductive period of females, female sex steroids promote the glucocorticoid responses to stressful stimuli, while after ovariectomy (and perhaps also in normal menopause) estrogen is inhibitory to the glucocorticoid stress response.

Since the repression of both 'stress-related' genes – such as pro-opiomelanocortin (POMC) and corticotropin-releasing hormone (CRH) – and of proinflammatory genes – such as IL-1 and IL-6 – involves glucocorticoid receptors (GR), sex differences in GR expression would ultimately affect GR-induced suppression of these genes. Little information exists on sex differences in GR expression of immune cells, but in general, brain and spleen glucocorticoid binding are regulated similarly, and in the pituitary and in the brain, females show less gluco-corticoid binding than males (Turner, 1990). Ovariectomy increases the number of GR binding sites in the hypothalamus (Turner & Weaver, 1985) that can be reversed by dexamethasone (Pfeiffer et al., 1991) suggesting that the increase in GR is due to lower glucocorticoid levels following ovariectomy. However, E_2 administration to long-term ovariectomized rats also increases GR mRNA (Redei et al., 1994). Estrogen may regulate GR directly as well as through regulating basal and stress-induced glucocorticoid levels.

In extrapolating these data to the prevalence of both autoimmune illnesses and affective disorders in human females, we could postulate the following hypothesis. In cycling females, higher basal levels of glucocorticoids may permanently down-regulate the expression of GR (as it has been observed) and therefore decrease the efficacy of glucocorticoids in regulating glucocorticoid-responsive genes, even if the glucocorticoid response to acute stimuli is higher in the female than in the male. This effect may lead to increased susceptibility to autoimmune illnesses due to the decreased suppression of glucocorticoid-regulated 'stress' and pro-inflammatory genes.

Mechanism of glucocorticoid regulation of immune function

The anti-inflammatory therapeutic effect of glucocorticoids is thought to be medi-ated by multiple mechanisms including such different mechanisms as the repres-sion of metalloprotease genes such as collagenase (Jonat et al., 1990); the inhibition of the pro-inflammatory IL-1β (Lee & Tsou, 1988); or the increase of the immu-nosuppressor cytokine IL-10 (Gayo et al., 1998). In each case, however, glucocorti-coids affect gene expression at the transcriptional level.

Glucocorticoid receptor is a member of a superfamily of ligand-activated hormone receptors that function as transcriptional modulators. The hormone-bound GR binds to specific sequences (glucocorticoid responsive elements, GREs) in the 5' flanking regions of target genes and alters transcriptional activity. Glucocorticoids are involved in the negative regulation of many genes including POMC (Drouin et al., 1989) and proliferin (Mordacq & Linzer, 1989). This inhibi-tion may occur via putative 'negative GREs', sequences upstream from glucocorti-coid-regulated genes that differ from GREs and may overlap with transcriptional activation sites.

Recent studies have described a mechanism whereby the GR can interfere with the activity of another transcription factor, AP-1, by direct protein–protein inter-action (Diamond et al., 1990). The AP-1 transcription factor complex is composed of Jun and Fos oncoproteins. Glucocorticoid receptors can interact with an AP-1 transcription heterodimer (Fos/Jun) or homodimer (Jun/Jun) to either inhibit or activate the transcription of glucocorticoid-responsive genes. An additional mechanism for glucocorticoid-induced inhibition of gene expression may involve NF-ATp, a transcription factor expressed in T-cells following their stimulation (Shaw et al., 1988). It was shown to bind the IL-2 promoter together with an IL-2 AP-1 motif (Jain et al., 1992). The GR may mediate the suppression of IL-2 expression via impairment of the cooperativity between NF-ATp and AP-1 enhancer elements (Vacca et al., 1990). Furthermore, it has recently been shown that glucocorticoids induce the production of IκBα, a cytoplasmic inhibitor of NF-κB, thereby reducing the amount of NF-κB that can translocate to the nucleus and subsequently decrease cytokine production (Auphan et al., 1995, Scheinman et al., 1995). Taken together, these findings show that all genes containing a negative GRE or AP-1 binding site or an NF-ATp site in their promoter region may be suppressed by glucocorticoids.

The expression of several pro-inflammatory and pro-autoimmune lymphokines including IL-1β (Lee & Tsou, 1988), IL-2 (Rao, 1994), IL-3, IL-6 (Ray et al., 1990), IFN-γ (Almawi et al., 1991), and TNF (Tsujimoto et al., 1988) are suppressed by glucocorticoids through any of the mechanisms described above. Interestingly, whereas the NF–ATp complex that is thought to drive IL-2 expression contains an AP-1 component, the NF–ATp complex alone can drive IL-4 expression without the AP-1 complex (Rooney et al., 1994). This suggests that mechanisms mediated by protein kinase-C, calcium, or AP-1 may serve to specify the differential cytokine expression by subsets of T-helper cells and their respective cellular functions in the immune response.

In addition to the findings that high levels of glucocorticoids can regulate immune function through their suppressive effects on the expression of several cytokines, recent reports also suggest that decreased levels of glucocorticoids or a lack of glucocorticoid receptors can also permanently impair T-cell function. In transgenic adult mice expressing GR antisense, an increase in the percentage of immature double positive and helper T-cells and a decrease in the number of suppressor-cytotoxic T-cells were found (Morale et al., 1995). These phenotypic changes are also reflected in a higher lymphocyte proliferative response to T-cell mitogens. In another study, transgenic mice were generated that express antisense transcripts to GR, specifically in immature double negative thymocytes (King et al., 1995). In these animals, there was a dramatic loss of double positive thymocytes (Ashwell et al., 1996) suggesting that glucocorticoid stimulation is required for normal progression of CD4$^-$CD8$^-$ to CD4$^+$CD8$^+$ cells.

Glucocorticoid regulation of thymic development can apparently also occur through locally produced glucocorticoids as thymic epithelial cells can produce corticosterone in response to ACTH (Vacchio et al., 1994). This thymic production of corticosterone suggests the existence of local thymic CRH–ACTH–corticosterone regulation since both ACTH and CRH are synthesized locally in the thymus.

Mechanism of sex steroid regulation of immune function

Clinical, physiological, and experimental data clearly suggest a sexual dimorphism in the immune function (Ansar et al., 1985). Females seem to have a more vigorous immune response, higher immunoglobulin concentrations, and better resistance against certain viral and parasitic infections. However, the majority of patients suffering from autoimmune diseases are also female (Ahmed & Talal, 1989). In contrast, males seem to be more susceptible than females to certain infectious diseases (Green, 1992), but less susceptible to autoimmune diseases. The predominance in infectious diseases was suggested to stem from a higher prevalence of relative immune deficiency in males (Schegel et al., 1969).

The higher female/male susceptibility ratio is seen in most, but not all, autoimmune illnesses: the adult form of Hashimoto's thyroiditis, 25–50:1; systemic lupus erythematosus (SLE), 9:1; rheumatoid arthritis (RA) and multiple sclerosis 2–3:1, but not in insulin dependent diabetes mellitus (Beeson, 1994). The female preponderance is more pronounced during the childbearing years than in the periods preceding or following the reproductive years. This latter finding, together with the increased susceptibility ratio in females, argues for the involvement of sex steroids in the etiology or the manifestation of these autoimmune illnesses.

Estrogen is the obvious candidate to attribute the female prevalence in most autoimmune illnesses. Estrogen, however, seems to have opposing effects in autoimmunity, and it has been suggested that autoimmune diseases can be divided into two categories on the basis of their responsiveness to estrogen. In the first group, which includes SLE, the autoimmunity involves polyclonal B-cell activation. In the much larger second group, which includes rheumatoid arthritis, Hashimoto's thyroiditis, and multiple sclerosis, T-cell-mediated mechanisms seem to induce the autoimmune process.

The role of sex steroids has been extensively investigated in human SLE as well as in an animal model of SLE, the NZB/W mice. Female SLE patients have abnormal metabolism of androgens and decreased levels of testosterone (T), dihydrotestosterone (DHT), and dihydroepiandrosterone (DHEA; Lahita et al., 1990). The disease is exacerbated during pregnancy and by treatment with oral contraceptives. Therapeutic regimens aimed at increasing the androgen/estrogen ratio, such as the medication Danazol, lead to clinical improvement (Dougados et al., 1990). The mechanism may involve activating T-suppressor cells, thus leading to decreased antibody production. In the SLE animal model, the disease progresses more rapidly in NZB/W female mice than in males, and DHT treatment of ovariectomized mice ameliorates the disease and restores suppressor function and IL-2 production (Ahmed & Talal, 1989). In contrast to SLE, estrogens seem to ameliorate the clinical symptoms of rheumatoid arthritis rather than aggravate it. Rheumatoid symptoms subside during pregnancy, oral contraceptive treatment, or with estrogen replacement therapy. The elevated levels of IL-1 and IL-2 reported in the joint fluid of RA patients (Wood et al., 1983; Nouri et al., 1984) suggest that both macrophages and a subset of T-helper cells are activated.

Cellular events induced by sex steroids

Increased production of IL-2 or increased responsiveness to IL-2 has been observed in a number of clinical autoimmune illnesses such as SLE, myasthenia gravis, and multiple sclerosis. Elevated levels of IL-1, IL-2 and IL-6 have also been reported in the joint fluid of patients with RA and other inflammatory diseases (Wood et al., 1983; Nouri et al., 1984; Hirano et al., 1988). Since excessive production of these immunostimulatory cytokines has been implicated in the pathogenesis of RA (Arend & Dayer, 1990), the female prevalence of this disease may be directly related to the effects of sex steroids on the synthesis and secretion of these cytokines.

A phenomenon of dose-dependent stimulatory or inhibitory effects of estrogen on IL-1 production in cycling and ovariectomized females, respectively, is very similar to the biphasic effects of estrogen on plasma glucocorticoid production. Serum levels of IL-1 are elevated during the periovulatory (high estrogen) phase of the menstrual cycle (Cannon & Dinarello, 1985) but IL-1 production from monocytes is increased in menopause, and this increase is reversed by estrogen/progesterone replacement (Pacifici et al., 1989). Interestingly, IL-1 release from peripheral blood mononuclear cells (PBMC) is also increased after oophorectomy (Pioli et al., 1992). A further complexity is indicated by the finding that IL-1 production by human monocytes in vitro is stimulated by physiological concentrations of estrogen (Polan et al., 1988) and inhibited by higher doses of the steroid. A similarly complex regulation is found in rats, where peritoneal macrophages synthesize and secrete increased amounts of IL-1 in response to estrogen (Hu et al., 1988). Furthermore, macrophages from adult female rats produce more IL-1 than those from males; ovariectomy reduces IL-1 production, but this can be reversed by estrogen replacement.

Expression of the IL-6 gene is readily induced by inflammation-associated cytokines such as IL-1 (Isshiki et al., 1990). Thus, it is not surprising that the biological activities of IL-6 are closely interrelated to those of IL-1 (Kishimoto, 1989). Production of IL-6 from PBMC is also increased after oophorectomy (Pioli et al., 1992), although high doses of estrogen are necessary to stimulate IL-6 production in vitro (Li et al., 1993).

IL-2 is produced by a subset of T-cells. Functional T-cell subsets have been defined by their surface markers and the patterns of lymphokines produced: T-helper-1 (Th1) and T-helper-2 (Th2). Th1 cells produce IL-2, tumor necrosis factor-β and interferon-γ and serve as effector cells for cell mediated immunity and delayed-type hypersensitivity. The Th2 cells produce cytokines IL-4, IL-5, IL-6, and IL-10 and regulate antibody formation (Mossman & Coffman, 1989). Stimulated lymphocytes of female mice elicits a higher IFN-γ response than in male mice both in vivo and in vitro (McFarland & Bigley, 1989), an effect that may result from estrogen stimulating IFN-γ production. Female mice seem to produce more IL-4 than males; perhaps the result of decreased levels of testosterone in females. Daynes and colleagues have shown that DHT, derived from testosterone, can inhibit the production of IL-4, IL-5, and IFN-γ but not of IL-2 from activated T-cells (Araneo et al., 1991).

The potential mechanisms whereby sex hormones may modulate a predisposition for autoimmunity includes the direct and indirect effects of sex steroids on immunoregulatory T-lymphocytes. The direct effects on transcriptional regulation of steroid responsive genes involve interaction of steroid hormone receptors and other transcriptional factors with cis-acting sequences. Alternatively, estrogen can act indirectly through alteration of the expression of glucocorticoid receptors (GR), thereby altering the response to glucocorticoids as described above.

Direct effects of sex steroids on immune function

The primary criterion for a direct effect of sex steroids on immune cells is the presence of steroid receptors in these cells. Estrogen receptors have been found in human peripheral blood mononuclear cells, CD8$^+$ (suppressor/cytotoxic) T-lymphocytes (Stimson, 1988), thymic, and spleen cells (Danel et al., 1983), but not in CD4$^+$ (helper/inducer) lymphocytes (Cohen et al., 1983) or B-cells. Androgen receptors have been found in human thymus (Grossman et al., 1983) but not in peripheral T-cells (Cohen et al., 1983; see Table 14.1). Androgen receptor binding and expression have been found recently in rat thymic epithelial cells, and the thymolytic actions of androgens are mediated through these receptors (Kumar et al., 1995).

In order for these steroids to have a direct effect on any component of the immune function, their activated receptors would directly regulate transcription of genes important in T-cell function. Among the previously mentioned proinflammatory or T-cell derived lymphokines only IFN-γ has been shown to date to have estrogen responsive elements in its promoter region. In a transient expression assay, estradiol markedly increased the activity from the IFN-γ promoter in lymphoid cells that express estrogen receptor (Fox et al., 1991). Although IFN-γ is made by CD4$^+$ and CD8$^+$ cells, only CD8$^+$ cells have estrogen receptors. Thus, it seems that direct hormonal effects on these cells can contribute to the gender differences found in some autoimmune disorders.

Table 14.1. Direct effects of sex steroids on immune function

Steroid receptors	ER	AR	PR
Thymus	+	+	?
Spleen	+	+	?
Macrophages	+/?	?	?
T-cells	−	−	−
CD4+	−	−	−
CD8+	+	−	−
B-cells	−	−	?

Source: Adapted from Cohen et al., 1983; Grossman et al., 1983

Even in the absence of estrogen responsive elements (ERE), lymphokine genes can be regulated by estrogen or other steroids through trans-acting elements or a cascade-type regulation (Beato, 1989). One model of steroid regulation of gene expression proposes that the liganded steroid receptor binds to regulatory sequences in 'early genes' that code for transcriptional factors. These factors then act to regulate expression of 'delayed structural' genes (Spelsberg et al., 1987). Such a cascade model could provide an enhanced level of fine-tuning of cell-specific gene regulation even in the absence of trans-acting elements.

For example, estrogen increases the expression of c-jun and c-fos in a variety of tissues, including rat uterus (Weisz & Rosalles, 1990; Weisz et al., 1990) and rat anterior pituitary (Szijan et al., 1992) suggesting that the estrogen receptor (ER) acts on upstream regulatory elements. Since a Jun–Fos heterodimer or a Jun–Jun homodimer can bind to an AP-1 site in the promoter region, estrogen may enhance transcription from genes having an AP-1 site. In order for this to occur, the cell must have the ER, as well as express c-fos and c-jun (both of which must contain ERE in their promoter regions), while the target gene must contain an AP-1 site. Two potential EREs were located in the human c-fos promoter of HeLa cells (Weisz & Rosalles, 1990). EREs and other hormone-response elements were found in the 3'-flanking region of the mouse c-fos gene (Hyder et al., 1998). If all the previous criteria are fulfilled, then estrogen or other steroid receptors can regulate a wider array of genes in a tissue-specific manner than is currently thought.

Aging

The lifespan of the different cell types responsible for maintaining the communication between the neuroendocrine and immune systems is a function of genetic components (expression) and environmental influences. Most cell types of related organisms have similar lifespans despite different physiological environments, indicating the importance of the genetic program. The cellular aging process may involve subtle, but cumulative, changes in transcription and expression that leads to progressive cellular failure (Vellanoweth et al., 1994).

Cellular aging or senescence refers to the declining ability of a cell to proliferate in vitro (Goldstein, 1990) with senescent cells arresting prior to DNA replication at the G1/S phase (Rittling et al., 1986). The expression of genes involved in DNA synthesis and the activity of different cell-specific and ubiquitous transcription factors may underlie the age-related changes in gene expression and cellular activity seen in cellular senescence. The most important mechanism that regulate the onset of senescence are the telomeres (tips of the chromosomes), which shorten with each round of cell division until they are shortened beyond a critical level to induce senescence (Singh & Gupta, 1998). Cancer cells, however, can undergo an infinite number of divisions by increasing telomerase activity which can restore the telomere length, and thereby the cells do not undergo senescence. Inserting the telomerase gene into senescent human cells can lead to cells that can be characterized as young and healthy (Fossel, 1998). Interestingly, the proto-oncogene c-myc induces telomerase activity (Fujimoto & Takahashi, 1997), and estrogen is known to induce c-myc expression (Murphy et al., 1987). Estrogen, therefore, may play a role in balancing telomerase activity between cellular senescence and malignancy.

Several cell-cycle genes are expressed at normal levels in aged fibroblasts. However, there is a decrease in the expression of others, such as the G1/S-specific thymidine kinase. This may be the result of the diminished activity of a specific CCAAT-binding protein, CBP/tk that is involved in the regulation of the thymidine kinase genes in human fibroblasts during senescence (Pang & Chen, 1993).

Alternatively, increased expression of genes, such as sdi-1 (senescent cell-derived inhibitors) may occur in senescent cells. This increase in transcription paralleled the onset of a senescent phenotype and the loss of cell proliferation (Noda et al., 1994). The protein product of this gene was identical to another protein that was positively regulated by the tumor suppressor transcription factor p53 (Harper et al., 1993; El-Deiry et al., 1993; Xiong et al., 1993). Therefore, cellular aging may reflect a loss of regulation of p53, which may inhibit growth in senescent cells via action on sdi-1 and suppression of cyclin-dependent kinases.

AP-1 activity is necessary to initiate DNA synthesis and to progress from the G1 to S phase in cell division. However, senescent fibroblasts express ten-fold lower levels of c-fos mRNA (Seshadri & Campisi, 1990), therefore, the resulting AP-1 complexes may consist of low stochiometric Fos/Jun ratios (Riabowol et al., 1992). This may explain the diminished AP-1 activity since Jun–Jun homodimers are less active than the Fos–Jun heterodimer. The role of the AP-1 complex may also be seen in senescent T-lymphocytes where there is a general decline in T-cell function and proliferative capacity (Thoman, 1985) reflected by a decline in AP-1 DNA binding activity in vivo (Sikora et al., 1992) as well as a decrease in IL-2 expression (Nagel et al., 1988). However, because all cells do not require c-fos for growth, the reduced proliferation seen in senescence may result from the interaction of other tissue-specific factors with cell cycle modulators such as the tumor suppressors p53 or retinoblastoma gene products.

Several groups have examined the DNA-binding activities of other transcription factors at the prepubertal, adult, and senescent stages. The transcription factor Sp1 is found in many mammalian cell types. Studies have shown that nuclear extracts from aged rat brain and liver have 60–fold less binding activity to Sp1 sites, which may actually reflect post-translational modifications rather than a diminished level of Sp1 transcription. In addition, Sp1–responsive genes decrease in expression during senescence (Ammendola et al., 1992). Likewise, the binding activity of the transcription factor CREB declines with age (Singh & Kanungo, 1993). This profile is not universal: while AP-1 was found to be (normally) low during immaturity, rise in adulthood, and decline markedly during senescence, the transcription factors NF-1 and C/EBP showed no change in activity with senescence (Vellanoweth et al., 1994). It seems that, in addition to gene defects that lead to human diseases, an age-related decline in functions are associated with changes in transcription factors that can regulate these 'disease' genes. Cellular aging may represent an unmasking of disease genes to which the organism was already predisposed.

An alternative but not exclusive mechanism is related to the increased production of the 'immunosuppressive' cortisol in aging and to the dramatic decreases that occur in the levels of the 'immunoprotective' DHEA. The age-dependent decrease in the production of DHEA is correlated with increased IL-6 production (Straub et al., 1998), and this increased IL-6 may contribute to the presence of inflammatory and age-related illnesses such as rheumatoid arthritis.

Areas for further study

In this review, we have presented a limited number of examples illustrating the sex difference in cellular immune function. We have also attempted to describe at least some of the cellular and molecular mechanisms that underlie this sexual dimorphism, including new and more general principles describing the regulation of gene expression by steroids. The interaction between the brain, endocrine, and immune systems is a newly emerging interdisciplinary area. Adding the complexities of gender and aging issues makes it an unmanageable area for basic science explorations. Therefore, we have developed a scientific outline that may lead to further understanding of these complex issues. Further elucidation of the etiology of the sexual dimorphism in immune function requires molecular analysis of sex steroid receptors in immune cells and of their interaction with transcription factors and regulatory sequences necessary to confer responsiveness to sex steroids in cytokine gene expression. It is furthermore important to determine how sex steroids regulate the expression of glucocorticoid receptors and whether this regulation is cell- or tissue-specific.

This basic analysis can be extended to multiple animal studies to identify the mediators of sexual differentiation of the immune system and their relationship to the sexual differentiation of the brain: first, to characterize the immune function of male and female animals during development and in aging; second, to develop animal models of mood disorders showing high sex predominance and to characterize their immune function; and third, to elucidate the relationship between the stress response and immune function in young, adult, and aged male versus female animals. Clinically, one can ask how the hormonal milieu affects the immune response in healthy men and women of all ages. Then, elucidating the effect of mood disorders on the immune competence of aged men and women would clarify whether those with mood disorders are substantially more susceptible to infectious diseases or neoplasia. Finally, establishing the role of estrogen replacement on immunocompetence in postmenopausal women with mood disorders would address a health issue of increasing importance given that the elderly is the fastest growing segment of the population.

REFERENCES

Ahmed, S. & Talal, N. (1989). Sex hormones and autoimmune rheumatic disorders. *Scandinavian Journal of Rheumatology*, **18**, 69–76.

Almawi, W., Lipman, M., Stevens, A., Zanker, B., Hadro, E. & Strom, T. J. (1991). Abrogation of glucocorticoid-mediated inhibition of T-cell proliferation by the synergistic action of IL-1, IL-6, and IFN gamma. *Immunology*, **146**, 3523.

Ammendola, R., Mesuraca, M., Russo, T. & Cimino, F. (1992). Sp1 DNA binding efficiency is highly reduced in nuclear extract from aged rat tissue. *Journal of Biological Chemistry*, **267**, 17944–8.

Ansar, A., Penhale, S. & Talal, N. (1985). Sex hormones, immune responses, and autoimmune diseases. Mechanisms of sex hormone action. *American Journal of Pathology*, **121**, 531.

Araneo, B., Dowell, T., Diegel, M. & Daynes, R. A. (1991). Dihydrotestosterone exerts a depressive influence on the production of IL-4, IL-5 and γ-interferon, but not IL-2 by activated murine T-cells. *Blood*, **78**(3), 688–99.

Arend, W. & Dayer, J. (1990). Cytokines and cytokine inhibitors or antagonists in rheumatoid arthritis. *Arthritis and Rheumatism*, **33**, 305–15.

Ashwell, J. D., King, L. B. & Vacchio, M. S. (1996). Cross-talk between the T-cell antigen receptor and the glucocorticoid receptor regulates thymocyte development. *Stem Cells*, 14(5), 490–500.

Auphan, N., DiDonato, J. A., Rosette, C., Helmberg, A. & Karin, M. (1995). Immunosuppression by glucocorticoids: inhibition of NF-kappaB activity through induction of IkappaB synthesis. *Science*, 270, 286–90.

Beato, M. (1989). Gene regulation by steroid hormones. *Cell*, 56, 335–44.

Beeson, P. (1994). Age and sex associations of 40 autoimmune diseases. *American Journal of Medicine*, 96, 457–62.

Cannon, J. & Dinarello, C. (1985). Increases plasma interleukin-1 activity in women after ovulation. *Science*, 227, 1247–9.

Cohen, J., Danel, L., Cordier, G., Saez, S. & Revillard, J. (1983). Sex steroid receptors in peripheral T-cells: absence of androgen receptors and restriction of estrogen receptors to OKT8–positive cells. *Journal of Steroid Biochemistry*, 18, 559.

Danel, L., Souweine, G., Monier, J. & Saez, Z. (1983). Specific estrogen binding sites in human lymphoid cells and thymic cells. *Journal of Steroid Biochemistry*, 18(5), 559–63.

Diamond, M., Miner, J., Yoshinaga, S. & Yamamoto, K. (1990). Transcription factor interactions: selectors of positive or negative regulation from a single DNA element. *Science*, 249, 1266–72.

Dougados, M. (1990). Sex hormone metabolism in acute system lupus erythematosus. *Annales de Médécine Interne*, 14(3), 244–6.

Drouin, J., Trifiro, M., Plante, R., Nemer, M., Eriksson, P. & Wrange, O. (1989). Glucocorticoid receptor binding to a specific DNA sequence is required for hormone-dependent repression of pro-opiomelanocortin gene transcription. *Molecular and Cellular Biology*, 9(12), 5305–14.

El-Deiry, W., Tokino, T., Velcelescu, V., Levy, D., Parson, R. & Trent, J. (1993). WAF1, a potential mediator of p53 tumor suppression. *Cell*, 75, 817–25.

Fossel, M. (1998). Telomerase and the aging cell: implications for human health. *Journal of the American Medical Association*, 279(21), 1732–5.

Fox, H. S., Bond, B. L. & Parslow, T. G. (1991). Estrogen regulates the IFN-gamma promoter. *Journal of Immunology*, 146, 4362–67.

Fujimoto, K. & Takahashi, M. (1997). Telomerase activity in human leukemic cell lines is inhibited by antisense pentadecadeoxynucleotides targeted against c-myc mrna. *Biochemical and Biophysical Research Communications*, 241(3), 775–81.

Gayo, A., Mozo, L., Suarez, A., Tunon, A., Lahoz, C. & Gutierrez, C. (1998). Glucocorticoids increase IL-10 expression in multiple sclerosis patients with acute relapse. *Journal of Neuroimmunology*, 85(2), 122–30.

Genazzani, A. R., Lemarchand-Beraud, T. H., Aubert, M. L. & Felber, J. P. (1975). Pattern of plasma ACTH, hGH, and cortisol during menstrual cycle. *Journal of Clinical Endocrinology and Metabolism*, 41, 431.

Goldstein, S. (1990). Replicative senescence: the human fibroblast comes of age. *Science*, 249, 1129–33.

Green, M. (1992). The male predominance in the incidence of infectious diseases in children: a postulated explanation for disparities in the literature. *International Journal of Epidemiology*, 21(2), 381–6

Grossman, C., Sholiton, L. & Roselle, G. (1983). Dihydrotestosterone regulation of thymocyte function in the rat: mediation by serum factors. *Journal of Steroid Biochemistry*, 19, 1459–67.

Harper, J., Adami, G., Wei, N., Keyomarsi, K. & Elledge, S. (1993). The p21 cdk-interacting protein Cip1 is a potent inhibitor of G1 cyclin-dependent kinases. *Cell*, 75, 805–16.

Hirano, T., Matsuda, T., Turner, M., Miyasaka, N., Buchan, G., Tang, B., Sato, K., Shimizu, M., Maini, R., Feldmann, M. et al. (1988). Excessive production of IL-6/B cell stimulatory factor-2 in rheumatoid arthritis. *European Journal of Immunology*, 18, 1797.

Hu, S., Mitcho, Y. & Rath, N. (1988). Effect of estradiol on interleukin 1 synthesis by macrophages. *Journal of Immunopharmacology*, 10, 247.

Hyder, S. M., Chiappetta, C. & Stancel, G. M. (1998). The 3'-flanking region of the mouse c-fos gene contains a cluster of GGTCA hormone-response like elements. *Molecular Biology Reports*, 25(3), 189–191.

Isshiki, H., Akira, S., Tanabe, O. Nakajima, T. & Shimamoto, T. (1990). Constitutive and IL-1–inducible factors interact with the IL-1–responsive element in the IL-6 gene. *Molecular and Cellular Biology* 10, 2757–64.

Jablons, D. M., Mule, J. J., McIntosh, J. K., Seghal, P. B., May, L. T., Huang, C. M., Rosenberg, S. A., & Lotze, M. T. (1989). IL-6/Interferon-b2 as a circulating hormone. Induction by cytokine administration in man. *Journal of Immunology*, 142, 1542–7.

Jain, J., McCaffrey, P., Valge-Archer, V. & Rao, A. (1992). Nuclear factor of activated T-cells contains fos and jun. *Nature*, 356, 801–4.

Jonat, C., Stein, B., Ponta, H., Herrlich, P., & Rahmsdorf, H. (1990). Positive and negative regulation of collagenase gene expression. In *Proceedings of the Matrix Metalloproteinase Conference, Destin, Florida*, ed. H. Birkedal-Hansen, AZ. Werb, H. Welgus, & H. van Wart.

King, L. B., Vaccio, M. S., Dixon, K., Hunziker, R., Margulies, D.H. & Ashwell, J.D. (1995). A target glucocorticoid receptor antisense transgene increases thymocyte apoptosis and alters thymocyte development. *Immunity*, 3, 647–56.

Kishimoto, T. (1989). The Biology of Interleukin-6. *Blood*, 74(1), 1–10.

Kumar, N., Shan, L. X., Hardy, M. P., Bardin, C. W. & Sundaram, K. (1995). Mechanism of androgen-induced thymolysis in rats. *Endocrinology*, 136, 4887–93.

Lahita, R., Bradlow, H., Ginzler, E. & Pang, S. (1987). Low plasma androgens in women with systemic lupus erythematosus. *Arthritis and Rheumatism*, 30(3), 241–8.

Lee, S. & Tsou, A. (1988). Glucocorticoids selectively inhibit the transcription of the IL-1β gene and decrease the stability of IL-1b mRNA. *Proceedings of the National Academy of Sciences, USA*, 85, 1204–8.

Li, Z., Danis, V. & Brooks, P. (1993). Effect of gonadal steroids on the production of IL-1 and IL-6 by blood mononuclear cells in vitro. *Clinical and Experimental Rheumatology*, 11, 157–62.

Luisi, S., Tonetti, A., Bernardi, F., Casarosa, E., Florio, P., Monteleone, P., Gemignani, R., Petraglia, F., Luisi, M. & Genazzani, A. R. (1998). Effect of acute corticotropin releasing factor on pituitary–adrenocortical responsiveness in elderly women and men. *Journal of Endocrinological Investigation*, 21(7), 449–53.

McFarland, H. & Bigley, N. (1989). Sex dependent early cytokine production by NK-like spleen cells following infection with the D variant of encepahlomyocarditis virus. *Viral Immunology*, 2, 205.

Morale, M. C., Batticane, N., Gallo, F., Barden, N. & Marchetti, B. (1995). Disruption of hypo-thalamic–pituitary–adrenocortical system in transgenic mice expressing type II glucocorticoid receptor antisense ribonucleic acid permanently impairs T-cell function: effects on T-cell trafficking and T-cell responsiveness during postnatal development. *Endocrinology*, **136**, 3949–60.

Mordacq, J. & Linzer, D. (1989). Co-localization of elements required for phorbol ester stimula-tion and glucocorticoid repression of proliferin gene expression. *Genes and Development*, 3(6), 760–9.

Mossman, T. & Coffman, R. (1989). TH1 and TH2 cells: different patterns of lymphokine secre-tion lead to different functional properties. *Annual Review Immunology*, 7, 145–73.

Murphy, L., Murphy, L. & Freisen, H. (1987). Estrogen induction of n-myc and c-myc proto-oncogene expression in the rat uterus. *Endocrinology*, **120**, 1882–8.

Nagel, J., Chopra, R., Chresh, F., McCoy, M., Schneider, E. & Holbrook, N. (1988). Decreased proliferation, interleukin-2 synthesis, and interleukin-2 receptor expression are accompanied by decreased mRNA expression in PHA-stimulated cells from elderly donor. *Journal of Clinical Investigation*, **81**, 1096–102.

Noda, A., Ning, Y., Venable, S., Pereira-Smith, O. & Smith, J. (1994). Cloning of senescent cell-derived inhibitors of DNA synthesis using an expression screen. *Experimental Cell Research*, 211, 90–8.

Nouri, A., Panayi, G., & Goodman, S. (1984). Cytokines and chronic inflammation of rheumatic diseases I. The presence of interleukin-2 in synovial fluids. *Clinical and Experimental Immunology*, **58**, 402.

Pacifici, R., Rifas, L., McCracken, R., Vered, I., McMurtry, C., Avioli, L. & Peck, W. (1989). Ovarian steroid treatment blocks a postmenopausal increase in blood monocyte interleukin 1 release. *Proceedings of the National Academy of Sciences*, USA, 86(7), 2398–402.

Pang, J. & Chen, K. (1993). A specific CCAAT-binding protein, CBP/tk, may be involved in the regulation of thymidine kinase gene expression in human IMR-90 diploid fibroblasts during senescence. *Journal of Biological Chemistry*, **268**, 2909–16.

Pfeiffer, A., LaPointe, B. & Barden, N. (1991). Hormonal regulation of type II glucocorticoid receptor messenger ribonucleic acid in rat brain. *Endocrinology*, **129**, 2166–74.

Pioli, G., Basini, G., Pedrazzoni, M., Musetti, G., Ulietti, V., Bresciani, D., Villa, P., Bacchi, A., Hughes, D., Russell, G. & Passeri, M. (1992). Spontaneous release of IL-1 and IL-6 by periph-eral blood mononuclear cells after oophorectomy. *Clinical Science*, **83**, 503–7.

Polan, M., Daniele, A. & Kuo, A. (1988). Gonadal steroids modulate human monocyte IL-1 activ-ity. *Fertility and Sterility*, 49(6), 964–8.

Rao, A. (1994). NF-ATp: a transcription factor required for the co-ordinate induction of several cytokine genes. *Immunology Today* 15(6), 274–81.

Ray, A., LaForge, S. & Seghal, P. (1990). On the mechanisms for efficient repression of the IL-6 promoter by glucocorticoids: enhancer, TATA box, and RNA start site (inr motif) Occlusion. *Molecular and Cellular Biology*, 10(11), 5736–46.

Redei, E., Li, L., Halasz, I., McGivern, R. & Aird, F. (1994). Fast glucocorticoid feedback inhibi-tion of ACTH secretion in the ovariectomized rat: effect of chronic estrogen and progesterone. *Neuroendocrinology*, **60**, 113–23.

Riabowol, K., Schiff, J. & Gilman, M. (1992). Transcription factor AP-1 activity is required for initiation of DNA synthesis and is lost during cellular aging. *Proceedings of the National Academy of Sciences, USA*, **89**, 157–61.

Rittling, S., Brooks, K., Cristafolo, V. & Baserga, R. (1986). Expression of cell cycle-dependent genes in young and senescent WI-38 fibroblasts. *Proceedings of the National Academy of Sciences, USA*, **83**, 3316–20.

Rivier, C. (1994). Stimulatory effect of interleukin-1b on the hypothalamic–pituitary–adrenal axis of the rat: influence of age, gender and circulating sex steroids. *Journal of Endocrinology*, **140**, 365–72.

Rooney, J., Hodge, M., McCaffrey, P., Rao, A. & Glimcher, L. (1994). A common factor regulates both Th1– and Th2–specific cytokine gene expression. *EMBO Journal*, **13**(3), 625–33.

Scheinman, R. I., Cogswell, P.C., Lofquist, A. K. & Baldwin, A.S. (1995). Role of transcriptional activation of I kappa B alpha in mediation of immunosuppression by glucocorticoids. *Science*, **270**, 283–90.

Schlegel, R. J. & Bellanti, J. A. (1969). Increased susceptibility of males to infection. *Lancet*, **ii** (7625); 826–7.

Seshadri, T. & Campisi, J. (1990). Repression of c-fos transcription and an altered genetic program in senescent human fibroblasts. *Science*, **247**, 205–9.

Shaw, J., Utz, P., Durand, D., Toole, J., Emmel, E. & Crabtree, G. (1988). Identification of a putative regulator of early T-cell activation genes. *Science*, **241**, 202.

Sikora, E., Kaminska, B., Radziszewska, E. & Kaczmarek, L. (1992). Loss of transcription factor AP-1 DNA binding activity during lymphocyte aging *in vivo*. *FEBS Letters*, **312**, 179–82.

Singh, S. & Kanungo, M. (1993). Changes in expression and CRE binding proteins of the fibronectin gene during aging of the rat. *Biochemical and Biophysical Research Communications*, **193**, 440–5.

Singh, J. & Gupta, A. (1998). Senescence or malignancy: telomere, the ultimate decision maker. *Medical Science Research*, **26**(10), 651–7.

Spelsberg, T., Horton, M., Fink, K., Goldberger, A., Rories, C., Gosse, B. & Rasmussen, K. (1987). A new model for steroid regulation of gene transcription using chromatin acceptor sites and regulatory genes and their products. In *Recent Advances in Steroid Hormone Action*, ed. V. K. Moudgil, pp. 59–83. New York: Walter de Gruyter and Co.

Spinedi, E., Suesciun, M. O., Hadid, R., Daneva, T., & Gaillard, R. (1992). Effects of gonadectomy and sex hormone therapy on the endotoxin-stimulated hypothalamo-pituitary-adrenal axis: evidence for a neuroendocrine–immunological sexual dimorphism. *Endocrinology*, **131**, 2430–6.

Stimson, W. H. (1988). Estrogen and human T-lymphocytes: presence of specific receptors in the T-suppressor/cytotoxic subset. *Scandinavian Journal of Immunology* **28**, 345.

Straub, R. H., Konecna, L., Hrach, S., Rothe, G., Kreutz, M., Scholmerich, J., Falk, W. & Lang, B. (1998). Serum dehydroepiandrosterone (DHEA) and DHEA sulfate are negatively correlated with serum interleukin-6 (IL-6), and DHEA inhibits IL-6 secretion from mononuclear cells in man *in vitro*: possible link between endocrinosenescence and immunosenescence. *Journal of Clinical Endocrinology and Metabolism*, **83**(6), 2012–17.

Szijan, I., Parma, D. & Engel, N. (1992). Expression of c-myc and c-fos protooncogenes in the anterior pituitary gland of the rat. Effect of estrogen. *Hormone and Metabolic Research*, 24(4), 154–7.

Thoman, M. (1985). Role of IL-2 in the age-related impairment of immune function. *Journal of American Geriatrics Society*, 33, 781–7.

Tsujimoto, M., Okamura, N. & Adachi, H. (1988). Dexamethasone inhibits the cytotoxic activity of tumor necrosis factor. *Biochemical and Biophysical Research Communications*, 153, 109.

Turner, B. & Weaver, D. (1985). Sexual dimorphism of glucocorticoid binding in rat brain. *Brain Research*, 343, 16.

Turner, B. B. (1990). Sex difference in glucocorticoid binding in rat pituitary is estrogen dependent. *Life Sciences*, 46, 1399–406.

Vacca, A., Martinotti, S., Screpanti, I., Maroder, M. & Felli, M. P. (1990). Transcriptional regulation of the IL-2 gene by glucocorticoid hormones. Role of steroid receptor and antigen-responsive 5- flanking sequences. *Journal of Biological Chemistry* 265(14), 8075–80.

Vacchio, M. S., Papadopoulos, V. & Ashwell, J. D. (1994). Steroid production in the thymus: implications for thymocyte selection. *Journal of Experimental Medicine*, 179, 1835–46.

Vellanoweth, R., Supakar, P. & Roy, A. (1994). Transcription factors in development, growth, and aging. *Laboratory Investigation*, 70(6), 784–99.

Viau, V. & Meaney, M. J. (1991). Variations in the hypothalamic-pituitary-adrenal response to stress during the estrous cycle in the rat. *Endocrinology*, 129, 2503–11.

Weisz, A. & Rosales, R. (1990). Identification of an estrogen response element upstream of the human c-fos gene that binds the estrogen receptor and the AP-1 transcription factor. *Nucleic Acids Research*, 18(17), 5097–106.

Weisz, A., Cicatiello, L., Persico, E., Scalona, M. & Bresciani, F. (1990). Estrogen stimulates transcription of c-jun proto-oncogene. *Molecular Endocrinology*, 4(7), 1041–50.

Wood, D., Ihrie, E., Dinarello, C. & Cohen, P. (1983). Isolation of an interleukin-1 from human joint effusions. *Arthritis and Rheumatism*, 26, 975.

Xiong, Y., Hannon, G., Zhang, H., Casso, D., Kobayashi, R. & Beach, D. (1993). p21 is a universal inhibitor of cyclin kinases. *Nature*, 366, 701–4.

Zumoff, B., Fukushima, D. K., Weitzman, E. D., Kream, J. & Hellman, L. (1974). The sex differences in plasma cortisol concentration in man. *Journal of Clinical Endocrinology and Metabolism*, 39, 805–8.

Part IV

Hormones and gender differences in psychotropic drug metabolism

15

Gender differences in psychotropic drug metabolism

Bruce G. Pollock

Introduction

A consideration of the problem of gender differences in psychotropic drug metabolism recapitulates many of the same concerns of geriatric clinical psychopharmacology. Older women are the greatest consumers of all classes of psychotropics, and there is evidence that the elderly in general, and women in particular, experience a higher frequency of adverse drug reactions (Hurwitz, 1969; Domecq et al., 1980; Makkar et al., 1993; Warren et al., 1994). Yet drugs undergo phase one and early phase two testing predominantly in young male volunteers, a trend that has strongly increased over the past two decades (Schmucker & Vesell, 1993). This was to some extent mandated in 1977 by prior Food and Drug Administration guidelines which restricted enrollment of 'women of childbearing potential,' and reinforced, by the rather circular logic, that 'gender differences in pharmacokinetics are not worth studying systematically, yet just in case there is a variance due to gender, it should be excluded as a variable.' This of course prevented the accumulation of the necessary data to actually determine whether gender is indeed an issue in drug metabolism and response. Moreover, when women were included in early drug studies, they were usually young and there was seldom stratification by sex according to alcohol use, smoking, or use of oral contraceptives. Only three or four published studies in the area have controlled for menstrual phases. In addition, it is now recognized that single dose pharmacokinetic studies are not sufficient to examine nonlinear clearance phenomena.

Most importantly, where information on gender differences in pharmocokinetics is available, it is not being used in clinical practice. High-risk prescribing has been reported to occur most often with psychotropics, to be much higher for women than for men, and to increase with age until 75 to 84 years (Tamblyn et al., 1994). High-risk prescriptions include the use of questionable drug combinations, excessive treatment duration and drugs relatively contraindicated for the elderly, such as long-half-life benzodiazepines and highly anticholinergic antidepressants.

For women aged 16 to 39 who were prescribed psychotropic drugs, the relative risk of a fatal myocardial infarction was 17 times greater than those not taking a psychotropic (Thorogood et al., 1992). It is possible that physicians tend to ascribe physical symptoms such as chest pain in younger women to psychogenic causes, resulting in the prescription of a psychotropic. Nonetheless, gender-associated pathophysiologic differences urgently require exploration. Women are more at risk for digitalis toxicity and have a predisposition to prolonged cardiac repolarization (longer average QT_c intervals than men) and torsade de pointes arrhythmias, particularly when prescribed cardiovascular drugs (Warren et al., 1994; Makkar et al., 1993).

Of all physicians, psychiatrists have been among the most sensitive in recognizing gender differences in the phenomenology and treatment response of illness. These differences have most often been attributed to psychosocial factors. More recently elucidated sex differences in previously gender-neutral conditions may face exploration in depth with the application of neuroscience. For example, women suffering from Alzheimer's disease have been found to have differing patterns of psychiatric disturbance and regional brain glucose metabolism compared to male patients (Cohen et al. 1993; Siegel et al. 1994). In order to begin elucidation of possible differences in drug response, however, it is essential that drug concentrations be kinetically described for all pertinent subgroups.

Non-metabolic factors affecting drug disposition

Clearance vs. half-life

Although clinicians commonly compare medications in terms of their half-lives, it is clearance that has a direct bearing on the concentration of a drug at steady-state. The fact that half-life is directly proportional to a drug's apparent volume of distribution is also frequently overlooked. The age-related increase in the proportion of adipose tissue is magnified in women, from an average of 33% in younger subjects to 48% in the old, vs. 18% to 36% in men (Greenblatt et al., 1982). This fact alone will increase the half-life of lipid soluble drugs such as diazepam. Confronted by the lack of published pharmacokinetic data for bupropion in the elderly, we conducted a small study in five elderly women. We found that the volume of distribution was twice that reported in young males (79.3 l/kg) and that the plasma half-life was correspondingly lengthened to a much greater proportion than clearance was reduced, which was about 80% of that found in the young (Sweet et al., 1995).

Gastric effects

In general, women secrete less gastric acid than men, which causes women to experience increased absorption of weak bases (the majority of psychotropics). This effect is counterbalanced by gender associated reductions in gastric emptying which are exacerbated by estrogen and progesterone (Hutson et al., 1989). Importantly, alcohol dehydrogenase has been found to be significantly less in females than males, increasing the bioavailability of alcohol in women and placing them at increased risks for the complications of alcoholism (Frezza et al., 1990).

Oral contraceptives and the menstrual cycle also affect gastrointestinal transit. Estrogen and progesterone slow gastric emptying, particularly of liquids. Interestingly, transit times are longer after Day 15 than in the proceeding follicular phase (Wald et al., 1981), yet gender differences in gastric emptying persist into the menopause, even in those women not on hormonal supplementation.

Protein binding

Imipramine and a number of benzodiazepines have been found to be less protein bound in women than men (Kristensen, 1983; Wilson, 1984). It is possible that gender differences in lipoproteins, particularly apolipoprotein B, and/or alpha-1 acidglycoprotein are responsible. During pregnancy, a further reduction of protein binding occurs for many drugs (Perucca & Crema, 1982). Nonetheless, any differences in protein binding would be more of an issue for therapeutic drug monitoring since the free drug concentration quickly reequilibrates, but the total drug concentration (free and bound) is measured in most assays (Greenblatt et al., 1986).

Metabolic differences

Phase one and phase two metabolism

Male rats are the most frequently used experimental animals in drug toxicity tests. However, clear gender differences in rat drug metabolism have been known for at least 60 years, when it was observed that female rats required half the male dose of amobarbital for anesthesia (Nicholas & Barron, 1932). This pattern of an increased metabolism in male rats has been observed in other psychotropics including opiates, diazepam, and imipramine (Skett et al., 1980). The pattern of a slower female metabolism in rats is reversed for mice and more difficult to discern in humans.

The pattern of gender-related differences is observed only in adult rats. There has been considerable work demonstrating the effect of androgens on imprinting the hypothalamic–pituitary–hepatic axis. The patterns of growth hormone and somatostatin secretion have also been found to be determinants of the female or male metabolic types (Gustafsson et al., 1983).

There is a remarkable paucity of human data on gender differences in drug metabolism given the details on gender issues in rat drug metabolism that are currently available and those that continue to be elucidated (Kato & Yamazoe, 1992).

It is likely that the numerous uncontrolled confounding factors within grouped data, such as genetic polymorphisms, cigarette smoking, alcohol use, menstrual cycle phase, and oral contraceptive use, have often averaged out gender differences.

As more is learned about the diversity of the cytochrome P450 enzymes responsible for oxidative metabolism, a structure is emerging for categorizing gender-associated differences in phase-one metabolism (Pollock, 1994;). Although the data are very limited, no gender- or age-associated differences have been found for debrisoquine hydroxylase (CYP 2D6; Pollock et al., 1992). This isozyme, which is responsible for the metabolism of at least 30 clinically used medications, is non-inducible and displays a marked genetic polymorphism.

S-Mephenytoin hydroxylase (P450 2C19) activity is also subject to genetic polymorphism. In a study of 166 healthy white subjects, S-mephenytoin 4–hydroxylation was found to be modestly (34%) less in men who were younger than 50 years old (May et al., 1994). The demethylation of tertiary tricyclic antidepressants and diazepam and the oxidation of desmethyldiazepam are dependent on this isozyme. Consistent with increased CYP 2C19 activity in women, the total and unbound clearance of diazepam has been found to be greater in women (Greenblatt et al., 1980). Nonetheless, the metabolism of the 2C19 substrates methylphenobarbital, piroxicam, and propranolol appear higher in men than women (Hooper & Qing, 1990; Rugstad et al., 1986; Walle et al., 1989).

CYP 3A4 is quantitatively the most important cytochrome P450 isozyme: it makes up at least 60% of the liver's total P450 content and is responsible for the metabolism of the majority of clinically important medications (Nemeroff et al., 1996). Medications metabolized by this isozyme include calcium antagonists, terfenadine, astemizole, triazolam, alprazolam, zolpidem, midazolam, and cisapride. CYP 3A4 is believed to be the principal isozyme responsible for conversion of 17α-ethinyl estradiol into its major and more rapidly excreted 2–OH-estradiol metabolite (Guengerich, 1990) and there is evidence that CYP 3A4 activity is greater in younger women than in men and postmenopausal women. These gender and age-related pharmacokinetic differences have been demonstrated in studies of the CYP 3A4 substrates erythromycin, prednisolone, tirilazad, verapamil, and alfentanil (Watkins, 1994; Harris et al., 1996; Hulst et al., 1994; Schwartz et al., 1994; Rubio & Cox, 1991).

Interestingly, nefazodone levels have been reported to be 50% higher in older women as compared to younger subjects and older men (Barbhaiya et al., 1996). If P450 3A4 activity is increased in younger women, it would result in shorter half-lives of triazolam and alprazolam, which might further increase their addictive liabilities. In contrast, the possible decline in CYP 3A4 activity in postmenopausal women might make them more liable to adverse effects with these medications. Of considerable relevance to aging is the evidence that 3A4 induction may have an anti-atherogenic effect by increasing HDL cholesterol apolipoprotein A-1 (Luoma, 1988), while 3A4 inhibition may negate the beneficial effects of hypolipidemic drugs such as gemfibrozil (Tam, 1991). Moreover, declining 3A4 activity in older women may account for significant increases in cholesterol found in menopausal women but not in men of the same age (Akahoshi et al., 1996).

Although gender-related differences have not yet been reported for CYP 1A1/2, higher plasma levels in women have been reported for the 1A1–2 drug substrates tacrine, clozapine, and fluvoxamine, suggesting the need for closer examination (Ford et al., 1993; Hartter et al., 1993). In this regard it should be noted that the careful pharmacokinetic studies that examined the use of caffeine as a metabolic probe for this isozyme included very few women (Cheng et al., 1990; Fuhr & Rost, 1994). Moreover the activity of this isozyme has been found to be reduced in women receiving contraceptive medication and in pregnant women (Lambert et al., 1983). Adequate tacrine plasma levels are the most robust indicator of treatment response and adverse effects (Ford et al., 1993; Schneider & Farlow, 1995). Pertinent to estrogen's possible inhibition of CYP 1A2 is the recent report of estrogen replacement enhancing response to tacrine (Schneider et al., 1996). This may be a result of estrogen amplifying tacrine's very modest bioavailability (25%).

CYP 1A1 has been found in breast tumors, and the 1A1 Msp1 allele is significantly associated with breast cancer in black women, but not in white women (Murray et al., 1991; Taioli et al., 1995). Both CYPs 3A4 and 1A1/2 are believed to be the major enzymes responsible for estrogen metabolism (Aoyama et al., 1990). Metabolism by two alternative and competing pathways results in the inactive 2–hyroxyestrogen and the active 16a-hydroxy metabolite. Because 16a-hydroxy-estrogen has been implicated in carcinogenesis, it has been proposed that the balance between the production of these metabolites may be pertinent to the development of breast cancer. In this regard, the finding that the mean ratio of 2–OH/16–OH-estrogen is 60% lower in black women, as compared to white women, is concerning (Taioli et al., 1996).

Interestingly, phase two reactions have been considered less subject to the extensive genetic and environmentally determined variations apparent in phase one metabolism. Yet, a number of studies have demonstrated a sex difference in the elimination of drugs undergoing glucuronidation. For example, plasma clearances of oxazepam and temazepam have been found to be greater in males than females. While no gender difference has been found in the plasma clearance of lorazepam, the use of oral contraceptives increases clearance.

Effects of exogenous estrogen

Estrogen reduces alpha 1–acid glycoprotein concentrations, increasing the proportion of free drug and inhibiting cytochrome P450 metabolism. Estrogen also inhibits monoamine oxidase activity while progesterone increases it. Work on early oral contraceptive preparations found a tendency for phase one metabolism to be impaired (Homeida et al., 1978) and for phase two glucuronidation to be induced (Stoehr et al., 1984). Oral contraceptives have been demonstrated to affect the metabolism of benzodiazepines and antidepressants (Abernethy et al., 1982; 1984). Given the increasing use of estrogens in the menopause for prevention of cardiovascular disease or osteoporosis, it is remarkable that no attention has been paid to possible affects on the metabolism of psychotropics. Transdermal estrogen, for example, has been found to decrease levels of some anticoagulants, placing women with a history of thrombosis at additional risk (Greendale & Judd, 1993). An added concern is the possibility of tumor production when giving dopamine antagonists to women taking concurrent estrogen (ThyagaRajan et al., 1993). Experimental data have found that haloperidol in combination with estrogen increases expression of protooncogenes in the rat anterior pituitary, but this did not occur with haloperidol alone (Chernavsky et al., 1993).

Menstrual cycle effects

The elimination of the oxidative probe, antipyrine, has been found to vary over the menstrual cycle (Kellerman & Luyten-Kellermann, 1978). The only study that has systematically explored menstrual cycle effects with a psychotropic found that a significant increase in methaqualone metabolism occurs at mid-cycle. The metabolic data in men were similar to the Day 1 female data. In women, the Day 1 clearance doubled on Day 15 (Wilson et al., 1982). Two intriguing case reports with antidepressants also reveal a doubling of the plasma levels of trazodone and desipramine at mid-cycle (Kimmel et al., 1992). If more data were available to guide practice, this might imply that patients on maintenance antidepressants are more at risk for relapse prior to menses or toxicity during the follicular phase. Research is also needed to examine if the variations in plasma serotonin over the menstrual cycle have specific implications for treatment with selective serotonin reuptake inhibitors (SSRIs). For example, plasma serotonin has been found to be greatest during the periovulatory period, which could be raised further by SSRIs. This may have implications for women with compromised vasculature (Hindberg & Naesh, 1992).

Gender differences in the course and phenomenology of schizophrenia may hold important leads to etiology and therapeutics (Seeman, 1983). It has been noted in schizophrenic women on maintenance antipsychotic medication that psychopathology scores were significantly lower during their midluteal phases (Hallonquist et al., 1993), possibly a result of estrogen's inhibition of neuroleptic metabolism or its neuroleptic-like action. This finding reinforces the need to study periodic vs.

constant dosing of antipsychotics in younger women as well as the need to improve therapeutics to address the female predominance in late-onset schizophrenia.

Effects of pregnancy

For obvious reasons, drug trials are not carried out in pregnant women. Expectant mothers, nonetheless, are not excluded from drug therapy. There is evidence of increased metabolism of anticonvulsants such as phenytoin, phenobarbitone, and carbamazepine (Dam et al., 1977), leading, perhaps, to a reported increased incidence of seizures (Knight & Rhind, 1975). During pregnancy the dosage of several psychotropics must be increased to maintain therapeutic levels. Lithium clearance increases by 30% to 50% (Weinstein, 1980), and nortriptyline doses must be increased by approximately 1.6 times to maintain equivalent plasma levels during the second half of pregnancy (Wisner et al., 1993). Raised progesterone concentrations may lead to induction of hepatic enzymes, such as CYP 3A4. In addition, decreased protein binding and increased volume of distribution may be relevant factors. Interestingly, the CYP 1A2 substrate, caffeine, may undergo a significant reduction of clearance during pregnancy (Aldridge et al., 1981). Other 1A2 substrates have not been studied, but particular care should be given when clozapine and fluvoxamine are deemed necessary.

Summary

As early as the introduction of analytical methods for determining plasma levels of tricyclic antidepressants, researchers noted that steady-state imipramine and nortriptyline concentrations were higher in females (Moody et al., 1967; Hammer & Sjoqvist, 1967). When a large population database of plasma levels was recently examined, clomipramine metabolic clearance was clearly shown to be diminished in young women (Gex-Fabry et al., 1990). The serotonergic antidepressant fluvoxamine, metabolized by CYP 1A2, has also been found to have higher plasma levels in women, even after weight-adjusting (Hartter et al., 1993). Nefazodone, a CYP 3A4 substrate, demonstrates reduced metabolism in postmenopausal women. Conversely, trazodone, metabolized by CYP 2D6, has shown no sex differences in clearance or plasma levels, but it does have a larger volume of distribution in women, leading to an increased plasma half-life.

Lithium as a polar compound would be expected to have a smaller volume of distribution in women, and this may contribute to the more frequent production of hypothyroidism in women. An additional concern in older women is the possibility that lithium-induced hyperparathyroidism may exacerbate osteoporosis (Baastrup et al., 1978; Nordenstrom et al., 1992).

In view of the large number of prescriptions for benzodiazepines given to women, it is worth noting that the elimination half-life for those benzodiazepines undergoing oxidation is prolonged in women. This is despite their enhanced metabolic clearance because of their increased volumes of distribution (Greenblatt et al., 1980). Nonetheless, the more water-soluble benzodiazepines, such as oxazepam, which have smaller volumes of distribution, have reduced metabolic clearance (glucuronidation) in women with prolonged half-lives (Divoll et al., 1981).

Consistent with gender differences found earlier for chlorpromazine, increased plasma levels of fluphenazine (Simpson et al., 1990), fluspirilene (Chouinard et al., 1986), and thiothixene (Ereshefsky et al., 1991) have been found in women on equivalent doses as men. Moreover, the CYP 1A2 drug clozapine has exhibited plasma levels that are almost twice as high in women, with excessive concentrations leading to seizures rather than tardive dyskinesia (Haring et al., 1989).

Recommendations

Systematic studies should be done at all phases of clinical trials with gender comparisons and matched for age and race as well as the traditional variables of alcohol, smoking, and illness. These studies should include both pharmacokinetic/dynamic and clinical parameters. More research is urgently needed on how pregnancy, the menstrual cycle, hormonal therapy, and age affects psychotropic drugs. As noted by Barry (1986), women live one-third of their lives after menopause, yet there is a notable gap in data concerning the effects of hormone replacement on drug clearance. Some of these studies could be organized by drug metabolic phenotyping approaches (e.g. what is the effect of a given dose of a conjugated estrogen on P450 1A2?).

It is to be hoped that the FDA Guidelines for the Study and Evaluation of Gender Differences in the Clinical Evaluation of Drugs (Federal Register, July 22, 1993) will increase our database. Nonetheless, past experience with geriatric concerns mandates that NIH provide leadership and that academia take an active role.

ACKNOWLEDGMENT

Supported by USPHS Grants MH-01509 and MH-52247.

REFERENCES

Abernethy, D. R., Greenblatt, D. J., Divoll, M., Arendt, R., Ochs, H. & Shader, R. I. (1982). Impairment of diazepam metabolism by low-dose estrogen-containing oral contraceptive steroids. *New England Journal of Medicine*, **306**, 791–2.

Abernethy, D. R., Greenblatt, D. J. & Shader, R. I. (1984). Imipramine disposition in users of oral contraceptive steroids. *Clinical Pharmacology Therapeutics*, **35**, 792–7.

Akahoshi, M., Soda, M., Nakashima, E., Shimaoka, K., Seto, S. & Yano, K. (1996). Effects of menopause on trends of serum cholesterol, blood pressure, and body mass index. *Circulation*, **94**, 61–6.

Aldridge, A., Bailey, J. & Neims, A. H. (1981). The disposition of caffeine during and after pregnancy. *Seminars in Perinatology*, **5**, 310–14.

Aoyama, T., Korzekwa, K., Nagata, K., Gillete, J., Gelboin, H. V. & Gonzalez, F. J. (1990). Estradiol metabolism by complementary deoxy ribonucleic acid-expressed human cytocrome P450s. *Endocrinology*, **126**, 3101–6.

Baastrup, P. C., Christiansen, C. & Transbol, I. (1978). Calcium metabolism in lithium treated patients. *Acta Psychiatrica Scandinavica*, **57**, 124–8.

Barbhaiya, R. H., Buch, A. B. & Greene, D. S. (1996). A study of the effect of age and gender on the pharmacokinetics of nefazodone after single and multiple doses. *Journal of Clinical Psychopharmacology*, **16**, 19–25.

Barry, P. P. (1986). Gender as a factor in treating the elderly. *NIDA Research Monograph*, **65**, 65–9.

Cheng, W. S. C., Murphy, T. L., Smith, M. T., Cooksley, W. G., Halliday, J. W. & Powell, L. W. (1990). Dose-dependent pharmacokinetics of caffeine in humans: Relevance as a test of quantitative liver function. *Clinical Pharmacology Therapeutics*, **47**, 516–24.

Chernavsky, A. C., Valerani, A. V. & Burdman, J. A. (1993). Haloperidol and oestrogens induce c-myc and c-fos expression in the anterior pituitary gland of the rat. *Neurology Research*, **15**, 339–43.

Chouinard, G., Annable, L. & Steinberg, S. (1986). A controlled clinical trial of fluspirilene, a long-acting injectable neuroleptic, in schizophrenic patients with acute exacerbation. *Journal of Clinical Psychopharmacology*, **6**, 21–6.

Cohen, D., Eisdorfer, C., Gorelick, P., Luchins, D., Freels, S., Semla, T., Paveza, G., Shaw, H. & Ashford, J. W. (1993). Sex differences in the psychiatric manifestations of Alzheimer's disease. *Journal of the American Geriatric Society*, **41**, 229–32.

Dam, M., Christiansen, J., Munck, O. & Mygind, K. I. (1977). Antiepileptic drugs: metabolism in pregnancy. *Clinical Pharmacokinetics*, **2**, 427–36.

Divoll, M., Greenblatt, D. J., Harmatz, J. S. & Shader, R. I. (1981). Effect of age and gender on disposition of temazepam. *Journal of Pharmaceutical Science*, **70**, 1104–7.

Domecq, C., Naranjo, C. A., Ruiz, I. & Busto, U. (1980). Sex-related variations in the frequency and characteristics of adverse drug reactions. *International Journal of Clinical Pharmacology Therapeutics and Toxicology*, **18**, 362–6.

Ereshefsky, L., Saklad, S. R., Wantanabe, M. D., Davis, C. M. & Jann, M. W. (1991). Thiothixene pharmacokinetic interactions: a study of hepatic enzyme inducers, clearance inhibitors, and demographic variables. *Journal of Clinical Psychopharmacology*, **11**, 296–301.

Ford, J. M., Truman, C. A., Wilcock, G. K. & Roberts, C. J. C. (1993). Serum concentrations of tacrine hydrochloride predict its adverse effects in Alzheimer's disease. *Clinical Pharmacology Therapeutics*, 53, 691–5.

Frezza, M., di Padova, C., Pozzato, G., Terpin, M., Baraona, E. & Lieber, C. S. (1990). High blood alcohol levels in women. The role of decreased gastric alcohol dehydrogenase activity and first-pass metabolism. *New England Journal of Medicine*, 322, 95–9.

Fuhr, U. & Rost, K. L. (1994). Simple and reliable CYP1A2 phenotyping by the paraxanthine/caffeine ratio in plasma and in saliva. *Pharmacogenetics*, 4, 109–16.

Gex-Fabry, M., Balant-Gorgia, A. E., Balant, L. P. & Garrone, G. (1990). Clomipramine metabolism: model-based analysis of variability factors from drug monitoring data. *Clinical Pharmacokinetics*, 19, 241–55.

Greenblatt, D. J., Abernethy, D. R. & Shader, R. I. (1986). Pharmacokinetic aspects of drug therapy in the elderly. *Therapy Drug Monitor*, 8, 249–55.

Greenblatt, D. J., Allen, M. D., Harmatz, J. S. & Shader, R. I. (1980). Diazepam disposition determinants. *Clinical Pharmacology Therapeutics*, 27, 301–12.

Greenblatt, D. J., Sellers, E. M. & Shader, R. I. (1982). Drug Disposition in old age. *New England Journal of Medicine*, 306, 1081–8.

Greendale, G. A. & Judd, H. L. (1993). The menopause: health implications and clinical management. *Journal of the American Geriatrics Society*, 41, 426–36.

Guengerich, F. P. (1990). Inhibition of oral contraceptive steroid-metabolizing enzymes by steroids and drugs. *American Journal of Obstetrics and Gynecology*, 163, 2159–63.

Gustafsson, J-A., Mode, A., Norstedt, G. & Skett, P. (1983). Sex steroid induced changes in hepatic enzymes. *Annual Review of Physiology*, 45, 51–60.

Hallonquist, J. D., Seeman, M. V., Lang, M. & Rector, N. A. (1993). Variation in symptom severity over the menstrual cycle of schizophrenics. *Biological Psychiatry*, 33, 207–9.

Hammer, W. & Sjoqvist, F. (1967). Plasma levels of monomethylated tricyclic antidepressants during treatment with imipramine-like compounds. *Life Sciences*, 6, 1895–903.

Haring, C., Meise, U., Humpel, C., Saria, A., Fleischhaker, W. W. & Hinterhuber, H. (1989). Dose-related plasma levels of clozapine: Influence of smoking behavior, sex and age. *Psychopharmacology*, 99, S38–S40.

Harris, R. Z., Tsunoda, S. M., Mroczkowski, P., Wong, H. & Benet, L. Z. (1996). The effects of menopause and hormone replacement therapies on prednisolone and erythromycin pharmacokinetics. *Clinical Pharmacology Therapeutics*, 59, 429–35.

Hartter, S., Wetzel, H., Hammes, E. & Hiemke, C. (1993). Inhibition of antidepressant demethylation and hydroxylation by fluvoxamine in depressed patients. *Psychopharmacology*, 110, 302–8.

Hindberg, I. & Naesh, O. (1992). Serotonin concentrations in plasma and variations during the menstrual cycle. *Clinical Chemistry*, 38, 2087–9.

Homeida, M., Halliwell, M. & Branch, R. A. (1978). Effects of an oral contraceptive on hepatic size and antipyrine metabolism in premenopausal women. *Clinical Pharmacology Therapeutics*, 24, 228–32.

Hooper, W. D. & Qing, M. S. (1990). The influence of age and gender on the stereoselective metabolism and pharmacokinetics of mephobarbital in humans. *Clinical Pharmacology Therapeutics*, 48, 633–40.

Hulst, L. K., Fleishaker, J. C., Peters, G. R., Harry, J. D., Wright, D. M. & Ward, P. (1994). Effect of age and gender on tirilazad pharmacokinetics in humans. *Clinical Pharmacology Therapeutics*, 55, 378–84.

Hurwitz, N. (1969). Factors predisposing to adverse drug reactions. *British Medical Journal*, i(643), 536–9.

Hutson, W. R., Roehrkasse, R. L. & Wald, A. (1989). Influence of gender and menopause on gastric emptying and motility. *Gastroenterology*, 96, 11–17.

Kato, R. & Yamazoe, Y. (1992). Sex-specific cytochrome P450 as a cause of sex- and species-related differences in drug toxicity. *Toxicology Letters*, 64/65, 661–7.

Kellermann, G. H. & Luyten-Kellermann. (1978). Antipyrine metabolism in man. *Life Sciences*, 23, 2485–90.

Kimmel, S., Gonsalves, L., Youngs, D. & Gidwani, G. (1992). Fluctuating levels of antidepressants premenstrually. *Journal of Psychosomatic Obstetrics and Gynaecology*, 13, 277–80.

Knight, A. H. & Rhind, E. G. (1975). Epilepsy and pregnancy: a study of 153 pregnancies in 59 patients. *Epilepsia*, 16, 99–110.

Kristensen, C. B. (1983). Imipramine serum protein binding in healthy subjects. *Clinical Pharmacology Therapeutics*, 34, 689–94.

Lambert, G. H., Kotake, A. N. & Schoeller, D. (1983). The CO_2 breath tests as monitors of the cytochrome P450 dependent mixed function oxygenase system. In *Developmental Pharmacology*, ed. S. M. McLeod, A. B. Okey & S. P. Spielberg, pp. 119–45. New York: Alan R. Liss.

Luoma, P. V. (1988). Microsomal enzyme induction, lipoproteins and atherosclerosis. *Pharmacology and Toxicology*, 62, 243–49.

Makkar, R. R., Fromm, B. S., Steinman, R. T., Meissner, M. D. & Lehmann, M. H. (1993). Female gender as a risk factor for torsades de pointes associated with cardiovascular drugs. *Journal of the American Medical Association*, 270, 2590–7.

May, D. G., Porter, J., Wilkinson, G. R. & Branch, R. A. (1994). Frequency distribution of dapsone N-hydroxylase, a putative probe for P450 3A4 activity, in a white population. *Clinical Pharmacology Therapeutics*, 55, 492–500.

Moody, J. P., Tait, A. C. & Todrick, A. (1967). Plasma levels of imipramine and desmethylimipramine during therapy. *British Journal of Psychiatry*, 113, 183–93.

Murray, G. I., Foster, C. O., Barnes, T. S., Weaver. R. J., Ewen, S. W. B., Melvin, W. T. & Burke, M. D. (1991). Expression of cytochrome P4501A in breast cancer. *British Journal of Cancer*, 63, 1021–3.

Nemeroff, C. B., DeVane, C. L. & Pollock, B. G. (1996). Newer antidepressants and the cytochrome P450 system. *American Journal of Psychiatry*, 153, 311–20.

Nicholas, G. S. & Barron, D. H. (1932). The use of sodium amytal in the production of anesthesia in the rat. *Journal of Pharmacology and Experimental Therapy*, 46, 125–9.

Nordenstrom, J., Strigard, K., Perbeck, L., Willems, J., Bagedahl-Strindlund, M. & Linder, J. (1992). Hyperparathyroidism associated with treatment of manic-depressive disorders by lithium. *European Journal of Surgery*, 158, 207–211.

Perucca, E. & Crema, A. (1982). Plasma protein binding of drugs in pregnancy. *Clinical Pharmacokinetics*, 7, 336–52.

Pollock, B. G. (1994). Recent developments in drug metabolism of relevance to psychiatrists. *Harvard Review of Psychiatry*, 2, 204–13.

Pollock, B. G., Altieri, L., Kirshner, M., Yeager, A., Houck, P. & Reynolds, C. F. (1992). Debrisoquine hydroxylation phenotyping in geriatric psychopharmacology. *Psychopharmacology Bulletin*, **28**, 163–8.

Rubio, A. & Cox, C. (1991). Sex, age and alfentanil pharmacokinetics. *Clinical Pharmacokinetics*, **21**, 81–2.

Rugstad, H. E., Hundal, O., Holme, I., Herland, O. B., Husby, G. & Giercksky, K. E. (1986). Piroxicam and naproxen plasma concentrations in patients with osteoarthritis: relation to age, sex, efficacy and adverse events. *Clinical Rheumatology*, **5**, 389–98.

Schmucker, D. L. & Vesell, E. S. (1993). Underrepresentation of women in clinical drug trials. *Clinical Pharmacology Therapeutics*, **54**, 11–15.

Schneider, L. S. & Farlow, M. R. (1995). Predicting response to cholinesterase inhibitors in Alzheimer's disease. *CNS Drugs*, **4**, 114–24.

Schneider, L. S., Farlow, M. R., Henderson, V. W. & Pogoda, J. M. (1996). Effects of estrogen replacement therapy on response to tacrine in patients with Alzheimer's disease. *Neurology*, **46**, 1580–4.

Schwartz, J., Capili, H. & Daugherty, J. (1994). Aging of women alters S-verapamil pharmacokinetics and pharmacodynamics. *Clinical Pharmacology Therapeutics*, **55**, 509–17.

Seeman, M. V. (1983). Interaction of sex, age, and neuroleptic dose. *Comprehensive Psychiatry*, **24**, 125–8.

Siegel, B., Shihabuddin, L. & Buchsbaum, M. (1994). Gender differences in regional brain glucose utilization in Alzheimer's disease and normal aging (abstract). *Neuropsychopharmacology*, **10** (Suppl 3S/Part 2), 24.

Simpson, G. M., Yadalam, K. G., Levinson, D. F., Stephanos, M. J., Sing Lo, E. E. & Cooper, T. B. (1990). Single dose pharmacokinetics of fluphenazine after fluphenazine decanoate administration. *Journal of Clinical Psychopharmacology*, **10**, 417–21.

Skett, P., Mode, A., Rafter, J., Sahlin, L. & Gustafsson, J-A. (1980). The effects of gonadectomy and hypophysectomy on the metabolism of imipramine and lidocaine by the liver of male and female rats. *Biochemical Pharmacology*, **29**, 2759–62.

Stoehr, G. P., Kroboth, P. D., Juhl, R. P., Wender, D. B., Philips, J. P. & Smith, R. B. (1984). Effect of oral contraceptives on triazolam. temazepam, alprazolam and lorazepam kinetics. *Clinical Pharmacology Therapeutics* **36**, 683–90.

Sweet, R. A., Pollock, B. G., Wright, B., Kirshner, M. & DeVane, C. (1995). Single and multiple dose bupropion pharmacokinetics in elderly patients with depression. *Journal of Clinical Pharmacology*, **35**, 876–84.

Taioli, E., Garte, S. J., Trachman, J., Garbers, S., Sepkovic, D. W., Osborne, M. P., Mehl, S. & Bradlow, H. L. (1996). Ethnic differences in estrogen metabolism in healthy women. *Journal of the National Cancer Institute*, **88**, 617.

Taioli, E., Trachman, J., Chen, X., Toniolo, P. & Garte, S. J. (1995). A CYP1A1 restriction fragment length polymorphism is associated with breast cancer in African-American women. *Cancer Research*, **55**, 3757–8.

Tam, S. P. (1991). Effects of gemfibrizol and ketoconazole on human apolipoprotein A1, B and E levels in two hepatoma cell lines, HepG2 and Hep3B. *Atherosclerosis*, **91**, 51–61.

Tamblyn, R. M., McLeod, P. J., Abrahamowicz, M., Monette, J., Gayton, D. C., Berkson, L.,

Dauphinee, W. D., Grad, R. M., Huang, A. R., Isaac, L. M., Schnarch, B. S. & Snell, L. S. (1994). Questionable prescribing for elderly patients in Quebec. *Canadian Medical Association Journal*, **150**, 1801–9.

Thorogood, M., Cowen, P., Mann, J., Murphy, M. & Vessey, M. (1992). Fatal myocardial infarction and use of psychotropic drugs in young women. *Lancet*, **340**, 1067–8.

ThyagaRajan, S., Meites, J. & Quadri, S. K. (1993). Underfeeding-induced suppression of mammary tumors: counteraction by estrogen and haloperidol. *Proceedings of the Society of Experimental and Biological Medicine*, **203**, 236–42.

Wald, A., Van Thiel, D. H., Hoechstetter, L., Gavaler, J. S., Egler, K. M., Verm, R., Scott, L. & Lester, R. (1981). Gastrointestinal transit: the effect of the menstrual cycle. *Gastroenterology*, **80**, 1497–500.

Walle, T., Walle, U. K., Cowart, T. D. & Conradi, E. C. (1989). Pathway-selective sex differences in the metabolic clearance of propranolol in human subjects. *Clinical Pharmacology Therapeutics*, **46**, 257–63.

Warren, J. L., McBean, A. M., Hass, S. L. & Babish, J. D. (1994). Hospitalizations with adverse events caused by digitalis therapy among elderly Medicare beneficiaries. *Archives of Internal Medicine*, **154**, 1482–7.

Watkins, P. B. (1994). Noninvasive tests of CYP3A enzymes. *Pharmacogenetics*, **4**, 171–84.

Weinstein, M. R. (1980). Lithium treatment of women during pregnancy and in the post-delivery period. In *Handbook of Lithium Therapy*, ed. F. N. Johnson. Baltimore: Baltimore University Park Press.

Wilson, K. (1984). Sex-related differences in drug disposition in man. *Clinical Pharmacokinetics*, **9**, 189–202.

Wilson, K., Oram, M., Horth, C. E. & Burnett, D. (1982). The influence of the menstrual cycle on the metabolism and clearance of methaqualone. *British Journal of Clinical Pharmacology*, **14**, 333–9.

Wisner, K. L., Perel, J. M. & Wheeler, S. B. (1993). Tricyclic dose requirements across pregnancy. *American Journal of Psychiatry*, **150**, 1541–2.

16

The influence of progesterone on the pharmacokinetics and pharmacodynamics of gamma-aminobutyric acid-active drugs

Patricia D. Kroboth and James W. McAuley

Introduction

The question of how hormones affect response to drugs is closely related to the separate question of how the aging process influences response to drugs. One can readily acknowledge that the production and secretion of gonadal hormones change with the aging process through childhood, puberty, and adult life, including the young adult, middle age, and late life. Additionally, exogenous administration of hormones is important, particularly for women. Many women take oral contraceptives during mid-life, and they often take hormone replacement therapy in late life. The latter leads to a possible confounding of the aging process and hormone administration with benzodiazepine administration.

We first addressed the potential for hormones to affect drug pharmacokinetics and response in 1982, when we designed a study to determine whether oral contraceptives interact with benzodiazepines. Intrigued by the difference in response between the women who took oral contraceptives and the control women who did not, we turned to the literature on estrogen and progesterone. In doing so, questions progressively became focused on progesterone, its neurosteroid metabolites, and aging. The chapter provides an overview of the combined pharmacokinetic and pharmacodynamic approach and its application to the evaluation of the influence of aging and hormones on drug response.

As indicated in Fig. 16.1, there is a link between drug dose and drug effect (Holford & Sheiner, 1981). Pharmacokinetics relates the dose of a drug to drug concentration, where concentrations of the drug are affected by changes in drug metabolism. Pharmacodynamics relates drug concentration to response and extends to the study of receptors and their modulators.

The schematic identifies the importance of using both pharmacokinetic and pharmacodynamic approaches to assess whether hormones, aging, or other factors affect drug response. Hormones and the aging process can each potentially affect

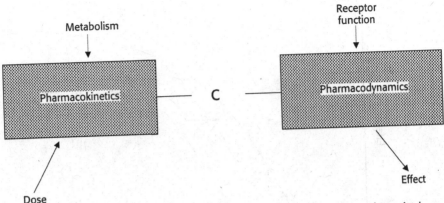

Figure 16.1. This schematic demonstrates the roles of pharmacokinetics and pharmacodynamics in linking dose administered plasma concentration (c) and response. It also shows the links between metabolism and receptor function to pharmacokinetics and pharmacodynamics, respectively. (Adapted from Holford & Sheiner, 1981.)

drug response by altering pharmacokinetics, pharmacodynamics, or both. Identification of factors that alter not only the pharmacokinetics, but also the effect–concentration relationship, is critical to predicting and controlling variability in response to drug, and therefore, critical to optimizing the safety and efficacy of drug therapy.

In Chapter 15, Pollock describes the role that specific enzymes have in metabolizing drugs. Briefly, a decrease in drug metabolism results in increased drug concentration, which in turn increases the therapeutic effect, the side effects, or both. However, an assumption implicit in this statement is that the factors that increase concentration do not perturb the effect-concentration relationship, but instead only cause movement upward along the effect vs. concentration curve. A second assumption is that the maximum responses have not already been achieved.

These assumptions are not always valid, however. Hormones and aging have the potential not only to alter metabolism, but also to alter the physiology such that the effect–concentration relationship is shifted to the right or left. That is, both pharmacokinetics and pharmacodynamics can be affected both by a change in hormone concentration and by aging. In the context of this manuscript, the term pharmacodynamics is used exclusively to describe the relationship between drug concentration and drug response. A number of factors can perturb the effect–concentration relationship and cause a change in the position of the curve. The curves in Fig. 16.2 were simulated using the sigmoid E_{max} model, which relates the observed effect to the maximum effect (E_{max}), concentration (C), the concentration that elicits 50% of the maximum effect (EC_{50}), and the slope (s). Any factor

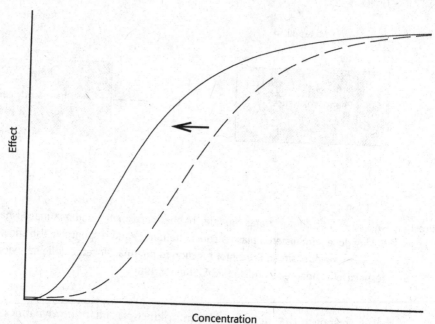

Figure 16.2. Simulated sigmoid E_{max} curves that demonstrate the theoretical relationship between intensity of effect and drug concentration. The solid curve on the left has a lower EC_{50} (concentration that elicits 50% of the maximum response) than the dashed curve, indicating increased sensitivity. The figure demonstrates that, if concentration stays constant, and a hormone or other entity increases sensitivity as indicated by the left shift, a greater effect will be elicited.

that increases sensitivity to drug lowers the EC_{50}, shifting the curve to the left. The example of the shift in Fig. 16.2 shows that a given concentration will elicit a greater response for the curve on the left.

Influence of aging on benzodiazepine pharmacokinetics and pharmacodynamics

The importance of evaluating the impact of aging on both pharmacokinetics and pharmacodynamics is demonstrated by data from young and elderly men (Bertz et al., 1997). Table 16.1 shows that the elderly have a lower alprazolam clearance than the young. However, in addition to the effect of aging on pharmacokinetics, Table 16.1 shows that aging also affects the pharmacodynamics of alprazolam. Sedative, psychomotor, and memory effects relative to alprazolam concentration after a single dose were studied. The approach allowed quantification of both pharmacokinetic and pharmacodynamic changes. The lower EC_{50} values in the elderly men indicate that aging increases sensitivity to effects of alprazolam.

Table 16.1. Alprazolam pharmacokinetics in young and elderly adults

	C_{max} (ng/ml)	β (h^{-1})	$t_{1/2\beta}$ (h)	Clearance (l/kg)	EC50 for DSST (ng/ml)
Young ($n = 26$)	44.9 ± 12.3	0.060 ± 0.156	12.5 ± 3.7	0.058 ± 0.017	36.5 ± 11.1
Elderly ($n = 13$)	50.7 ± 5.5	0.045 ± 0.147	16.7 ± 4.8	0.046 ± 0.019	25.0 ± 3.9
P value	0.12	0.01	0.005	0.05	0.0009

Source: (Abstracted from Bertz et al. 1997).

The conclusion from these data is that aging decreases the clearance of alprazolam and, through a separate mechanism increases sensitivity to alprazolam 2 mg administered intravenously. Curiously, Greenblatt et al. showed no difference in sensitivity when they administered alprazolam 1 mg by mouth (Kaplan et al., 1998). The mechanism responsible for the increased sensitivity in the elderly is still unknown.

From the data, however, it is reasonable to postulate that, although aging may not affect the metabolism of some benzodiazepines (e.g. those that are metabolized through conjugation), it potentially increases sensitivity to other benzodiazepines since response is mediated by receptor interaction. Likewise, the data quantify and lend credence to the clinical belief that the 'usual dosage range' for the elderly is generally lower than for younger adults.

An important note about these data is that they are from healthy young and elderly men. The objective was to assess the influence of aging on benzodiazepine pharmacokinetics and pharmacodynamics in an approach that was not confounded by gender or by fluctuating hormones.

Influence of oral contraceptives on benzodiazepine pharmacokinetics and pharmacodynamics

Using both pharmacokinetic and pharmacodynamic principles, we evaluated the influence of oral contraceptives on benzodiazepine response. Lorazepam and temazepam are metabolized by conjugation while alprazolam and triazolam are metabolized by hydroxylation. The working hypothesis was that oral contraceptives would affect the clearance of the latter two benzodiazepines differently. Changes in concentrations alone, however, did not address the question of whether sedation or psychomotor effects would be altered. Thus, we designed a study to evaluate pharmacokinetics and pharmacodynamics of these four drugs in a total of 48 women.

The results indicated a pharmacokinetic interaction between oral contraceptives

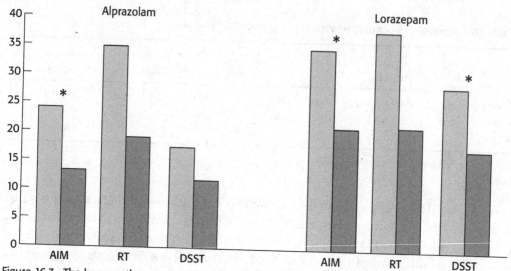

Figure 16.3. The bars are the mean ratios of maximum observed effect/logarithm of the maximum observed concentration for women taking oral contraceptives (light bars) and control women (darker bars). Data are for the aiming test (AIM), reaction time test (RT), and digit symbol substitution test (DSST). The asterisks denote $P < 0.05$. (Adapted from Kroboth et al., 1985).

and benzodiazepines, with an increase or decrease in clearance depending upon the benzodiazepine and its metabolic pathway. Clearances of triazolam and alprazolam were higher in control women than in those taking oral contraceptives by factors of 1.47 and 1.27, respectively; however, only the difference in alprazolam clearance was statistically significant. (Subsequently, another group reported that low-dose estrogen oral contraceptives did not affect metabolism of alprazolam (Scavone et al., 1988).) Clearance of temazepam was higher in the oral contraceptive group by a factor of 1.62; clearance was unchanged in the lorazepam group. Notable, however, is the observation that peak benzodiazepine concentrations did not differ between the oral contraceptive-taking and control women for any of the four drugs (Stoehr et al., 1984).

The surprise result of the study was that there was a pharmacodynamic interaction in addition to the pharmacokinetic interaction. Fig. 16.3 shows that when corrections were made for concentration differences, women taking oral contraceptives experienced greater psychomotor impairment than control women (Kroboth et al., 1985).

These results generated questions not only about which hormones are responsible for the altered pharmacodynamics, but also about the mechanism for the alteration. The information we gleaned from subsequent studies (described below) from our laboratory, and from others regarding progesterone metabolites, cannot explain the observations in this study. Synthetic progesterones in oral contraceptives do not have the structure–activity relationships required to modulate the GABA$_A$ receptor.

GABA$_A$ receptor complex

Gamma-aminobutyric acid (GABA) is the major inhibitory neurotransmitter, and it is present in about 30% of mammalian central nervous system synapses. Two major subtypes of GABA receptors are well characterized. GABA$_A$ receptors are sensitive to the convulsant alkaloid bicuculline; GABA$_B$ receptors are bicuculline-insensitive. Recently, a third subtype, GABA$_C$, has also been identified in the retina (Johnston, 1996). The latter two subtypes are not modulated by neurosteroids, and so they are not a focus of this discussion.

Activation of GABA$_A$ receptors by synaptically released GABA stimulates a transient increase in chloride ion conductance that usually results in membrane hyperpolarization and thus reduces the probability of action potential generation. It is on this basis that GABA$_A$ receptor agonists have an inhibitory effect on the central nervous system. This receptor has recently been reviewed by Costa (1998). The function of the GABA$_A$ receptor is allosterically modulated by several anxiolytic-hypnotic drugs, including benzodiazepines and barbiturates, that act to enhance and prolong GABA$_A$-mediated synaptic inhibition (Costa, 1991; Zorumski & Isenberg, 1991).

Neurosteroids

In the 1980s, the work of many individuals, including Majewska and Paul at NIMH demonstrated that selected naturally occurring steroids modulate the GABA$_A$ receptor complex through rapid, non-classical steroid mechanisms. This is in contrast to the classical steroid action, thought to be due to an interaction with intracellular receptors and gene-controlled changes in protein synthesis (McEwen, 1991). These potent steroids include the ring-A reduced metabolites of progesterone and deoxycorticosterone: allopregnanolone and tetrahydrocorticosterone (THDOC), both of which can be formed by neurons and glial cells (Jung-Testas et al., 1989), on which basis they are known as neurosteroids. For a greater description, see reviews by Baulieu (1997), Lambert et al. (1996), and Wilson (1996).

Several observations suggest that steroids play a physiological role in brain excitability regulation, including a role in aggression (Canonaco et al., 1990), postpartum depression (Majewska et al., 1989), epilepsy (Laidlaw, 1956), and premenstrual syndrome (Majewska, 1987). For example, THDOC has been shown to be an effective hypnotic (Mendelson et al., 1987) and anxiolytic (Crawley et al.,

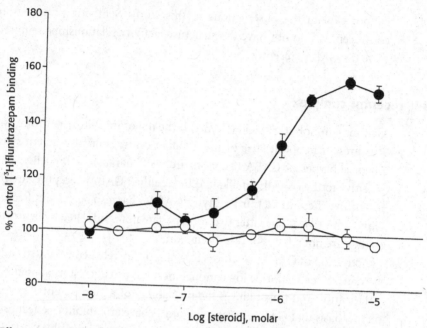

Figure 16.4. Effect of progesterone (open circle) and allopregnanolone (closed circles) on specific [³H]flunitrazepam binding to rat cortical membranes. Data are mean (±SE) from at least four animals. (Adapted from McAuley et al., 1993.)

1996) in animals; and allopregnanolone has been shown to be an effective anxiolytic (Wieland et al., 1991), anticonvulsant (Belelli et al., 1989), analgesic (Kavaliers & Wiebe, 1987), and anesthetic in both animals (Mok & Krieger, 1990) and humans (Unseld et al., 1990). Brain and plasma concentrations of allopregnanolone and THDOC have been shown to rapidly increase after a brief exposure to swim stress, which suggests these endogenous modulators may play a role in the adaptive response to stress (Purdy et al., 1991). Additionally, using specific [³H]flunitrazepam binding as a marker, allopregnanolone enhances benzodiazepine binding to the GABA$_A$ receptor (Majewska et al, 1986; Harrison et al., 1987; Gee et al., 1988; McAuley et al., 1993). As observed in Fig. 16.4, progesterone has no effect, but allopregnanolone significantly enhances binding. These observations are consistent with a physiological role for allopregnanolone and other neurosteroids in the regulation of brain excitability and, potentially, with a clinical role in response to a benzodiazepine.

Medroxyprogesterone acetate (MPA, Provera), a synthetic derivative of progesterone, is commonly prescribed in combination with estrogen supplementation for hormonal replacement in postmenopausal women. MPA and progesterone are structurally similar and have similar metabolic pathways (Aufrere & Benson, 1976; Martin et al., 1980). There is limited information in humans that MPA and/or its metabolites interact at the GABA$_A$ receptors. Suggestion of interaction at the

GABA$_A$ receptor is found in a report by Mattson and colleagues; when MPA was added to existing anticonvulsant regimens, 11 of 14 women with uncontrolled seizures had significantly fewer seizures (Mattson et al., 1984). Based on the similarity between MPA and progesterone, our objective was to determine whether MPA and/or its ring-A reduced metabolites interact with the GABA$_A$ receptor (McAuley et al., 1993). While known modulators of specific [^{3}H]flunitrazepam binding demonstrated expected effects in frozen and fresh rat cortical tissue, allopregnanolone enhanced [^{3}H]flunitrazepam binding only in fresh, not frozen, tissue. Neither the dihydro-metabolite nor the tetrahydro-metabolite affected binding. MPA partially inhibited [^{3}H]flunitrazepam binding by 40%. The clinical implication of this unexpected finding is unknown. Additionally, five test-drugs were used to assess the effect of gender and hormonal status on [^{3}H]flunitrazepam binding. Neither gender nor hormonal status influenced binding. Thus, ring-A reduced metabolites of progesterone but not of MPA enhanced [^{3}H]flunitrazepam binding. The clinical implications of these in vitro results were subsequently evaluated in postmenopausal women (see below).

Effects of exogenously administered progesterone

Postmenopausal women and GABA-active drugs

Subsequently, we conducted a study to determine whether the in vitro observation that allopregnanolone enhances benzodiazepine binding to the GABA$_A$ receptor translates to increased benzodiazepine effects in vivo. Sedative, psychomotor, and memory effects of triazolam were evaluated in postmenopausal women with and without administration of oral progesterone (McAuley et al., 1995). Triazolam was chosen as the in vivo probe because of its high affinity for the GABA$_A$ receptor (Sethy et al., 1983), its short half-life, its lack of important active metabolites, and its availability for intravenous administration for investigational purposes.

Sixteen women were randomly assigned to one of two treatment groups: micronized progesterone 300 mg p.o. plus triazolam i.v. (triazolam plus progesterone) or placebo p.o. plus triazolam i.v. (triazolam). Micronized progesterone 300 mg is the dose used clinically for hormone replacement (Hargrove et al., 1989). After an overnight fast, women ate a light breakfast at 7:15 am; an intravenous catheter was placed in the forearm of each woman and at 8:30 am, a dose of micronized progesterone 300 mg or placebo was administered. Triazolam was administered 2.5 hours later as an intravenous infusion at a rate of 0.025 mg/min until a predetermined effect was observed or 20 minutes had elapsed (0.5 mg administered), whichever occurred first. Fig. 16.5 shows the observed data and fitted line for the continuous performance test (CPT) scores vs. triazolam concentration for a patient in the triazolam plus progesterone group.

Table 16.2 summarizes results from fitting the sigmoid E_{max} model to effect vs.

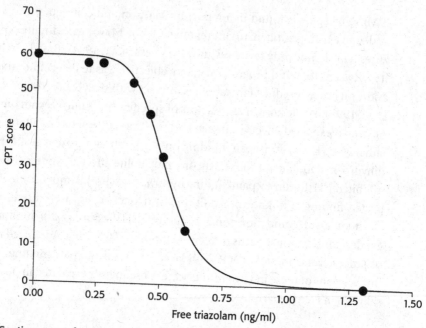

Figure 16.5. Continuous performance test (CPT) scores vs. unbound triazolam concentration data for one subject in the triazolam plus progesterone group; the subject received triazolam infused to a predetermined maximal response. The solid line depicts the predicted curve generated from sigmoid E_{max} model parameter estimates; symbols are observed data. (Adapted from McAuley et al., 1995)

free triazolam concentration data for the triazolam and triazolam plus progesterone treatments. The data from the 16 postmenopausal women demonstrate that the concurrent administration of progesterone significantly enhances the psychomotor, memory and sedative effects of triazolam. Results from digit symbol substitution (DSST), CPT, and hand–eye (HE) are presented. In essence, progesterone administration shifted the triazolam effect–concentration curve to the left, indicating enhanced sensitivity.

Another important observation from this study is that the progesterone-induced increase in triazolam sensitivity is dependent on progesterone concentration. Three women in the triazolam plus progesterone group had progesterone concentrations that were substantially higher than those of the other five. Fig. 16.6 shows the ratio of area under the effect curve, area under the triazolam concentration (AUC) curve for the no progesterone, progesterone AUC<300 ng/ml, and AUC>300 ng/ml groups. Statistical comparison was not done because the numbers of subjects per group were so small. Curiously, the highest concentrations of progesterone and the greatest response to triazolam were observed in the three women who had the longest duration since the onset of menopause.

Table 16.2. Sensitivity estimates (EC_{50} in ng/ml) from fitting the sigmoid E_{max} model to effect vs. free triazolam concentration data for the two treatment groups.[a, b]

	DSST	CPT	Hand–Eye
TRZ	0.492 ± 0.085[c]	0.590 ± 0.130	0.574 ± 0.091[d]
	(0.390 to 0.625)	(0.460 to 0.763)	(0.476 to 0.704)
TRZProg	0.396 ± 0.080	0.441 ± 0.120	0.387 ± 0.144
	(0.278 to 0.496)	(0.306 to 0.648)	(0.128 to 0.636)
p value	0.044	0.038	0.017

Notes:
[a] Data are presented as mean (SD $\pm$ range).
[b] Data are from eight women unless otherwise noted.
[c] Data are from seven women.
[d] Data are from six women.
Source: Abstracted from McAuley et al., (1995).

There was no evidence for an effect of progesterone administration on the pharmacokinetics of triazolam. By relating concentrations to responses, we have learned that progesterone affects benzodiazepine response in a dose-dependent way. At this point, we can also say that it is likely that this has occurred via the neuroactive metabolites of progesterone which have been shown in vitro to modulate the $GABA_A$ receptor complex.

Premenopausal women

The influence of progesterone alone on psychomotor performance and on indices of fatigue has been evaluated in 24 premenopausal women (Freeman et al., 1992). In a four-way crossover study, Freeman et al. gave single doses of placebo, progesterone 300 mg, 600 mg, and 1200 mg and assessed responses during the next 6 hours. Progesterone 1200 mg produced significant fatigue and decreased performance on digit symbol substitution and immediate recall. The lower doses did not produce notable effects.

Influence of endogenous progesterone on GABA-active drugs

Based on in vitro benzodiazepine receptor binding results, information regarding the rapid membrane effects of neuroactive steroids at the $GABA_A$ receptor complex, and the extent of progesterone-enhanced triazolam effects in postmenopausal women, we designed a crossover study to determine whether alprazolam pharmacodynamics are influenced by the menstrual cycle, specifically endogenous

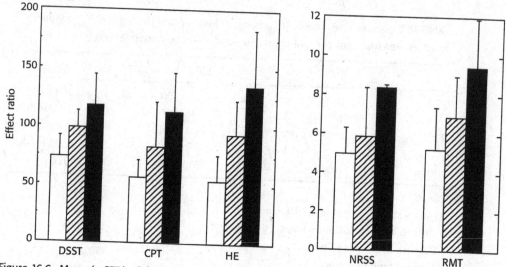

Figure 16.6. Mean (±STD) of the ratio of area under the effect curve: area under the plasma concentration curve for digit symbol substitution test (DSST), continuous performance test (CPT), hand–eye co-ordination (HE), nurse-rated sedation score (NRSS), and Randt memory tests (RMT) for three groups: triazolam (no fill), triazolam with progesterone AUC <300 ng/ml (cross-hatched) and triazolam with progesterone AUC >300 ng/ml (solid fill). (McAuley et al., 1995.)

progesterone concentration fluctuations (McAuley & Friedman, 1999). We hypothesized that women would have more psychomotor impairment from the alprazolam during the mid-luteal phase because of the high levels of progesterone as compared to the mid-follicular phase.

Fig. 16.7 demonstrates that fluctuations of endogenous progesterone across the menstrual cycle do not influence alprazolam pharmacodynamics. Despite the fact that progesterone concentrations were higher in the mid-luteal than in the mid-follicular phase, no differences were observed in either DSST, CSS, card sorting, or sedation scores after a single oral dose of alprazolam 2 mg on these two occasions. The mid-luteal and mid-follicular progesterone serum concentrations measured in our patients are within the expected ranges for premenopausal women (Aufrere & Benson, 1976). The lack of changes during the menstrual cycle in demonstrable cognitive impairment and pharmacokinetics following alprazolam implies that dose adjustment based on menstrual timing is not required.

Recently, de Wit and Rukstalis reported that the sedative effects of triazolam were not greater during the luteal phase, when levels of progesterone and allopregnanolone were high, as compared with follicular and ovulatory phases (de Wit & Rukstalis, 1997). They observed little differences in their subjective and behavioral responses after a low dose of triazolam as compared with a placebo. Because they

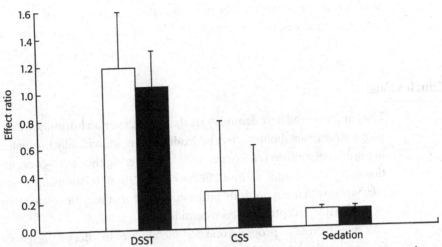

Figure 16.7. Mean ($\pm$ STD) effect ratios for digit symbol substitution test (DSST) ($P = 0.2771$), card sorting skills (CSS) ($P = 0.2066$), and sedation ($P = 0.3770$) for the mid-luteal (closed bars) and mid-follicular (open bars) groups. (Adapted from McAuley & Friedman, 1999.)

did not show pharmacokinetic data, they were unable to calculate effect ratios that normalize data to an effect per unit of concentration.

Despite a large increase in progesterone concentrations in the luteal phase, as compared with the follicular phase, the same proportionate increase in allopreg-nanolone concentrations was not observed in two other studies that measured serum concentrations of this neurosteroid (de Wit & Rukstalis, 1997). It is unknown whether CNS concentrations of allopregnanolone capable of modulating the GABA$_A$ receptor complex were achieved in our nine premenopausal women. Although the ratios of progesterone metabolites to the parent drug are greater in the CNS of rats than in the blood (Bixo & Backstrom, 1990), our data and that reported by de Wit suggest that endogenous neurosteroids do not play a major role in enhancing impairment induced by acutely administered benzodiazepines.

Influence of aging on allopregnanolone concentrations

Genazzani and colleagues (1998) recently assessed allopregnanolone concentrations by gender, menstrual cycle phase, and age in normal men and women. They measured serum allopregnanolone as well as progesterone and dehydroepiandrosterone (DHEA) concentrations in 189 premenopausal women, 112 postmenopausal women, and 46 men ranging in age from 19 to over 60 years. An age-related decrease in allopregnanolone was observed only in men. In women, there was a decrease in progesterone concentrations that was not paralleled by a decrease in allopregnanolone concentrations. DHEA concentrations decreased with age in men and in women.

Conclusions

The data reviewed here demonstrate that aging, ovarian hormones, and specifically progesterone metabolites affect benzodiazepines individually through either altering drug metabolism (clearance) and/or by altering the effect–concentration relationship. The change in the effect–concentration relationship occurs through mechanisms that are not fully understood, but that may be related to modulation of the $GABA_A$ receptor by neurosteroids.

While the role of progesterone and metabolites in affecting response to drug is far from understood, a pattern appears to be emerging. Reports from two studies indicate that exogenously administered progesterone affects GABA-mediated responses in a concentration-dependent way (McAuley et al., 1995; Freeman et al., 1992). However, the fluctuations in endogenous concentrations of progesterone that normally occur during the menstrual cycle do not seem important in modulating GABA-mediated responses elicited by administration of GABA agonist (de Wit & Rukstalis, 1997; McAuley & Friedman, 1999). Notable, however, is the fact that, in each of these studies, the responses assessed were those other than the therapeutic effect. The impact of combined use of progesterone and a benzodiazepine on therapeutic outcome in either pre- or postmenopausal women is unknown.

An important direction for the future is to study patients who are at most risk from benzodiazepine side effects, and who may also benefit from benzodiazepine therapy. Older patients with anxiety disorders are particularly at risk for adverse effects of benzodiazepines. As indicated, aging decreases clearance and, in one study, increased sensitivity to a single dose of alprazolam 2 mg. Finding the appropriate low dose for optimal treatment minimizes adverse effects. Response measures in such a study should include therapeutic response as well as balance, psychomotor function, and a measure such as saccadic eye movements as a sensitive indicator of GABA-activity.

A third direction for future study is to collect limited numbers of blood samples and responses from community or institution-based patients taking benzodiazepines for anxiety disorders. Application of population pharmacokinetic and pharmacodynamic analyses using nonlinear mixed effect models provides information about factors that affect response in patients.

Ultimately, application of the combined pharmacokinetic and pharmacodynamic approach should also be applied to other therapeutic classes to better understand the role of hormones and aging as they affect response to other psychotherapeutic agents.

ACKNOWLEDGMENT

This work was supported by NIH Grant MH55756.

REFERENCES

Aufrere, M. B. & Benson, H. (1976). Progesterone: an overview and recent advances. *Journal of Pharmaceutical Sciences*, **65**, 783–800.

Baulieu, E-E. (1997). Neurosteroids: of the nervous system, by the nervous system, for the nervous system. *Recent Progress in Hormone Research*, **52**, 1–32.

Belelli, D., Bolger, M. B. & Gee, K. W. (1989). Anticonvulsant profile of the progesterone metabolite 5α-pregnane-3α-ol-20-one. *European Journal of Pharmacology*, **166**, 325–9.

Bertz, R. J., Kroboth, P. D., Kroboth, F. J., Reynolds, I. J., Salek, F., Wright, C. E. & Smith, R. B. (1997). Alprazolam in young and elderly men: Sensitivity and tolerance to psychomotor, sedative and memory effects. *Journal of Pharmacology and Experimental Therapeutics*, **281**, 1317–29.

Bixo, M. & Backstrom, T. (1990). Regional distribution of progesterone and 5α-pregnane-3,20–dion in rat brain during progesterone-induced 'anesthesia'. *Psychoneuroendocrinology*, **15**, 159–62.

Canonaco, M., Valenti, A. & Maggi, A. (1990). Effects of progesterone on [35S]t-butylbicyclophosphorothionate binding in some forebrain areas of the female rat and its correlation to aggressive behavior. *Pharmacology, Biochemistry and Behavior*, **37**, 433–8.

Costa, E. (1991). The allosteric modulation of GABA$_A$ receptors: seventeen years of research. *Neuropsychopharmacology*, **4**, 225–35.

Costa, E. (1998). From GABA$_A$ receptor diversity emerges a unified vision of GABAergic inhibition. *Annual Review of Pharmacology and Toxicology*, **38**, 321–50.

Crawley, J. N., Glowa, J. R., Majewska, M. D. & Paul, S. M. (1996). Anxiolytic activity of an endogenous adrenal steroid. *Brain Research*, **398**, 382–5.

de Wit, H. & Rukstalis, M. (1997). Acute effects of triazolam in women: relationsips with progesterone, estradiol and allopregnanolone. *Psychopharmacology*, **130**, 69–78.

Freeman, E. W., Weinstock, L., Rickels, K., Sondheimer, S. J. & Coutifaris, C. (1992). A placebo-controlled study of effects of oral progesterone on performance and mood. *British Journal of Clinical Pharmacology*, **33**, 293–8.

Gee, K. W., Bolger, M. B., Brinton, R. E., Coirini, H. & McEwen, B. S. (1988). Steroid modulation of the chloride ionophore in rat brain: structure–activity requirements, regional dependence and mechanism of action. *Journal of Pharmacology and Experimental Therapeutics*, **246**, 803–12.

Genazzani, A. R., Petraglia, F., Bernardi, F., Casarosa, E., Salvestroni, C., Tonetti, A., Nappi, R. E., Luisi, S., Palumbo, M., Purdy, R. H. & Luisi, M. (1998). Circulating levels of allopregnanolone in humans: gender, age, and endocrine influences. *Journal of Clinical Endocrinology and Metabolism*, **83**, 2099–103.

Hargrove, J. T., Maxson, W. S. & Wentz, A. C. (1989). Absorption of oral progesterone is influenced by vehicle and particle size. *American Journal of Obstetrics and Gynecology*, **161**, 948–51.

Harrison, N. L., Majewska, M. D., Harrington, J. W. & Barker, J. L. (1987). Structure–activity relationships for steroid interacion with the γ-aminobutyric acid$_A$ receptor complex. *Journal of Pharmacology and Experimental Therapeutics*, **241**, 346–52.

Holford, N. H. G. & Sheiner, L. B. (1981). Understanding the dose–effect relationship: clinical application of pharmacokinetic–pharmacodynamic models. *Clinical Pharmacokinetics*, **6**, 429–53.

Johnston, G. A. (1996). GABA$_C$ receptors: relatively simple transmitter-gated ion channels? *Trends in Pharmacological Sciences*, **17**, 301–37.

Jung-Testas, I., Hu, Z. Y., Baulieu, E. E. & Robel, P. (1989). Neurosteroids: biosynthesis of pregnenolone and progesterone in primary cultures of rat glial cells. *Endocrinology*, **125**, 2083–90.

Kaplan, G. B., Greenblatt, D. J., Ehrenberg, B. L., Goddard, J. E., Harmatz, J. S. & Shader, R. I. (1998). Single dose pharmacokinetics and pharmacodynamics of alprazolam in elderly and young subjects. *Journal of Clinical Pharmacology*, **38**, 14–21.

Kavaliers, M. & Wiebe, J. P. (1987). Analgesic effects of the progesterone metabolite: 3α-hydroxy-5α-pregnan-20-one, and possible modes of action in mice. *Brain Research*, **415**, 393–8.

Kroboth, P. D., Smith, R. B., Stoehr, G. P. & Juhl, R. P. (1985). Pharmacodynamic evaluation of the benzodiazepine–oral contraceptive interaction. *Clinical Pharmacology Therapeutics*, **38**, 525–32.

Laidlaw, J. (1956). Catamenial epilepsy. *Lancet*, **ii**, 1235–7.

Lambert, J. J., Belelli, D., Hill-Venning, C., Callachan, H. & Peters, J. A. (1996). Neurosteroid modulation of native and recombinant GABA$_A$ receptors. *Cellular and Molecular Neurobiology*, **16**, 155–74.

Majewska, M. D. (1987). Steroids and brain activity: essential dialogue between body and mind. *Biochemistry and Pharmacology*, **36**, 3781–8.

Majewska, M. D., Ford-Rice, F. & Falkay, G. (1989). Pregancy-induced alteration of GABA$_A$ receptor sensitivity in maternal brain: an antecedent of post-partum 'blues'? *Brain Research*, **482**, 397–401.

Majewska, M. D., Harrison, N. L., Schwartz, R. D., Barker, J. L. & Paul, S. M. (1986). Steroid hormone metabolites are barbiturate-like modulators of the GABA receptor. *Science*, **232**, 1004–7.

Martin, F., Järvenpää, P., Kosunen, K., Somers, C., Lindstrom, B. & Adlercreutz, H. (1980). Ring-A reduction of medroxyprogesterone acetate [17α-acetoxy-6α-methyl-4 pregnene-3,20-dione (MPA)] in biological systems. *Journal of Steroid Biochemistry*, **12**, 491–7.

Mattson, R. H., Cramer, J. A., Caldwell, B. V. & Siconolfi, B. C. (1984). Treatment of seizures with medroxyprogesterone acetate: preliminary report. *Neurology*, **34**, 1255–8.

McAuley, J. W. & Friedman, C. I. (1999). Influence of endogenous progesterone on alprazolam pharmacodynamics. *Journal of Clinical Psychopharmacology*, **19**, 233–9.

McAuley, J. W., Kroboth, P. D., Stiff, D. D. & Reynolds, I. J. (1993). Modulation of [$_3$H]Flunitrazepam binding by natural and synthetic progestational agents. *Pharmacology, Biochemistry and Behavior*, **45**, 77–83.

McAuley, J. W., Reynolds, I. J., Kroboth, F. J., Smith, R. B. & Kroboth, P. D. (1995). Orally administered progesterone enhances sensitivity to triazolam in postmenopausal women. *Journal of Clinical Psychopharmacology*, 15, 3–11.

McEwen, B. S. (1991). Non-genomic and genomic effects of steroids on neural activity. *Trends in Pharmacological Sciences*, 12, 141–7.

Mendelson, W. B., Martin, J. V., Perlis, M., Wagner, R., Majewska, M. D. & Paul, S. M. (1987). Sleep induction by an adrenal steroid in the rat. *Psychopharmacology* 93, 226–9.

Mok, W. M. & Krieger, N. R. (1990). Evidence that 5α-pregnan-3α-ol-20-one is the metabolite responsible for progesterone anesthesia. *Brain Research*, 533, 42–5.

Purdy, R. H., Morrow, A. L., Moore, P. H. & Paul, S. M. (1991). Stress-induced elevations of γ-aminobutyric acid type A receptor-active steroids in the rat brains. *Neurobiology*, 88, 4553–7.

Scavone, J. M., Greenblatt, D. J., Locniskar, A. & Shader, R. I. (1988). Alprazolam pharmacokinetics in women on low-dose oral contraceptives. *Journal of Clinical Pharmacology*, 28, 454–7.

Sethy, V. H., Russell, R. R. & Daenzer, C. L. (1983). Interaction of triazolobenzodiazepines with benzodiazepine receptors. *Journal of Pharmaceuticals and Pharmacology*, 35, 524–6.

Stoehr, G. P., Kroboth, P. D., Juhl, R. P., Wender, D. B., Phillips, J. P. & Smith, R. B. (1984). Effect of oral contraceptives on triazolam, temazepam, alprazolam, and lorazepam kinetics. *Clinical Pharmacology Therapeutics*, 36, 683–90.

Unseld, E., Ziegler, G., Gemeinhardt, A., Janssen, U. & Klotz, U. (1990). Possible interaction of fluoroquinolones with the benzodiazepine GABA$_A$–receptor complex. *British Journal of Clinical Pharmacology*, 30, 63–70.

Wieland, S., Lan, M. D., Mirasedeghi, S. & Gee, K. W. (1991). Anxiolytic activity of the progesterone metabolite 5α-pregnane-3α-ol-20-one. *Brain Research*, 565, 263–8.

Wilson, M. A. (1996). GABA physiology: modulation by benzodiazepines and hormones. *Critical Reviews in Neurobiology*, 10, 1–37.

Zorumski, C.F. & Isenberg, K. E. (1991). Insights into the structure and function of GABA-benzodiazepine receptors: ion channels and psychiatry. *American Journal of Psychiatry*, 148, 162–73.

Index